Head and Neck Cancer Rehabilitation

T0249684

Head and Neck Cancer Rehabilitation

Edited by

Adrian Cristian, MD MHCM FAAPMR

*Chief, Cancer Rehabilitation Miami Cancer Institute,
Baptist Health South Florida,
Miami, FL, United States*

*Clinical Professor, Department of Translational Medicine,
FIU Herbert Wertheim College of Medicine,
Miami, FL, United States*

ELSEVIER

Elsevier
Radarweg 29, PO Box 211, 1000 AE Amsterdam, Netherlands
125 London Wall, London EC2Y 5AS, United Kingdom
50 Hampshire Street, 5th Floor, Cambridge, MA 02139, United States

Copyright © 2025 Elsevier Inc. All rights are reserved, including those for text and data mining, AI training, and similar technologies.

Publisher's note: Elsevier takes a neutral position with respect to territorial disputes or jurisdictional claims in its published content, including in maps and institutional affiliations.

No part of this publication may be reproduced or transmitted in any form or by any means, electronic or mechanical, including photocopying, recording, or any information storage and retrieval system, without permission in writing from the publisher. Details on how to seek permission, further information about the Publisher's permissions policies and our arrangements with organizations such as the Copyright Clearance Center and the Copyright Licensing Agency, can be found at our website: www.elsevier.com/permissions.

This book and the individual contributions contained in it are protected under copyright by the Publisher (other than as may be noted herein).

Notices

Knowledge and best practice in this field are constantly changing. As new research and experience broaden our understanding, changes in research methods, professional practices, or medical treatment may become necessary.

Practitioners and researchers must always rely on their own experience and knowledge in evaluating and using any information, methods, compounds, or experiments described herein. In using such information or methods they should be mindful of their own safety and the safety of others, including parties for whom they have a professional responsibility.

To the fullest extent of the law, neither the Publisher nor the authors, contributors, or editors, assume any liability for any injury and/or damage to persons or property as a matter of products liability, negligence or otherwise, or from any use or operation of any methods, products, instructions, or ideas contained in the material herein.

ISBN: 978-0-443-11806-7

For information on all Elsevier publications visit our website at
https://www.elsevier.com/books-and-journals

Publisher: Sarah E. Barth
Acquisitions Editor: Humayra R. Khan
Editorial Project Manager: Billie Jean Fernandez
Production Project Manager: Gomathi Sugumar
Cover Designer: Matthew Limbert

Typeset by TNQ Technologies

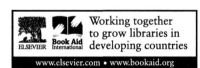

This book is dedicated to:
Eliane, my soul mate, best friend, and greatest supporter, who
personifies the true meaning of kindness and compassion,
Alec and Chloe who add joy and meaning to my life,
Steluta, Cali, Daniela, and Rasela, who taught me the importance of
hard work and empathy,
Drs. Jerry Weissman, David Bressler, Adam Stein, Steve Flanagan,
and Kristjan Ragnarsson, who taught me the holistic multidisciplinary
approach of rehabilitation medicine,
Dr. Maria Beatriz Currier for her leadership and encouragement,
My colleagues at the Miami Cancer Institute, who inspire me with
their hard work and dedication, and
My patients for their tremendous courage and perseverance in the face
of adversity.

Contents

CHAPTER 7   Oral complications from head and neck cancer
Alessandro Villa, DDS, PhD, MPH and Michele Lodolo, DDS

CHAPTER 8   Physical therapy for head and neck cancer
Dessislava Dakova, MSPT, CLT Physical Therapist

Contributors

Marielle Araujo, MD
Department of Physical Medicine and Rehabilitation, Northwell Heath, Zucker School of Medicine at Hofstra University, Hempstead, NY, United States

Deepti A. Chopra, MD
Department of Psychiatry, University of Texas MD Anderson Cancer Center, Houston, TX, United States

Meghan B. Crawley, MD
Florida International University, Herbert Wertheim College of Medicine, Miami, FL, United States; Miami Cancer Institute, Baptist Health South Florida, Miami, FL, United States

Adrian Cristian, MD, MHCM, FAAPMR
Cancer Rehabilitation, Miami Cancer Institute, Baptist Health South Florida, Miami, FL, United States; Department of Translational Medicine, FIU Herbert Wertheim College of Medicine, Miami, FL, United States

Carsyn Cunningham, MA
Department of Head & Neck Surgery, University of Texas MD Anderson Cancer Center, Houston, TX, United States

Christian M. Custodio, MD
Clinical Rehabilitation Medicine, Memorial Sloan Kettering Cancer Center, New York, NY, United States

Dessislava Dakova, MSPT, CLT Physical Therapist
Oncology Rehabilitation at South Miami Hospital, Miami, FL, United States

Chanel Davidoff, DO
Physical Medicine and Rehabilitation, Donald and Barbara School of Medicine at Hofstra/Northwell Health, Hempstead, NY, United States

Jack B. Fu, MD
Department of Palliative, Rehabilitation & Integrative Medicine, University of Texas MD Anderson Cancer Center, Houston, TX, United States

Daniel Gonzalez, MSV
Miami Cancer Institute, Miami, FL, United States

Carolina Gutiérrez, MD
Department of Physical Medicine and Rehabilitation, The University of Texas Health Science Center at Houston, Houston, TX, United States

Lydia Henderson, MD
Shirley Ryan AbilityLab, Chicago, IL, United States; Department of Physical Medicine and Rehabilitation, Northwestern University Feinberg School of Medicine of Medicine, Chicago, IL, United States

Katherine Hutcheson, PhD
University of Texas MD Anderson Cancer Center, Houston, TX, United States

Michelle Issac, MD
Palliative Medicine Attending Physician, Miami Cancer Institute, Baptist Health South Florida, Miami, FL, United States

Noah S. Kalman, MD, MBA
Radiation Oncology, Miami Cancer Institute, Baptist Health South Florida, Miami, FL, USA

Noah Kalman, MD
Herbert Wertheim College of Medicine, Miami, FL, United States

Ryan Kelly, MD
Shirley Ryan AbilityLab, Chicago, IL, United States; Department of Physical Medicine and Rehabilitation, Northwestern University Feinberg School of Medicine of Medicine, Chicago, IL, United States

Cristina Kline-Quiroz, DO
Cancer Rehbilitation Medicine, Department of Physical Medicine and Rehabilitation, Vanderbilt University Medical Center, Nashville, TN, United States

Krytal Lee, DO
Cancer Rehabilitation Medicine, Department of Physical Medicine and Rehabilitation, Northwell Health, Zucker School of Medicine at Hofstra University, Hempstead, NY, United States

Victor F. Leite, MD
University of Sao Paulo, Sao Paulo, Brazil; Hospital Israelita Albert Einstein, São Paulo, SP, Brazil

Michele Lodolo, DDS
University of California San Francisco (UCSF), San Francisco, CA, United States

Price Lucks, MS
Department of Head & Neck Surgery, University of Texas MD Anderson Cancer Center, Houston, TX, United States

Patrick Martone, DO
Cancer Rehabilitation Medicine, Department of Physical Medicine and Rehabilitation, Northwell Health, Zucker School of Medicine at Hofstra University, Bay Shore, NY, United States

Keelin McKenna
Herbert Wertheim College of Medicine, Miami, FL, United States

Suleyki Medina, MD
Palliative Medicine Attending Physician, Miami Cancer Institute, Baptist Health South Florida, Miami, FL, United States

Zunli Mo, PhD
Miami Cancer Institute, Miami, FL, United States

Romer B. Orada, DO
Miami Cancer Institute, Baptist Health South Florida, Miami, FL, United States

Mary E. Owens, MEd, CCC-SLP
Miami Cancer Institute, Miami, FL, United States

Guilherme Rabinowits, MD
Herbert Wertheim College of Medicine, Miami, FL, United States

John C. Rasmussen, PhD
Brown Foundation Institute of Molecular Medicine, The University of Texas Health Science Center at Houston, Houston, TX, United States

Casey Richardson, MA, CCC-SLP
Atos Medical, Houston, TX, United States

Nicole Rittman, RD, CSO, LDN
Miami Cancer Institute, Miami, FL, United States

Ishan Roy, MD, PhD
Shirley Ryan AbilityLab, Chicago, IL, United States; Department of Physical Medicine and Rehabilitation, Northwestern University Feinberg School of Medicine of Medicine, Chicago, IL, United States; Robert H. Lurie Comprehensive Cancer Center, Chicago, IL, United States

Hani Samarah, BS, BS
Florida International University, Herbert Wertheim College of Medicine, Miami, FL, United States

Eileen H. Shinn, PhD
Department of Behavioral Science, University of Texas MD Anderson Cancer Center, Houston, TX, United States

Alessandro Villa, DDS, PhD, MPH
Miami Cancer Institute, Baptist Health South Florida, Miami, FL, United States; Herbert Wertheim College of Medicine, Florida International University (FIU), Miami, FL, United States

Eric W. Villanueva, MD
Shirley Ryan AbilityLab, Chicago, IL, United States; Department of Physical Medicine and Rehabilitation, Northwestern University Feinberg School of Medicine of Medicine, Chicago, IL, United States

Sreenija Yarlagadda, MD
Radiation Oncology, Miami Cancer Institute, Baptist Health South Florida, Miami, FL, USA

Geoffrey D. Young, MD, PhD, FACS
Florida International University, Herbert Wertheim College of Medicine, Miami, FL, United States; Miami Cancer Institute, Baptist Health South Florida, Miami, FL, United States

Introduction

1

Adrian Cristian, MD, MHCM, FAAPMR

Cancer Rehabilitation, Miami Cancer Institute, Baptist Health South Florida, Miami, FL, United States; Department of Translational Medicine, FIU Herbert Wertheim College of Medicine, Miami, FL, United States

Head and neck cancers comprise only a small percentage of all cancers in the United States and the world compared with other types of cancers. Their location and treatments pose unique challenges to those affected. These cancers arise from the oral cavity, pharynx, larynx, nasal cavity, sinuses, and salivary glands. The complex anatomy of this region is of vital importance to an individual's ability to breathe, eat, and communicate effectively as well as to their physical appearance. It is not unusual for those treated for head and neck cancers with surgery, radiation therapy, and systemic therapy to develop both short-term and late effects of cancer treatments. Swallowing dysfunction, odynophagia, dysgeusia, dysphonia, trismus, lymphedema of the face and neck, fatigue, malnutrition, and psychosocial distress are commonly reported. These in turn can have an adverse impact on an individual's ability to perform basic self-care, work, and enjoy those activities that add meaning to their lives.

This book provides a multidisciplinary and holistic approach to the care of head and neck cancer survivors. It aims to provide the reader with an understanding and appreciation of the pertinent anatomy, pathophysiology, clinical presentation, and treatments of these types of cancers as well as the common impairments associated with them. The goal is to provide clinicians caring for this fragile population with the knowledge to provide the best care possible to prevent or minimize the physical and psychosocial challenges facing head and neck cancer survivors and in doing so, improve the quality of their life.

Head and Neck Cancer Rehabilitation. https://doi.org/10.1016/B978-0-443-11806-7.00010-2
Copyright © 2025 Elsevier Inc. All rights are reserved, including those for text and data mining, AI training, and similar technologies.

Head and neck cancer

Keelin McKenna, Noah Kalman, MD, Guilherme Rabinowits, MD

Herbert Wertheim College of Medicine, Miami, FL, United States

Epidemiology

Head and neck cancer (HNC) is currently the seventh most common malignancy worldwide, accounting for more than 660,000 new diagnoses and 325,000 deaths each year.[1] In 2022, HNC accounted for approximately 4% of all cancer diagnoses in the United States, with an estimated 66,470 new diagnoses and 15,050 deaths.[2] Squamous cell carcinoma is the most common histological type and accounts for 90% of all head and neck malignancies.[1] These cancers frequently arise from the epithelial lining of the oral cavity, oropharynx, larynx, hypopharynx and, more rarely, from salivary glands and paranasal sinuses. The focus here is on squamous cell carcinomas arising from mucosal surfaces of the oral cavity, pharynx, and larynx.

HNC is usually more prevalent in the older population with a median age at diagnosis of 60 years old.[3] For decades, it has been understood that there is a strong association between squamous cell carcinoma of the head and neck and tobacco use.[3,4] It also seems that chronic, heavy alcohol use makes the carcinogenic effects of the tobacco more severe further increasing the risk of developing HNC.[5,6] Betel quid chewing, prevalent in areas outside of the United States, has also been shown to be a risk factor for HNC.[7] Luckily, due to the decreased use of tobacco products, the incidence of HNC has been declining globally.[8] However, there has been an increase in number of oropharyngeal squamous cell carcinoma cases due to human papillomavirus (HPV) infection.[9,10] This is becoming increasingly common in the younger populations of North America and Europe.[11] In the 1980s in the United States, 16.3% of oropharyngeal cancers were found to be HPV-positive. In the 2000s, this percentage has risen dramatically to 72.7%, in conjunction with the decrease in tobacco use.[10] HPV-positive oropharyngeal cancer has even surpassed cervical cancer and is now the number one HPV-related cancer in the United States.[10,12] Malignancy is most commonly associated with HPV 16, 18, 31, and 33, and over 90% of the oropharyngeal squamous cell carcinoma are due to oral sex exposure and are related to HPV 16.[13] The demographic of patients affected

Copyright © 2025 Elsevier Inc. All rights reserved, including those for text and data mining, AI training, and similar technologies.

has also shifted and is now most common in younger white males between the ages of 40–55.[10] This increase in prevalence is most likely due to a multitude of factors including increased awareness, knowledge about the association, and improved diagnostic testing for HPV. Luckily, patients with HPV-associated oropharyngeal cancer have a better prognosis since these tumors usually respond better to treatment, including radiation and chemotherapy, and the affected patients tend to have fewer comorbid conditions.[10,14] Conversely, patients with HPV-negative disease are often chronic alcohol and tobacco users and frequently have additional health concerns.

Prevention

The best prevention method for HPV-positive HNC is through vaccination. In 2020, Gardasil 9, which covers strains 6, 11, 16, 18, 31, 33, 45, 52, and 58, received extended approval indication by the US Food and Drug Administration (FDA) for the prevention of oropharyngeal and other head and neck cancers.[15,16] Gardasil 9 is administered in two or three doses depending on age of the patient. Ideal age for first dose is before the start of sexual activity, around age 9, but it has been approved for adults up to age 45 (Table 2.1).

Even though vaccination is an effective way to prevent malignancy, data has shown that only 54% of children between age 13 and 17 were up to date on vaccination.[17] Additionally, many individuals, including medical providers, are unaware of the connection between HPV and HNC, stressing the importance of bringing awareness to this association.[18]

Table 2.1 Center for disease control HPV vaccine recommendations.[58]

	Ages 9–26	Ages 27–45
General recommendations	Start at age 11 but can start as early as age 9.	Not indicated for everyone. Those at risk for HPV exposure through new sexual partners are likely to have the greatest benefit.
Number of doses and vaccination schedule	Two doses administered 6 –12 months apart if first vaccine is given before age 15 and no personal history of immunosuppression. Otherwise, three doses at month 0, 1–2, and 6.	Three doses administered at month 0, 1–2, and 6.

Patients should also be counseled and offered resources for the cessation of tobacco and alcohol use, and betel quid chewing, as these are known preventable risk factors for HNC.

Presentation and diagnosis

Head and neck cancers are often first discovered by dentists or primary care physicians at standard health maintenance visits. Patients most commonly present with an enlarging neck mass, dysphagia, odynophagia, hoarseness, oral/oropharynx mucosal abnormalities, throat/mouth pain, or weight loss and should be referred to an otolaryngologist or head and neck surgeon for a more thorough evaluation.[19] Even though many patients present with symptoms suggestive of an HNC, others are asymptomatic. The American Cancer Society and the US Department of Health and Human services recommend that physicians screen regularly for signs or symptoms of HNC at routine health visits.

As with every medical condition, a thorough history is the key to a proper diagnosis. When interviewing patients with suspected HNC, special attention should be given to toxic exposures, such as tobacco and alcohol use. Additionally, physicians should inquire about sexual practices to ascertain if they are at risk for HPV infection. Then, a thorough physical exam should be conducted, paying particular attention to the mucosal head and neck regions.

One of the most useful physical exam tools is visual inspection and palpation, especially for lesions localized in the oral cavity. This is especially useful in developing countries where this is a low-cost and accessible option.[20] For head and neck cancers that are located more distally in the oropharynx, hypopharynx, or larynx, inspection with a mirror examination or direct rigid or flexible laryngoscope (preferrable, if available, particularly to the nasal cavity and nasopharynx) is useful. This procedure can be done in the physician's office. After visual inspection, the physician should palpate the oral cavity and oropharynx feeling for any abnormalities.

After a thorough history and physical examination, further diagnostic tests and imaging may be warranted. For confirmation of a final diagnosis, a biopsy must be performed. This includes sampling the primary tumor site and/or biopsy of an abnormal lymph node. Fine needle aspiration is the method of choice for sampling lymph nodes.[21] Imaging studies are also recommended to determine the extent of disease. A cervical contrast-enhanced computed tomography (CT) or magnetic resonance imaging (MRI) can be performed to examine local spread. MRI is particularly useful in evaluating the tongue, perineural spread, skull base invasion, and intracranial extension.[22] Fluorodeoxyglucose-positron emission tomography/CT (FDG-PET/CT), if available, is commonly used to assess regional and distant metastatic spread.[23,24]

Patients who are diagnosed with HNC also require dental evaluation, particularly for those requiring radiation therapy, given risks of osteoradionecrosis, xerostomia, and teeth decay/cavities; speech language pathology therapy evaluation, given potential trismus, speech, and swallowing dysfunction caused by the cancer and its treatment; rehabilitation physicians given potential for muscle weakness/impairment and lymphedema; dietician to optimize their caloric intake and needs; and psychological or social evaluation, given anxiety/depression associated with the cancer diagnosis and its treatment.

Patients who present with an oropharyngeal squamous cell carcinoma should have their biopsy sample tested for HPV since a positive result has now staging, prognosis, and treatment implications. Although polymerase chain reaction (PCR) and in situ hybridization are frequently used for HPV evaluation and can be performed on a fresh frozen sample or formalin-fixed paraffin embedded tissue specimen, reverse transcriptase (RT) PCR amplification of viral E6/E7 messenger RNA is now considered the most accurate test for detecting functionally causal HPV within tumor specimens as it detects transcriptionally active HPV.[25,26]

Due to challenges in performing these tests, including limited availability and cost, p16 by immunohistochemistry (IHC) is often used as a surrogate marker for determining HPV status, since it is commonly overexpressed in HPV-related oropharyngeal squamous cell carcinoma.[27] Since other cancers, such as skin and lung cancers, can also overexpress p16, HPV testing should also be performed, particularly in the workup for unknown primary HNC, when a primary oropharyngeal tumor is not clearly identified.[28–31]

Staging

The TNM staging method is a well-recognized system for evaluating the extent of disease for all different types of cancer, including HNC. It is widely used by physicians as a systematic approach to treating patients with cancer. At diagnosis, this system helps to evaluate best treatment options and prognosis of the disease. It was first developed by Pierre Denoix in 1944 and includes the assessment of tumor characteristics (T), nodal spread (N), and distant metastases (M). In 1987, the first edition of the American Joint Committee on Cancer (AJCC) and the International Union Against Cancer (UICC) TNM classification system was published, utilizing Pierre Denoix's original concept. The AJCC/UICC classification system is now on its eighth edition, which introduced new classifications for HNC. Only the major changes from AJCC/UICC seventh to eighth edition will be discussed in the following.

Previously, for oral cavity cancer, the most important factor for the T stage was the tumor size. However, it is now known that depth of invasion (DOI) has important prognostic implications, including higher rate of metastasis to lymph nodes and decreased survival, in individuals with deeper tumors.[32,33] This factor has been added to the new edition so now patients with T1 tumors have a tumor size ≤ 2 cm with DOI ≤ 5 mm; T2 has a tumor size ≤ 2 cm with DOI >5 mm and ≤ 10 mm or tumor size >2 and ≤ 4 cm with DOI ≤ 10 mm; T3 has a tumor size >2 cm and ≤ 4 cm with DOI >10 mm or tumor size >4 cm with DOI ≤ 10 mm;

T4a tumor >4 cm with DOI >10 mm or tumor invades adjacent structures only (e.g., through cortical bone of mandible or maxilla, or involves the maxillary sinus or skin of the face); and T4b correlates to invasion of masticator space, pterygoid plates, or skull base and/or encases the internal carotid artery.[32,34]

For oral cavity cancer, the N category was also updated to contain extracapsular nodal extension (ENE).[32,34] This is an important prognostic factor in all mucosal head and neck squamous cell carcinoma cases, except for HPV-positive tumors, which remains less defined.[32,35,36] The updated criteria include N3b as any lymph node metastasis, regardless of size, with clinical/imaging findings concerning for ENE, or a single ipsilateral lymph node metastasis >3 cm with pathological ENE, or multiple (ipsilateral, contralateral, or bilateral) lymph nodes with pathological ENE, or a single contralateral lymph node, regardless of size, with pathological ENE. N1 consists of a single ipsilateral node metastasis ≤3 cm with no clinical/imaging findings concerning for ENE, but upstaged to N2 if, after surgery, that lymph node ≤3 cm is found to have pathological ENE. N2 consists of metastasis in a single ipsilateral lymph node >3 and ≤6 cm without ENE (N2a); metastasis in multiple ipsilateral lymph nodes ≤6 cm without ENE (N2b); metastasis in bilateral or contralateral lymph nodes ≤6 cm without ENE (N2c); N3a consists of a lymph node >6 cm without ENE.[32,34]

For the nasopharyngeal cancer, the eighth edition staging classification included a T0 for the Epstein—Barr virus (EBV) positive cervical lymph nodes with an unknown primary origin.[33,36]

One of the most interesting changes to the most current edition was the creation of a new category for HPV (or p16)-positive oropharyngeal squamous cell carcinoma, given the more favorable prognosis for these patients, even with advanced disease.[10,37] Previously, these cancers were staged based on their anatomic location but were realized to be a distinct subtype, showing drastically different behavior than their HPV-negative counterparts.[38] The Radiation Therapy Oncology Group (RTOG) 0129 was a phase 3 trial comparing two modified radiation fractionation regimens in combination with cisplatin in patients with locally advanced HNC.[37] Although there were no differences in terms of overall survival, progression-free survival, locoregional failure, and distant metastasis between the arms, the study demonstrated an improvement in 3-year overall survival for patients with HPV-positive oropharyngeal cancer in comparison with those with HPV-negative oropharyngeal cancer (82.4% vs. 57.1%, respectively; $P < .001$).[37] Even after adjusting for other factors, such as tobacco exposure or treatment group, HPV-positive patients had a 58% reduction in risk of death (hazard ratio, 0.42; 95% CI, 0.27—0.66). The better outcome was still maintained after a longer median follow-up, revealing an 8-year overall survival of 70.9% versus 30.2%; progression-free survival of 64.0% versus 23.3%; locoregional failure of 19.5% versus 52.4%; and distant metastasis of 10.3% versus 16.1% for HPV-positive and negative oropharyngeal squamous cell carcinoma patients, respectively.[39] These results were all statistically significant, except for the distant metastasis.

In the eighth AJCC staging edition for HPV-related oropharyngeal cancer, T0 includes the p16-positive cervical lymph nodes with an unknown primary origin; T4b was removed; clinical (c) N1 consists of ipsilateral node(s), none >6 cm; cN2 consists of contralateral or bilateral nodes, none >6 cm; cN3 consists of any node >6 cm. For the pathological (p) staging, the number of positive nodes stratifies the different pN stages, with pN1 consisting of 1−4 metastatic nodes, and pN2 consisting of >4 metastatic nodes.[32,36] Clinical and pathological prognostic stage groups have changed in a way that clinical (c) stage I now includes tumors ≤ cT2 (tumor size ≤4 cm) with none, one, or more ipsilateral metastatic nodes; and stage II with ≤ cT3 (tumor size >4 cm or extension to the lingual surface of the epiglottis) and/or bilateral or contralateral metastatic nodes; reserving the stage III for those with cT4 (tumor invasion to larynx, extrinsic tongue muscle, medial pterygoid, hard palate, mandible or beyond) or cN3 disease and clinical and pathological stage IV for those with distant metastasis (M1). Pathological (p) stage I includes tumors ≤ pT2 and ≤ pN1; stage II with ≤ pT2 and pN2 or pT3/4 and ≤ pN1; stage III with pT3/4 and pN2.[32,36]

The staging for the other head and neck cancer subsites remains relatively similar.

Treatment

Given the complexity of these cancers, these patients should be evaluated and treated at a high-volume, tertiary cancer center, where a multidisciplinary dedicated HNC team is available for decision-making and treatment planning to optimize the outcome and quality of life of these patients. The head and neck oncology multidisciplinary team should consist of a medical oncologist, radiation oncologist, head and neck surgical oncologist, head and neck reconstructive surgeon, dentist, prosthodontics, speech language pathologist, cancer rehabilitation physician, dietician, psychosocial therapist, and an oncology nurse. These are the key players on the management of these patients to optimize organ function pre-, during, and post-cancer treatment.

Treatment—Surgery

Surgery is often used by itself for early-stage HNC, or in combination with radiation therapy (or chemoradiation therapy) for those with more advanced disease, or with adverse features on surgical pathology report (lymphovascular space invasion, perineural invasion, lymph node metastasis, ENE, close or positive surgical margins). Although primary surgery and definitive radiation therapy are both options for early-stage disease, resulting in similar rates of local control and survival for many HNC subsites, primary surgery remains preferable for tumors arising in the oral cavity.

Advances in surgery include minimally invasive surgery such as transoral robotic surgery and transoral laser microsurgery with a better functional outcome and less morbidity in comparison to prior surgical techniques requiring mandibulotomy and transmandibular approach to gain access to the tumor site.[40–42] In addition, modified radical neck dissection (levels I–V) is becoming less frequent and now replaced by selective neck dissection (levels II–IV) or supraomohyoid neck dissection (levels I–III) with significant less morbidity.

Finally, advances in technology and three-dimensional surgical simulators now allow for advanced surgical planning, which results in better outcomes, as well as more successful reconstruction.[43] Preoperative high-resolution CT associated with 3D printers can create accurate models that allow the surgeon to better visualize the tumor and associated anatomical landmarks. This has led to more successful resection, graft harvesting, and reconstruction.

However, head and neck surgery is not without complications. When operating in the neck, there is risk of air embolus formation, pneumothorax, or a chyle leak, usually due to injury to the internal jugular vein, lungs, or lymphatics, respectively.[44] Additionally, there is risk of injury to the surrounding neural structures, including spinal accessory nerves, branches of the facial nerve, and the phrenic nerves. This can lead to decreased muscle function and weakness. Finally, a large percentage of morbidity and mortality is due to injury or prolonged occlusion of the carotid arteries, leading to deprivation of oxygen to the brain.[44] After operating in the oral cavity, patients are most at risk of having speech and swallowing problems postoperatively, which can significantly impair their quality of life.[45] These complications emphasize the importance of comprehensive rehabilitation efforts following surgical intervention.

Treatment—Radiation therapy

Radiation therapy is one of the main treatment modalities for HNC. It is used in the curative intent treatment of early-stage disease, in combination with surgery and/or chemotherapy for locally advanced disease, and in the palliative setting for those with incurable, metastatic disease.

A major implication in the treatment of HNC is the close proximity of a multitude of important structures. Damage to these structures, such as the brainstem, spinal cord, optic pathways, salivary glands, and swallowing structures, can drastically decrease a patient's quality of life.[46] Radiation-related toxicities include dermatitis, skin fibrosis, mucositis, carotid stenosis/plaques, esophageal stenosis, trismus, dysgeusia, xerostomia, osteoradionecrosis, teeth decay/cavities, occipital scalp hair loss, and lymphedema.

Modern advances in radiation therapy include imaging guided radiation therapy that allows for reduction of dose to organs/structures at risk for irradiation while preserving the target volume dose coverage, and adaptive radiation therapy to optimize the delivered dose distribution to the changing anatomy.[47] Another advance in radiation therapy is the use of protons instead of photons in situations where the normal tissue constrains cannot be met with the use of photon-based therapy given the proton's steeper distal fall-off dose.[48]

Multiple studies looking into treatment deintensification have been performed in an attempt to decrease both acute and long-term toxicities without sacrificing the excellent survival outcome of HPV-positive oropharyngeal squamous cell carcinoma patients.

Treatment—Systemic therapy

There are currently three major systemic treatment options available for HNC: traditional chemotherapy, targeted therapy, and immunotherapy.

Several ground-breaking trials have helped shape the way chemotherapy is delivered. The RTOG 91−11 trial investigated the optimal timing of adding chemotherapy to radiation therapy as an alternative to total laryngectomy for patients with locally advanced laryngeal cancer.[49] The RTOG 9501 and the European Organization for Research and Treatment of Cancer (EORTC) 22931 clinical trials investigated the outcomes of patients that had received postoperative cisplatin in combination with radiation therapy in comparison with radiation alone.[50,51] The RTOG 91−11 results revealed that larynx preservation and locoregional control were significantly improved with concomitant cisplatin and radiation therapy in comparison with induction chemotherapy followed by radiation therapy and to radiation therapy alone arms.[49] The laryngectomy-free survival (the primary endpoint of this study) was similar between the chemotherapy arms, and better in comparison with radiation alone, making concurrent chemoradiation therapy with cisplatin the standard of care treatment for locally advanced HNC patients. The RTOG 9501 and EORTC 22931 studies' results found that the combination chemoradiation therapy with cisplatin resulted in significantly better locoregional control and disease-free survival in comparison with radiation therapy alone for those with microscopic surgical margins or ENE, making adjuvant chemoradiation therapy with cisplatin standard of care treatment for HNC with these high-risk features on surgical pathology.[50,51] Despite the benefits seen with the combination, the addition of chemotherapy increased the toxicity of the treatment in comparison with radiation alone. Chemotherapy-related toxicities include increased mucositis, neurotoxicity, ototoxicity, nephrotoxicity, myelosuppression, electrolyte imbalance, nausea and vomiting, and skin rash.

Cetuximab is the only targeted therapy approved in HNC. It is a monoclonal antibody directed against epidermal growth factor receptor (EGFR). Over 90% of head and neck squamous cell carcinoma overexpress EGFR. It is approved in combination with radiation therapy for patients with locally advanced disease, as a single agent for patients with platinum refractory disease, or in combination with platinum and 5-fluorouracil (5FU) for those with incurable disease. These standard of care treatments were established due to several key studies. Bonner et al. performed a study to assess if the combination of cetuximab and radiation therapy was superior to radiation therapy alone in patients with locally advanced HNC.[52] Patients were randomized to cetuximab and radiation combination (211 patients) or radiation therapy alone (213 patients). The median duration of local disease control was 24.4 months for the combination therapy group versus 14.9 months for the radiation alone group. Additionally, overall survival was 49 months in the combination therapy group versus 29.3 months in the radiation alone group. There was no increase in adverse events, including mucositis, with the combination therapy when compared with the radiation therapy alone.[52]

Vermorken et al. conducted a trial to assess if cetuximab is a viable option for patients with disease refractory to platinum therapy.[53] One hundred and three HNC patients with disease progression on platinum therapy underwent weekly cetuximab. The response rate was 13%, disease control rate was 46%, and the median time to progression was 70 days. The treatment was well tolerated with the most common adverse reaction being rash. There was one treatment related death due to an infusion-related reaction.[53]

Vermorken at al. conducted a subsequent study to assess the activity of cetuximab in combination with platinum and 5FU in patients with incurable disease.[54] Four hundred and forty two eligible patients were randomized to platinum and 5FU with or without cetuximab. The median overall survival and the median progression-free survival increased from 7.4 and 3.3 months to 10.1 and 5.6 months, respectively, with the addition of cetuximab.[54]

In regard to immunotherapy, both pembrolizumab and nivolumab are monoclonal antibodies against programmed cell death 1 (PD1) receptor and approved for the use in the second line for HNC patients with incurable disease that failed platinum-based therapy. The Checkmate 141 clinical trial assessed the efficacy of nivolumab for the treatment of recurrent head and neck squamous cell carcinoma.[55] They randomized in a 2:1 ratio 361 patients to receive nivolumab or standard therapy (methotrexate, docetaxel or cetuximab). The median overall survival of those who received immunotherapy was better than for those who received standard of care therapy (7.5 vs. 5.1 months, respectively). The 6-month progression-free survival also improved from 9.9% in the control group to 19.7% in the immunotherapy group.[55]

The Keynote 040 study was similar in that it compared pembrolizumab to standard therapy (methotrexate, docetaxel, or cetuximab).[56] Overall survival for pembrolizumab was 8.4 months, compared with 6.9 months in the control group. The treatment was also well tolerated with fewer patients having severe adverse reactions in the immunotherapy group compared with the control group.

Pembrolizumab is also approved as first-line therapy as a single agent for patients with metastatic disease with programmed cell death ligand 1 (PD-L1) combined positive score (CPS) ≥ 1, and in combination with platinum and 5FU independent of the PD-L1 status. Of note, PD-L1 CPS appears to be a better predictor of immunotherapy response in HNC than tumor's PD-L1 expression only, since it takes into account the PD-L1 expression of lymphocytes and macrophages in addition to the tumor cells.

In the Keynote-048 clinical trial, 882 patients with incurable, recurrent, or metastatic head and neck squamous cell carcinoma were randomized to receive pembrolizumab alone, pembrolizumab plus platinum and 5FU, or cetuximab plus platinum and 5FU.[57] The median overall survival for the single agent pembrolizumab group with PD-L1 CPS ≥1 was superior in comparison with cetuximab plus chemotherapy group (12.3 vs. 10.3 months, respectively; $P = .0086$). That survival difference was further improved for those with CPS >20 (14.9 months in the single agent pembrolizumab vs. 10.7 months in the cetuximab plus chemotherapy group; $P = .0007$) but was noninferior in the total population (11.6 vs. 10.7 months). In contrast, pembrolizumab plus chemotherapy improved the overall survival in comparison with cetuximab plus chemotherapy in the total population (13 vs. 10.7 months; $P = .0034$), in those with PD-L1 CPS ≥20 (14.7 vs. 11 months; $P = .0004$) and in those with PD-L1 CPS ≥1 (13.6 vs. 10.4 months; $P < .0001$).[57]

Immunotherapy-related toxicities include fatigue, thyroiditis, skin rash, colitis, hepatitis, pneumonitis, myocarditis, hypophysitis, diabetes, and autoimmune disorder flares/exacerbations.

In summary, the toxicities caused not only by the different treatment modalities but also by the HNC itself can significantly impact the patients' quality of life. Basic functions such as talking, eating, swallowing, and breathing can easily be affected. Patients' appearance/cosmesis can also be affected secondary to surgical changes such as disfigurement and scar tissue formation; radiation-induced dermatitis, fibrosis, mucositis, lymphedema; and systemic therapy-induced rash, vitiligo, fluid retention, neurotoxicity, and ototoxicity. These toxicities can all lead to social isolation, physical pain, depression/anxiety, and suicidal ideation, so rehabilitation efforts, preferably starting at time of the diagnosis, are imperative in these patients. Referral to supportive services, including but not limited to cancer rehabilitation, speech and swallow therapy, psychosocial therapy, dietician, dentist should be made early on, preferentially prior cancer therapy initiation to help increase patients' functioning and quality of life throughout the treatment process. This is even more important now that the outcome of these patients is improving, not only by the advances on the different treatment modalities, but by the fact that the incidence of tobacco-related HNC is decreasing and the incidence of HPV-related oropharyngeal cancer is increasing. Early intervention is a must to optimize and maintain organ function so patients can not only live longer but also better.

References

1. Sung H, Ferlay J, Siegel RL, et al. Global cancer statistics 2020: GLOBOCAN estimates of incidence and mortality worldwide for 36 cancers in 185 countries. *CA A Cancer J Clin.* 2021;71:209−249. https://doi.org/10.3322/caac.21660.
2. Siegel RL, Miller KD, Fuchs HE, Jemal A. Cancer statistics, 2022. *CA A Cancer J Clin.* 2022;72:7−33. https://doi.org/10.3322/caac.21708.

3. Sturgis EM, Wei Q, Spitz MR. Descriptive epidemiology and risk factors for head and neck cancer. *Semin Oncol*. 2004;31:726−733. https://doi.org/10.1053/j.seminoncol. 2004.09.013.

4. Wyss A, Hashibe M, Chuang S-C, et al. Cigarette, cigar, and pipe smoking and the risk of head and neck cancers: pooled analysis in the international head and neck cancer epidemiology consortium. *Am J Epidemiol*. 2013;178:679−690. https://doi.org/10.1093/aje/kwt029.

5. Blot WJ, McLaughlin JK, Winn DM, et al. Smoking and drinking in relation to oral and pharyngeal cancer. *Cancer Res*. 1988;48:3282−3287.

6. Hashibe M, Brennan P, Benhamou S, et al. Alcohol drinking in never users of tobacco, cigarette smoking in never drinkers, and the risk of head and neck cancer: pooled analysis in the international head and neck cancer epidemiology consortium. *J Natl Cancer Inst*. 2007;99:777−789. https://doi.org/10.1093/jnci/djk179.

7. Su C-C, Yang H-F, Huang S-J, Lian I-B. Distinctive features of oral cancer in Changhua County: high incidence, buccal mucosa preponderance, and a close relation to betel quid chewing habit. *J Formos Med Assoc Taiwan Yi Zhi*. 2007;106:225−233. https://doi.org/10.1016/s0929-6646(09)60244-8.

8. Mourad M, Jetmore T, Jategaonkar AA, Moubayed S, Moshier E, Urken ML. Epidemiological trends of head and neck cancer in the United States: a SEER population study. *J Oral Maxillofac Surg*. 2017;75:2562−2572. https://doi.org/10.1016/j.joms.2017.05. 008.

9. Sturgis EM, Cinciripini PM. Trends in head and neck cancer incidence in relation to smoking prevalence: an emerging epidemic of human papillomavirus-associated cancers? *Cancer*. 2007;110:1429−1435. https://doi.org/10.1002/cncr.22963.

10. Chaturvedi AK, Engels EA, Pfeiffer RM, et al. Human papillomavirus and rising oropharyngeal cancer incidence in the United States. *J Clin Oncol*. 2011;29:4294−4301. https://doi.org/10.1200/JCO.2011.36.4596.

11. Mehanna H, Beech T, Nicholson T, et al. Prevalence of human papillomavirus in oropharyngeal and nonoropharyngeal head and neck cancer−systematic review and meta-analysis of trends by time and region. *Head Neck*. 2013;35:747−755. https://doi.org/10.1002/hed.22015.

12. Van Dyne EA, Henley SJ, Saraiya M, Thomas CC, Markowitz LE, Benard VB. Trends in human papillomavirus-associated cancers - United States, 1999-2015. *MMWR Morb Mortal Wkly Rep*. 2018;67:918−924. https://doi.org/10.15585/mmwr.mm6733a2.

13. Gillison ML. Human papillomavirus-associated head and neck cancer is a distinct epidemiologic, clinical, and molecular entity. *Semin Oncol*. 2004;31:744−754. https://doi.org/10.1053/j.seminoncol.2004.09.011.

14. Gillison ML, D'Souza G, Westra W, et al. Distinct risk factor profiles for human papillomavirus type 16-positive and human papillomavirus type 16-negative head and neck cancers. *J Natl Cancer Inst*. 2008;100:407−420. https://doi.org/10.1093/jnci/djn025.

15. GARDASIL9 (human papillomavirus 9-valent vaccine, recombinant). [Package insert]. Whitehouse Station, NJ; Merck & Co., Inc; Revised August 2020.

16. Gardasil. Available online: https://www.fda.gov/vaccines-blood-biologics/vaccines/gardasil-9.

17. Elam-Evans LD, Yankey D, Singleton JA, et al. National, regional, state, and selected local area vaccination coverage among adolescents aged 13-17 Years - United States, 2019. *MMWR Morb Mortal Wkly Rep*. 2020;69:1109−1116. https://doi.org/10.15585/mmwr.mm6933a1.

18. Mehta V, Holmes S, Master A, Leblanc B, Caldito LG, Bocchini J. Knowledge of HPV-related oropharyngeal cancer and use of human papillomavirus vaccines by Pediatricians in Louisiana. *J La State Med Soc*. 2017;169:37−42.

19. Mody MD, Rocco JW, Yom SS, Haddad RI, Saba NF. Head and neck cancer. *Lancet Lond Engl*. 2021;398:2289−2299. https://doi.org/10.1016/S0140-6736(21)01550-6.

20. Sankaranarayanan R, Ramadas K, Thomas G, et al. Trivandrum oral cancer screening study group effect of screening on oral cancer mortality in Kerala, India: a cluster-randomised controlled trial. *Lancet Lond Engl*. 2005;365:1927−1933. https://doi.org/10.1016/S0140-6736(05)66658-5.

21. Tandon S, Shahab R, Benton JI, Ghosh SK, Sheard J, Jones TM. Fine-needle aspiration cytology in a regional head and neck cancer center: comparison with a systematic review and meta-analysis. *Head Neck*. 2008;30:1246−1252. https://doi.org/10.1002/hed.20849.

22. Pfister DG, Spencer S, Adelstein D, et al. Head and neck cancers, version 2.2020, NCCN clinical practice guidelines in oncology. *J Natl Compr Cancer Netw JNCCN*. 2020;18: 873−898. https://doi.org/10.6004/jnccn.2020.0031.

23. Sun R, Tang X, Yang Y, Zhang C. (18)FDG-PET/CT for the detection of regional nodal metastasis in patients with head and neck cancer: a meta-analysis. *Oral Oncol*. 2015;51: 314−320. https://doi.org/10.1016/j.oraloncology.2015.01.004.

24. Rohde M, Nielsen AL, Johansen J, et al. Head-to-head comparison of chest X-ray/head and neck MRI, chest CT/head and neck MRI, and 18F-FDG PET/CT for detection of distant metastases and synchronous cancer in oral, pharyngeal, and laryngeal cancer. *J Nucl Med*. 2017;58:1919−1924. https://doi.org/10.2967/jnumed.117.189704.

25. Nuovo GJ. In situ detection of human papillomavirus DNA after PCR-amplification. *Methods Mol Biol Clifton NJ*. 2011;688:35−46. https://doi.org/10.1007/978-1-60761-947-5_4.

26. Galati L, Chiocca S, Duca D, et al. HPV and head and neck cancers: towards early diagnosis and prevention. *Tumour Virus Res*. 2022;14:200245. https://doi.org/10.1016/j.tvr.2022.200245.

27. Lewis JS, Beadle B, Bishop JA, et al. Human papillomavirus testing in head and neck carcinomas: guideline from the college of American pathologists. *Arch Pathol Lab Med*. 2018;142:559−597. https://doi.org/10.5858/arpa.2017-0286-CP.

28. Beadle BM, William WN, McLemore MS, Sturgis EM, Williams MD. P16 expression in cutaneous squamous carcinomas with neck metastases: a potential pitfall in identifying unknown primaries of the head and neck. *Head Neck*. 2013;35:1527−1533. https://doi.org/10.1002/hed.23188.

29. Conscience I, Jovenin N, Coissard C, et al. P16 is overexpressed in cutaneous carcinomas located on sun-exposed areas. *Eur. J. Dermatol. EJD*. 2006;16:518−522.

30. Chang SY, Keeney M, Law M, Donovan J, Aubry M-C, Garcia J. Detection of human papillomavirus in non-small cell carcinoma of the lung. *Hum Pathol*. 2015;46: 1592−1597. https://doi.org/10.1016/j.humpath.2015.07.012.

31. Prigge E-S, Arbyn M, von Knebel Doeberitz M, Reuschenbach M. Diagnostic accuracy of P16INK4a immunohistochemistry in oropharyngeal squamous cell carcinomas: a systematic review and meta-analysis. *Int J Cancer*. 2017;140:1186−1198. https://doi.org/10.1002/ijc.30516.

32. Amin MB,ES, Greene FL, et al., eds. *AJCC Cancer Staging Manual*. 8th ed. New York: Springer International Publishing: American Joint Commission on Cancer; 2017.

33. International Consortium for Outcome Research (Icor) in Head and Neck Cancer, Ebrahimi A, Gil Z, et al. Primary tumor staging for oral cancer and a proposed

modification incorporating depth of invasion: an international multicenter retrospective study. *JAMA Otolaryngol—Head Neck Surg*. 2014;140:1138−1148. https://doi.org/10.1001/jamaoto.2014.1548.

34. Zanoni DK, Patel SG. New AJCC: how does it impact oral cancers? *Oral Oncol*. 2020; 104:104607. https://doi.org/10.1016/j.oraloncology.2020.104607.

35. Wreesmann VB, Katabi N, Palmer FL, et al. Influence of extracapsular nodal spread extent on prognosis of oral squamous cell carcinoma. *Head Neck*. 2016;38(Suppl 1): E1192−E1199. https://doi.org/10.1002/hed.24190.

36. Zanoni DK, Patel SG, Shah JP. Changes in the 8th edition of the American joint committee on cancer (AJCC) staging of head and neck cancer: rationale and implications. *Curr Oncol Rep*. 2019;21:52. https://doi.org/10.1007/s11912-019-0799-x.

37. Ang KK, Harris J, Wheeler R, et al. Human papillomavirus and survival of patients with oropharyngeal cancer. *N Engl J Med*. 2010;363:24−35. https://doi.org/10.1056/NEJMoa0912217.

38. O'Sullivan B, Huang SH, Su J, et al. Development and validation of a staging system for HPV-related oropharyngeal cancer by the international collaboration on oropharyngeal cancer network for staging (ICON-S): a multicentre cohort study. *Lancet Oncol*. 2016; 17:440−451. https://doi.org/10.1016/S1470-2045(15)00560-4.

39. Nguyen-Tan PF, Zhang Q, Ang KK, et al. Randomized phase III trial to test accelerated versus standard fractionation in combination with concurrent cisplatin for head and neck carcinomas in the radiation therapy oncology group 0129 trial: long-term report of efficacy and toxicity. *J Clin Oncol*. 2014;32:3858−3866. https://doi.org/10.1200/JCO.2014.55.3925.

40. Genden EM, Kotz T, Tong CCL, et al. Transoral robotic resection and reconstruction for head and neck cancer. *Laryngoscope*. 2011;121:1668−1674. https://doi.org/10.1002/lary.21845.

41. Moore EJ, Olsen SM, Laborde RR, et al. Long-term functional and oncologic results of transoral robotic surgery for oropharyngeal squamous cell carcinoma. *Mayo Clin Proc*. 2012;87:219−225. https://doi.org/10.1016/j.mayocp.2011.10.007.

42. Nguyen AT, Luu M, Mallen-St Clair J, et al. Comparison of survival after transoral robotic surgery vs nonrobotic surgery in patients with early-stage oropharyngeal squamous cell carcinoma. *JAMA Oncol*. 2020;6:1555−1562. https://doi.org/10.1001/jamaoncol.2020.3172.

43. Zoabi A, Redenski I, Oren D, et al. 3D printing and virtual surgical planning in oral and maxillofacial surgery. *J Clin Med*. 2022;11:2385. https://doi.org/10.3390/jcm11092385.

44. Kerawala CJ. Complications of head and neck cancer surgery - prevention and management. *Oral Oncol*. 2010;46:433−435. https://doi.org/10.1016/j.oraloncology.2010.03.013.

45. Suarez-Cunqueiro M-M, Schramm A, Schoen R, et al. Speech and swallowing impairment after treatment for oral and oropharyngeal cancer. *Arch Otolaryngol Head Neck Surg*. 2008;134:1299−1304. https://doi.org/10.1001/archotol.134.12.1299.

46. Alterio D, Marvaso G, Ferrari A, Volpe S, Orecchia R, Jereczek-Fossa BA. Modern radiotherapy for head and neck cancer. *Semin Oncol*. 2019;46:233−245. https://doi.org/10.1053/j.seminoncol.2019.07.002.

47. Castelli J, Simon A, Lafond C, et al. Adaptive radiotherapy for head and neck cancer. *Acta Oncol Stockh Swed*. 2018;57:1284−1292. https://doi.org/10.1080/0284186X.2018.1505053.

48. Blanchard P, Gunn GB, Lin A, Foote RL, Lee NY, Frank SJ. Proton therapy for head and neck cancers. *Semin Radiat Oncol.* 2018;28:53−63. https://doi.org/10.1016/j.semradonc.2017.08.004.

49. Forastiere AA, Goepfert H, Maor M, et al. Concurrent chemotherapy and radiotherapy for organ preservation in advanced laryngeal cancer. *N Engl J Med.* 2003;349:2091−2098. https://doi.org/10.1056/NEJMoa031317.

50. Cooper JS, Zhang Q, Pajak TF, et al. Long-term follow-up of the RTOG 9501/intergroup phase III trial: postoperative concurrent radiation therapy and chemotherapy in high-risk squamous cell carcinoma of the head and neck. *Int J Radiat Oncol Biol Phys.* 2012;84:1198−1205. https://doi.org/10.1016/j.ijrobp.2012.05.008.

51. Bernier J, Domenge C, Ozsahin M, et al. Postoperative irradiation with or without concomitant chemotherapy for locally advanced head and neck cancer. *N Engl J Med.* 2004;350:1945−1952. https://doi.org/10.1056/NEJMoa032641.

52. Bonner JA, Harari PM, Giralt J, et al. Radiotherapy plus cetuximab for squamous-cell carcinoma of the head and neck. *N Engl J Med.* 2006;354:567−578. https://doi.org/10.1056/NEJMoa053422.

53. Vermorken JB, Trigo J, Hitt R, et al. Open-label, uncontrolled, multicenter phase II study to evaluate the efficacy and toxicity of cetuximab as a single agent in patients with recurrent and/or metastatic squamous cell carcinoma of the head and neck who failed to respond to platinum-based therapy. *J Clin Oncol.* 2007;25:2171−2177. https://doi.org/10.1200/JCO.2006.06.7447.

54. Vermorken JB, Mesia R, Rivera F, et al. Platinum-based chemotherapy plus cetuximab in head and neck cancer. *N Engl J Med.* 2008;359:1116−1127. https://doi.org/10.1056/NEJMoa0802656.

55. Ferris RL, Blumenschein G, Fayette J, et al. Nivolumab for recurrent squamous-cell carcinoma of the head and neck. *N Engl J Med.* 2016;375:1856−1867. https://doi.org/10.1056/NEJMoa1602252.

56. Cohen EEW, Soulières D, Le Tourneau C, et al. Pembrolizumab versus methotrexate, docetaxel, or cetuximab for recurrent or metastatic head-and-neck squamous cell carcinoma (KEYNOTE-040): a randomised, open-label, phase 3 study. *Lancet Lond Engl.* 2019;393:156−167. https://doi.org/10.1016/S0140-6736(18)31999-8.

57. Burtness B, Harrington KJ, Greil R, et al. Pembrolizumab alone or with chemotherapy versus cetuximab with chemotherapy for recurrent or metastatic squamous cell carcinoma of the head and neck (KEYNOTE-048): a randomised, open-label, phase 3 study. *Lancet Lond Engl.* 2019;394:1915−1928. https://doi.org/10.1016/S0140-6736(19)32591-7.

58. Meites E, Szilagyi PG, Chesson HW, Unger ER, Romero JR, Markowitz LE. Human papillomavirus vaccination for adults: updated Recommendations of the advisory committee on immunization practices. *MMWR Morb Mortal Wkly Rep.* 2019;68:698−702. https://doi.org/10.15585/mmwr.mm6832a3.

Radiation therapy in head and neck cancer

3

Sreenija Yarlagadda, MD and Noah S. Kalman, MD, MBA

Radiation Oncology, Miami Cancer Institute, Baptist Health South Florida, Miami, FL, USA

Epidemiology

Over 55,000 new head and neck cancer (HNC) cases and 14,000 cancer-related deaths are estimated to occur in the United States in 2023.[1] This incidence is anticipated to rise by 45% by 2040, with approximately 90% of HNCs being squamous cell carcinomas (SCCs) arising from the oral cavity, pharynx, and larynx.[2] Men are typically at two- to fourfold higher risk than women to develop HNC. Predisposing factors include exposure to tobacco-derived carcinogens and excessive alcohol consumption; specifically for oropharyngeal cancers, infection with human papillomavirus (HPV) stands out as a primary risk factor.

With increased awareness and advancements in treatment, the number of cancer survivors has been on the rise in the past decade.[3] However, HNC survivors are at substantial risk for functional and esthetic compromise; historically, HNC survivors have had the highest rates of suicide compared with other cancer survivors (almost two times).[4] This emphasizes the role of "rehabilitation" in attempting to reestablish impaired functions and improve patient's quality of life.

Assessment and workup

Many HNCs can arise from premalignant lesions, which are defined as morphologically altered tissue in which cancer is more likely to develop than in its apparently normal counterpart. Lesions typically present in the oral cavity as white patches (leukoplakia) or red patches (erythroplakia). A thorough history of tobacco exposure and careful physical examination of the oral cavity for these lesions remains the primary approach for early detection. However, a significant proportion of patients can also present without an apparent clinical history of a premalignant lesion.

Oral cavity tumors typically present as a persistent ulcer/mass commonly at the border of the tongue, buccal mucosa, gingiva, floor of mouth, or lower lip. Progressive pain, bleeding, and/or difficulty chewing are common presenting symptoms. Nonoral cavity lesions can present with dysphagia (difficulty swallowing), odynophagia (pain swallowing), referred otalgia (ear pain), epistaxis (nose bleeds), and/ or hoarseness of voice based on the site of origin of the lesion. At times, a painless

Head and Neck Cancer Rehabilitation. https://doi.org/10.1016/B978-0-443-11806-7.00004-7
Copyright © 2025 Elsevier Inc. All rights reserved, including those for text and data mining, AI training, and similar technologies.

17

neck lump can be the only complaint. A high index of suspicion is essential when the symptoms persist for more than 3 weeks and are progressing in severity.

The diagnosis of HNC must be established by histological examination with biopsy of the primary tumor or the suspicious neck mass. SCC is by far the most common histologic subtype, confirmed by cell morphology and p40 immunohistochemistry (IHC) staining. Oropharyngeal SCC or neck SCC with an unknown primary site mandates the evaluation of HPV status by the surrogate marker of p16 IHC testing and/or with HPV polymerase chain reaction (PCR) or in situ hybridization (ISH) testing to help determine staging and prognosis.[5] Although not included in the staging, determination of Epstein−Barr virus (EBV) status helps assess prognosis for nasopharyngeal carcinomas.

Direct inspection of the oral cavity, clinical nodal exam, fiber-optic nasopharyng-olaryngoscopy, and skin inspection (to rule a cutaneous primary tumor) are indicated to evaluate the extent of disease and to rule out a second primary tumor, as field cancerization can be seen in the upper aerodigestive tract. Staging evaluation includes cross-sectional imaging of the head and neck by computed tomography (CT) or magnetic resonance imaging (MRI) to characterize the locoregional extent of the disease and CT-chest or positron emission tomography (PET-CT) to rule out metastatic disease (PET is generally preferred). Once the appropriate pathological and imaging information has been obtained, TNM stage (extent of primary tumor [T], extent of spread to lymph nodes [N], and presence of metastasis [M]) of each patient is determined as published and periodically updated by the American Joint Committee on Cancer (AJCC).[6]

Principles of HNC management

As with all cancers, the primary intent of treatment needs to be determined upfront upon completion of staging: curative (aiming to cure the disease), or palliative (aiming to alleviate the symptoms and improve the quality of life rather than curing the underlying disease). Owing to the complex anatomy and compact structural organization, management of HNC becomes a rather challenging task requiring a multidisciplinary approach. Based on tumor factors such as histology, anatomic location, and disease stage, as well as patient-related factors such as age, performance status, and comorbid health conditions, the multidisciplinary team can determine the optimal treatment approach.

The principles of curative treatment in HNC have shifted from radical resection procedures to organ preservation approaches with a goal to achieve the highest possible cure rates while retaining the organ function as much as possible.[7] In the multimodality approach, the definitive treatment for most cancers is surgery and/or radiation therapy to remove or kill the tumor cells, respectively. Any treatment given after the definitive treatment is referred to as adjuvant (meaning "assistant"), and treatment given before the definitive treatment is referred to as neoadjuvant therapy.[8] Some early-stage tumors may be managed with radiation alone or surgery;

however, the majority of tumors require a combination of surgery, radiation therapy, and/or chemotherapy to achieve optimal disease control.

Surgical resection encompasses en bloc resection of the primary tumor as determined by clinical examination and radiographic imaging and neck exploration for regional lymphatics followed by reconstruction (as required). Neck exploration can be unilateral or bilateral dissection based on location and extent of the tumor. The role of sentinel lymph node biopsy is being investigated to minimize the postsurgical morbidity for clinically node-negative patients.[9] Specific factors to be looked into on histopathological assessment of the resected primary tumor include margin status, tumor size, tumor grade, perineural spread, lymphovascular invasion, depth of invasion, and worst pattern of invasion. Nodal factors include the number and size of involved lymph nodes, which nodal basins are involved, and the presence of extranodal extension. This information is used to determine the necessity of adjuvant treatment.

Radiation therapy (RT) provides oncological outcomes similar to surgical resection for certain sites of early stage (stage I and II) HNC, and it is a fundamental component of multimodality therapy for locally advanced disease (stage III, Iva, and IVb).[10] RT often is the preferred modality of treatment for early or locally advanced hypopharyngeal and laryngeal cancers, due to higher functional outcomes. Conventional RT is delivered in a daily fractionated regimen, consisting of 1.8−2 Gy per fraction, given for 5 days a week to a cumulative dose of 66−70 Gy in the primary setting and 50−66 Gy in the adjuvant setting. Adjuvant RT is indicated when adverse features are present after surgery.[11] RT can have short-term and long-term toxicities such as radiation dermatitis (dry skin), mucositis, xerostomia (dry mouth), dysphagia, trismus, dysgeusia, radiation fibrosis. To minimize the treatment-induced toxicities, various techniques have been adopted, which are further discussed later in the chapter.

Systemic therapy includes traditional chemotherapy, targeted therapy, and immunotherapy. Chemotherapy is typically used along with RT in the nonsurgical management of HNCs, referred to as concurrent chemoradiation therapy. Lower doses of chemotherapy are employed with the intent to potentiate the effect of RT. Systemic therapies are also used in the neoadjuvant setting to shrink the existing disease and improve the outcomes of locoregional therapy. Such therapy may also address disseminated micrometastases, but this is controversial.[12,13] In the adjuvant setting, systemic therapy is commonly indicated along with RT if high risk features such as positive margins or extranodal extension are identified.[11] Based on the systemic agent used, toxicities can vary between vomiting, neutropenia, infections, skin rash, to peripheral neuropathy.

Multidisciplinary care

HNC can cause substantial dysfunction in communication, nutrition, and breathing and thereby poses psychological challenges and social challenges. Studies reveal significant unmet needs of HNC survivors and their families, and they require comprehensive care at biopsychosocial level.[14] Management of HNC and monitoring of posttreatment survivorship phase should ideally involve multilevel interventions with health professionals of various disciplines, behavioral psychotherapy, workshops, and peer support groups.[15] A multidisciplinary team (MDT) consists of healthcare professionals with knowledge, experience, and clinical excellence in cancer care and include surgeons, radiation oncologists, medical oncologists, specialist nurses, physical medicine and rehabilitation, speech therapists, dieticians, pain management, dentists, and support staff. The effectiveness of multidisciplinary team in improving cancer outcomes is well established around the globe and is now considered the standard of care.[16]

A specialist nurse is someone with trained skills and experience in cancer care. For the patient and family, specialist nurses are often the cornerstone provider from diagnosis to posttreatment follow-up.[18] They offer assistance and guidance during postoperative care and radiation therapy. Patients with feeding tubes need guidance on managing the skin site, administering tube feedings, and flushing/cleaning the tube regularly. Postlaryngectomy patients would need to be trained by the specialist nurse regarding long-term stoma care: cleaning the stoma site, instilling saline solution, suction, and airway care. Postlaryngectomy patients also have to cope with their stoma (an opening created in the neck). They need to breathe through the stoma, learn new ways of communication, and also learn manage the stoma. This requires assisted training from specialist nurses, speech therapists, physical medicine and rehabilitation, and dieticians.

Dental health is important during HNC treatment. Dental procedures such as extractions and deep cleanings need to be avoided during chemotherapy cycles due to patient's relative immunosuppression. Furthermore, after radiation therapy, patients can be at risk of developing osteoradionecrosis after extractions and deep cleanings. Hence, all patients require dental evaluation and necessary therapeutic procedures prior to start of RT. Optimizing dental health before initiation of radiation is therefore critical in giving patients the best chance of maintaining long-term dental health.

For those HNC patients that require a temporary or permanent feeding tube, a dietitian provides the patients with support and advice about maintaining adequate dietary intake and choosing formulas that patients tolerate best. For those patients that maintain oral intake throughout treatment, dieticians provide similar advice regarding high-calorie high-protein foods to provide sufficient nutritional support despite common odynophagia/dysphagia symptoms.

Speech therapists offer assistance and recommendations regarding swallowing exercises and interventions to maintain/improve swallowing function. After laryngectomy, speech therapists train the patients with new ways of communication: some patients use valve inserted between trachea and esophagus (surgical voice restoration); some learn esophageal speech; and some need special equipment such as an electrolarynx.

During the course of treatment or in the survivorship phase, patients often require psychiatric and counseling services. Cognitive behavioral therapy—based approaches are emerging as potential new treatment paradigms for these patients.[17] After treatment completion, there can be a significant delay in returning to work, and patients might require social support as well.

Rehabilitation in HNC management occurs in various stages: "Preventive rehabilitation therapy" is started early after the diagnosis of cancer, where no significant physical impairment exists, but therapy is started to prevent functional loss; "restorative rehabilitation therapy" is directed at the comprehensive restoration of maximum function for patients who have a residual physical impairment and disability; and "supportive rehabilitation therapy" attempts to increase the self-care skills and mobility of the cancer patient with physical exercises. For example, regarding trismus (decreased mouth opening), a common tumor/treatment related toxicity, interventions can occur before, during, and after active treatment.

Treatment logistics

The multidisciplinary teams would typically meet every week to discuss and define individual optimal treatment strategies on per patient basis. After the initial cancer diagnosis confirmation and staging of the disease, along with treatment plan consensus, the MDT integrates help from the support teams. Once RT is indicated for HNC in a patient, the usual workflow is depicted in Fig. 3.1.

All patients require pre-RT dental evaluation from an HNC-experienced dentist and need to get elective dental procedures prior to starting RT, if required. Conventionally, RT is delivered in a fractioned regimen over a period of time (typically around 5—7 weeks). Usually, patients lie on the RT treatment couch in supine position (neck and shoulder positions are optimized based on location of the disease), and the same position needs to be maintained daily throughout the treatment course. The first procedure of RT planning is "CT simulation" where the patient is positioned on the couch and some immobilization devices (thermoplastic masks are molded for each patient in treatment position) are used to reproduce the same position with millimetric accuracy every day during treatment (Fig. 3.2). A CT scan is obtained in treatment position with immobilization devices in situ, and it is further reconstructed in three dimensions. This CT scan forms the reference for RT planning and delivery. The tumor (RT target) and the surrounding normal structures termed as organs at risk (OAR) are delineated on the CT slice by slice and prescription dose to be delivered is determined by the radiation oncologist (Fig. 3.3A). Once all the structures are delineated, medical dosimetrist creates an RT plan with an aim to deliver highest possible prescription dose to the target while minimizing the dose to OARs (Fig. 3.3B). This plan is reviewed by the radiation oncologist to ensure all the target and OAR dose constraints are adequately met and approves the plan. The patient comes back on the first day of treatment and RT is delivered once the position is ensured with immobilization devices and pre-RT imaging (X-ray or CT scan).

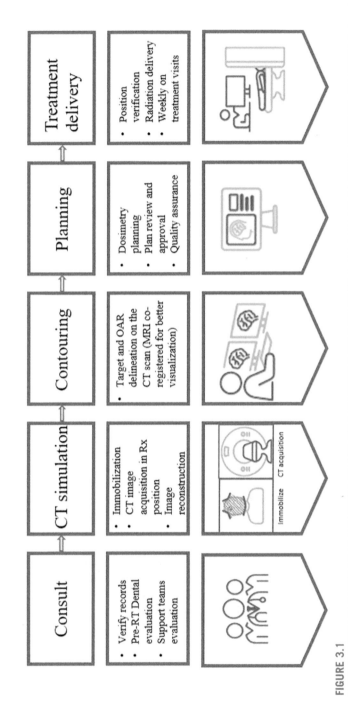

FIGURE 3.1

General RT workflow.

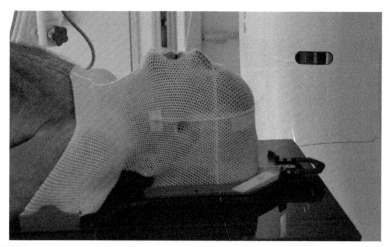

FIGURE 3.2

CT simulation with thermoplastic mask used as an immobilization device.

Added from Elsevier image bank.

This continues for 5—7 weeks, and the patient is reviewed weekly by the radiation oncologist, monitoring the weight, vitals, and labs when concurrent chemotherapy is being delivered.

Radiation toxicities—Organs at risk
Mechanism of radiation-induced toxicities (side effects)

With definitive RT, the primary goal is to achieve a balance between delivering the highest possible target (tumor) coverage with the lowest possible OAR doses. However, some inevitable dose is received by the surrounding OARs, which causes toxicities. These are classified as "acute toxicities" (during or immediate post-RT phase within 3 months) and "late toxicities" (>6 months post-RT). General mechanisms of radiation injury are identified to be production of free radicals, activation of inflammatory pathways, vascular endothelial dysfunction, and decreased normal tissue resilience and function.[19] The major mechanism of RT-induced cell injury is through production of free radicals such as superoxides and nitrogen species, which activate different signaling and inflammatory pathways. This damage caused by RT is fixed by oxygen making it irreversible and leading to cell injury/death. Tissues with rapidly dividing cells, including buccal mucosa, hair follicles, and gastrointestinal mucosa, are often the main source for acute RT-induced injury; cell depletion from RT leads to acute toxicities such as mucositis, alopecia, diarrhea, and vomiting. Inflammation, chronic oxidative stress, and damage to vasculature can lead to RT-

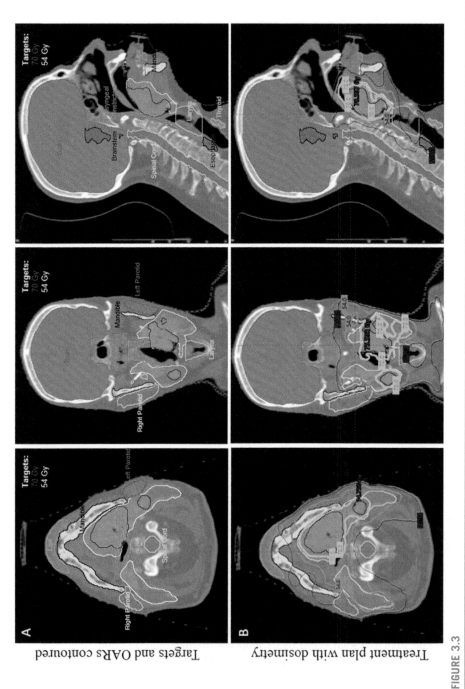

FIGURE 3.3

(A) A representative case of left-sided carcinoma oropharynx (extending to oral tongue) depicting the targets and OARs contoured on the CT in axial, coronal and sagittal planes. (B) Treatment plan of the same patient depicting dosimetry—gross disease treated to 70 Gy and prophylactic regions to 54 Gy in 35 fractions.

induced late toxicities.[20] The possible range of RT-induced toxicities is depicted in Fig. 3.4.

Organs at risk

OAR is defined as a normal tissue in or near the target volume whose presence influences treatment planning and/or prescribed dose.[21] These are categorized as "serial organ," where whole organ is a continuous unit and damage at one point can cause damage organ (spinal cord, gastrointestinal system); "parallel organ" where organ consists of several functional subunits, and if one subunit is damaged, rest of the organ can compensate for the loss (lung, liver); and "serial—parallel organ," which possesses features of both (kidney: glomerulus acts as parallel and tubules act as serial structure).[22] Each specific OAR has certain dose thresholds for an adverse event, and standard dose constraints are defined characterizing the probability of an adverse event occurrence when dose constraint is crossed. Typically, dose constraints to serial organs are mostly in the form of maximum absorbed dose as specified for 0.03cc of the tissue (D_{max}), whereas for parallel organs, mean dose (D_{mean}) and volume of tissue that receives at least the specified absorbed dose (V_D) is considered (V_{50} of larynx is the volume of larynx receiving more than 50 Gy). Dose constraint for spinal cord is $D_{max} < 50$ Gy (end point: myelopathy); for larynx is $D_{max} < 66$ Gy (end point: vocal dysfunction), $D_{mean} < 50$ Gy (end point: aspiration), $V_{50} < 27\%$ and $D_{mean} < 44$ Gy (end point: edema).[23]

Twenty-five OARs in HNC were identified, and standard delineation guidelines were defined.[24] Spinal cord and brainstem are the most critical OAR that carry utmost importance and can lead to paralysis when dose constraints are not obeyed. Salivary glands such as parotid and submandibular glands play a major role in xerostomia (dry mouth). Pharyngeal constrictors and the larynx are usually regarded as

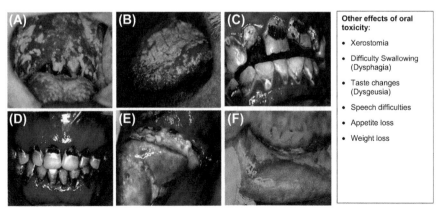

Other effects of oral toxicity:

- Xerostomia
- Difficulty Swallowing (Dysphagia)
- Taste changes (Dysgeusia)
- Speech difficulties
- Appetite loss
- Weight loss

FIGURE 3.4

The possible range of RT-induced toxicities.

Added from Elsevier image bank.

swallowing OARs with functional swallowing units in base and floor of tongue as well. Buccal mucosa can be delineated to optimize dose to minimize mucositis. Dose to mandible determines the risk of osteoradionecrosis.

Technology advancements and treatment deescalation

Prevention and mitigation of RT-induced normal tissue damage has been attempted in various ways, collectively termed as "radioprotection."

Intensity-modulated radiation therapy

The past few decades have seen tremendous evolution in the technology of imaging, RT planning and delivery. Intensity-modulated radiation therapy (IMRT) marked a paradigm shift in HNC treatment as it enables modulation of a number of fields and radiation intensity within each field. The feature of inverse planning helps dose sculpting of tumor while avoiding dose to OAR. This provides the advantages of relative conservation of normal tissue, improved tumor coverage, and escalation of dose delivered to the tumor.[25]

Radiation-induced dysphagia (swallowing impairment) has a significant negative impact on the quality of life and can present as a late toxicity. It is a broad spectrum of structural, mechanical, and neurological deficits that can vary between mild, restriction of diet and severe, aspiration of food into lungs.[26] Dysphagia-optimized IMRT (DO-IMRT) is a new technique that reduces RT dose to the pharyngeal constrictor muscles ($D_{mean} < 50$ Gy). In a phase 3, multicenter, randomized control trial, 112 patients were randomly assigned to DO-IMRT and standard IMRT groups. MD Anderson Dysphagia Inventory (MDADI) composite scores 12 months after RT were significantly higher for DO-IMRT group with mean difference of 7.2 (95% CI; 0.4−13.9; $P = .037$).[27]

Xerostomia (dry mouth) is another common RT-induced late effect that can be detrimental to quality of life and occurs due to damage to the salivary glands causing alterations in volume, consistency, and pH of saliva.[28] On stimulation, parotid glands produce 60%−65% saliva, submandibular glands (SMG) produce 20%−30%, and sublingual glands produce 2%−5%. At resting phase, 90% of salivary output is by SMG.[29] Limiting the mean dose of at least one parotid gland to <26−30 Gy can substantially reduce incidence and severity of xerostomia. PARSPORT trial compared parotid-sparing IMRT with conventional RT in pharyngeal carcinoma patients with 47 patients in each arm. At 12 and 24 months, grade 2 or worse xerostomia was 38%, 29% in parotid sparing-IMRT arm and 74%, 83% in standard RT arm, respectively, $P < .01$.[30] Surgical transfer of SMG to submental space to reduce RT dose to the gland was in practice before, but in this era of IMRT, this procedure is no longer necessary as IMRT can provide SMG dose reduction without invasive manipulation.[31]

Intensity-modulated proton therapy

While photons deposit radiation dose continually throughout their path in the tissue and exit dose, protons exhibit the "Bragg peak" depositing maximum dose at a specific depth with sharp dose fall-off and no exit dose. Intensity-modulated proton therapy (IMPT) is a complex and sophisticated technique of proton delivery that allows greater degree of freedom to produce optimized dose distributions. IMPT provides significant dosimetric advantage in HNC compared with any photon-based RT technique in target coverage and sparing OAR.[32] The clinical experience with IMPT in HNC is still new and is evolving rapidly.

Treatment deescalation

HPV-related oropharyngeal cancer (OPC) incidence has been on rise in the past decade and has also surpassed cervical cancer as the most common HPV-related cancer in the United States.[33] HPV-related OPC accounts for about 65% of OPC and has significantly better survival rates (3-year overall survival—82% vs. 57%) and is identified as a strong independent prognostic as well as predictive factor to surgery and chemoradiation therapy.[33,34] Consequently, various treatment deintensification strategies have been investigated to minimize toxicity in the long-term survivors while maintaining high cure rates. The phase 2 ECOG-1308 trial was a single arm study that evaluated role of tailoring RT dose postinduction chemotherapy (cisplatin, docetaxel, and cetuximab). Postchemotherapy, patients with complete clinical response received 54 Gy, while others received 69.3 Gy with weekly cetuximab. The 2-year locoregional control was 94% and 2-year OS was 93%.[35] Another randomized phase 2 trial compared dose deescalation to 60 Gy with or without concurrent weekly cisplatin chemotherapy and reported IMRT to 60 Gy with cisplatin to be the better strategy.[36] However, optimal treatment strategy is yet to be standardized in the near future.

Case studies
Oral cavity

In this example, a 65-year-old man who has smoked one pack of cigarettes daily since age 15 and drinks one to two beers per day presented to his dentist with a painful tongue lesion on the right anterior tongue. He used topical numbing agents for 2 weeks with no relief. On examination, the patient had poor dentition and a ~2 cm ulcer. In the office, the dentist obtained a biopsy that demonstrated p40 (+), p16 (−) moderately differentiated SCC. The patient was referred to a head and neck surgeon, who confirmed the clinical exam findings; there was also noted ~1 cm thickness of the primary lesion. No cervical lymphadenopathy was palpated. A CT neck with contrast and PET-CT were obtained, which confirmed a 2.5-cm primary tumor in the right anterior oral tongue without regional or distant spread of the disease (Fig. 3.5). Clinical staging was determined to be cT2N0M0.

The patient was then seen in multidisciplinary clinic with head and neck surgery, radiation oncology, and medical oncology. Recommendation was for partial glossectomy (with likely free flap reconstruction) and bilateral neck dissection as initial treatment. Prior to surgery, the patient had consults with speech therapy and nutrition. The patient completed a full dental evaluation given the potential high need of adjuvant RT, with 4 teeth extracted before surgery. Patient tolerated surgery well and had a prophylactic feeding tube placed during surgery. Pathology demonstrated a 2.3-cm primary tumor with 11 mm depth of invasion, worst pattern of invasion 4, with lymphovascular invasion present and perineural invasion absent; surgical margins were negative >5 mm. Of the 40 nodes that were sampled, one node in right level IB, measuring 6 mm, had disease spread; no extranodal extension was seen. Hence, the final staging was determined to be pT3N1.

Upon representation in multidisciplinary clinic, the patient was recommended adjuvant RT to the primary site and the involved nodal basin (60 Gy in 30 fractions) and bilateral elective neck levels IB-IV (54 Gy in 30 fractions) (Fig. 3.6). The patient was referred to pain management and cancer rehabilitation. The patient started RT 5 weeks after surgery. He experienced grade 3 mucositis, grade 2 dysgeusia and xerostomia, and grade 1 dermatitis, among other side effects. On completion of

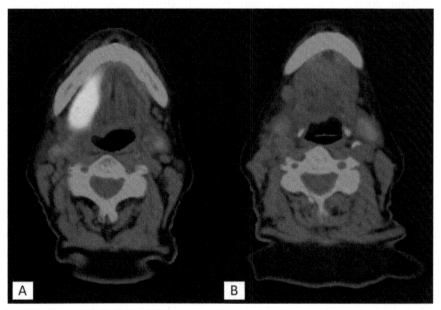

FIGURE 3.5

PET-CT axial images of right oral tongue SCC (A) with questionable ipsilateral level IB lymph node (B).

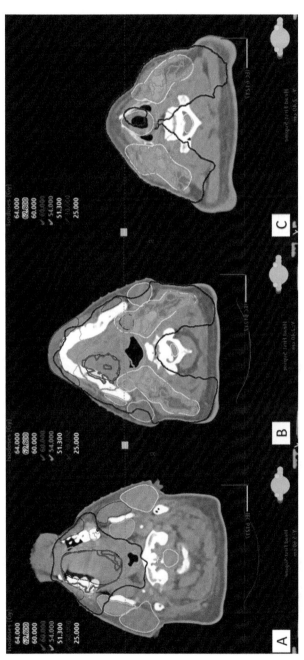

FIGURE 3.6

Treatment plan for the right oral tongue SCC patient. Isodose lines 60 Gy (pink), 54 Gy (orange), and 30 Gy (purple). OARs include panel A—parotid glands (green and yellow), masseters (green and pink), mandible (brown), lips (red), pharyngeal constrictors (orange), and spinal cord (green); panel B—submandibular glands (orange and blue); panel C—larynx (yellow).

RT, the feeding tube was removed after 6 weeks; he subsequently underwent a restaging PET-CT 3 months later, which showed no active disease.

HPV-positive oropharynx

In this example, a 55-year-old male who was a never smoker and never drinker noticed a left neck mass while shaving. His primary care physician gave him 2 weeks of antibiotics with minimal improvement. He then saw an otolaryngologist, who performed a nasopharyngolaryngoscopy. This exam showed an exophytic lesion in the left base of tongue that extended into the vallecula and was tethered to the epiglottis. An MRI neck with/without contrast and PET-CT were obtained which showed a 1.9-cm primary lesion in the vallecula and two left neck level II lymph nodes, largest of which was 2.2 cm (Fig. 3.7). A fine needle aspiration of the left neck demonstrated p40/p16 (+) SCC. Subsequent PCR testing confirmed HPV positivity of the specimen. Staging was determined to be cT3N1M0.

The patient was then seen in multidisciplinary clinic with head and neck surgery, radiation oncology, and medical oncology. Given the involvement of the epiglottis, surgical resection was not recommended. Recommendation was for definitive chemoradiation with concurrent cisplatin. RT would treat all gross disease to 70 Gy in 35 fractions, high risk areas ~1 cm around gross disease to 63 Gy in 35 fractions, and elective bilateral neck regions II—IV to 54 Gy in 35 fractions (Fig. 3.8).

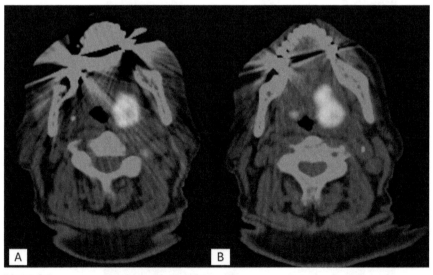

FIGURE 3.7

PET-CT axial images of left base of tongue SCC (A) with involved level II lymph node (B).

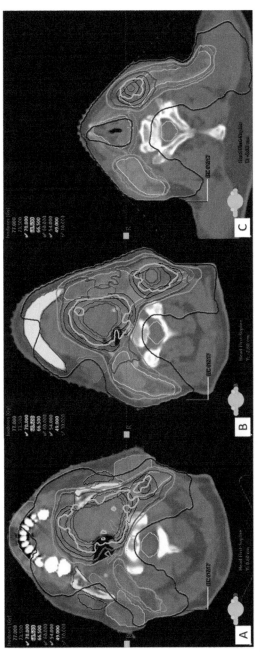

FIGURE 3.8

Treatment plan for the left base of tongue SCC. Isodose lines 70 Gy (green), 60 Gy (pink), 54 Gy (orange), and 30 Gy (purple). OARs include panel A—parotid glands (green and lavender), masseters (blue and purple), medial pterygoids (beige and purple), lips (lavender), mandible (brown), pharyngeal constrictors (blue), spinal cord (green); panel B—submandibular glands (orange and red); panel C—larynx (green).

Cisplatin 100mg/m^2 was planned on weeks 1, 4, and 7 during RT. The patient had consults with cancer rehabilitation, speech therapy, palliative care, and nutrition departments. The patient completed a full dental evaluation with no pretreatment intervention recommended.

The patient tolerated the planned course of chemoradiation therapy with expected side effects. He had grade 3 mucositis and grade 2 dysphagia, dermatitis, and dysgeusia. He had grade 1 weight loss of 7.5% body weight decrease. His blood counts decreased after the second cisplatin infusion, and the patient did not receive his third cycle; the patient also experienced grade 2 nausea and grade 1 neuropathy. Posttreatment follow-up and scans demonstrated the patient to be disease free 3 months after completion of treatment.

Nasopharynx

This example is a 45-year-old woman originally from Hong Kong who presented with epistaxis. She presented to her otolaryngologist who performed a nasopharyngolaryngoscopy, which demonstrated a 3-cm lesion centered in the right fossa of Rosenmuller. The patient also noted right-sided otalgia. No cervical adenopathy was noted. An MRI neck with/without contrast and PET-CT were obtained, which demonstrated a right nasopharyngeal lesion involving the parapharyngeal space, bilateral retropharyngeal lymph nodes, and a right level II lymph node (Fig. 3.9).

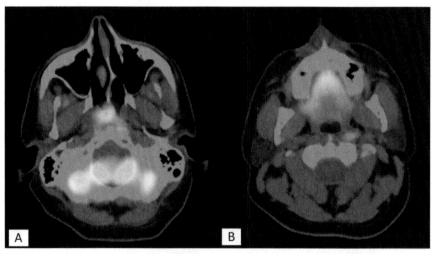

FIGURE 3.9

PET-CT axial images of nasopharyngeal carcinoma (A) with involved retropharyngeal lymph nodes (B).

No distant disease was noted. A direct laryngoscopy and biopsy demonstrated non-keratinizing carcinoma, EBV positive. Laboratory testing further revealed detectable EBV blood titers. Staging was determined to be cT2N1M0.

The patient was then seen in multidisciplinary clinic with head and neck surgery, radiation oncology, and medical oncology. Given nonbulky disease, neoadjuvant chemotherapy was not advised. Recommendation was for definitive chemoradiation with concurrent cisplatin. RT would treat all gross disease to 70 Gy in 33 fractions, high-risk areas ~ 1 cm around gross disease, the retropharyngeal lymph node basins, and the entire nasopharynx to 60 Gy in 33 fractions, and elective right neck regions IB–V/left neck regions II–V to 54 Gy in 33 fractions (Fig. 3.10). Cisplatin 100 mg/m^2 was planned on weeks 1, 4, and 7 during RT. The patient had consults with cancer rehabilitation, speech therapy, palliative care, and nutrition departments. The patient completed a full dental evaluation with no pretreatment intervention being recommended. The patient tolerated the planned course of chemoradiation therapy with expected side effects.

Patient education

Patients who are diagnosed with HNC need to be properly counseled regarding the prognosis of disease, potential toxicities of the treatment with realistic expectations of recovery, and the required changes in their lifestyle thereafter. Although it can seem overwhelming initially, this transparency would lead the patients and their families to cope with and adhere to the treatment in a better way. The manner and pace of this information delivery play a crucial role in patient's understanding. In this era of often unreliable medical information availability from the internet, patients need to have the accurate understanding from someone knowledgeable and experienced in treating similar conditions before. Written information booklets can be handed to them to reinforce the verbal explanations of care and will be a reference resource to go back each time when in doubt. Time frame–based counseling sessions would help in reducing distress and anxiety. Introducing prophylactic swallowing and other rehabilitation exercises that have been designed to increase the muscle power prior to start of RT may have the potential to improve swallowing and other functions.[37] The importance of food intake and potential need for placement of a feeding tube to maintain adequate weight also need to be explained to the patient upfront. Referral to cancer rehabilitation and palliative care may also assist in improving patient quality of life during and after therapy.

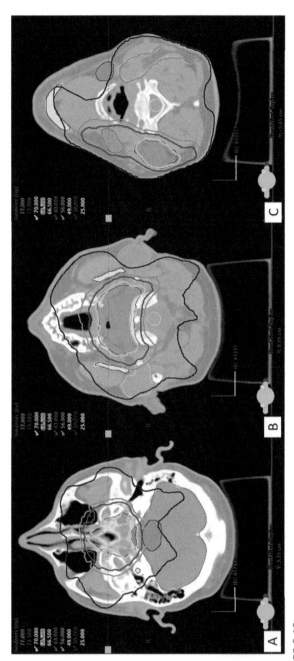

FIGURE 3.10

Treatment plan for the nasopharyngeal carcinoma. Isodose lines 70 Gy (green), 60 Gy (pink), 54 Gy (orange), and 30 Gy (purple). OARs include panel A—brain (pink), brainstem (brown), cochleas (red and pink); panel B—parotids (green and lavender), spinal cord (green); panel C—submandibular glands (orange and red), mandible (brown).

References

1. Siegel RL, Miller KD, Wagle NS, Jemal A. Cancer statistics, 2023. *CA Cancer J Clin.* 2023;73:17–48. https://doi.org/10.3322/caac.21763.
2. Sung H, Ferlay J, Siegel RL, et al. Global cancer statistics 2020: GLOBOCAN estimates of incidence and mortality worldwide for 36 cancers in 185 countries. *CA Cancer J Clin.* 2021;71:209–249. https://doi.org/10.3322/caac.21660.
3. Miller KD, Nogueira L, Devasia T, et al. Cancer treatment and survivorship statistics, 2022. *CA Cancer J Clin.* 2022;72:409–436. https://doi.org/10.3322/caac.21731.
4. Osazuwa-Peters N, Simpson MC, Zhao L, et al. Suicide risk among cancer survivors: head and neck versus other cancers. *Cancer.* 2018;124:4072–4079. https://doi.org/10.1002/cncr.31675.
5. Amin MB, Greene FL, Edge SB, et al. The eighth edition AJCC cancer staging manual: continuing to build a bridge from a population-based to a more "personalized" approach to cancer staging. *CA Cancer J Clin.* 2017;67:93–99. https://doi.org/10.3322/caac.21388.
6. Huang SH, O'Sullivan B. Overview of the 8th edition TNM classification for head and neck cancer. *Curr Treat Options Oncol.* 2017;18:40. https://doi.org/10.1007/s11864-017-0484-y.
7. Cognetti DM, Weber RS, Lai SY. Head and neck cancer: an evolving treatment paradigm. *Cancer.* 2008;113:1911–1932. https://doi.org/10.1002/cncr.23654.
8. West H, Jin J. Neoadjuvant therapy. *JAMA Oncol.* 2015;1:550. https://doi.org/10.1001/jamaoncol.2015.1241.
9. NRG Oncology. *Randomized Phase II/III Trial of Sentinel Lymph Node Biopsy versus Elective Neck Dissection for Early-Stage Oral Cavity Cancer.* clinicaltrials.gov; 2023.
10. Mody MD, Rocco JW, Yom SS, Haddad RI, Saba NF. Head and neck cancer. *Lancet.* 2021;398:2289–2299. https://doi.org/10.1016/S0140-6736(21)01550-6.
11. Pfister DG, Spencer S, Adelstein D, et al. Head and neck cancers, version 2.2020, NCCN clinical practice guidelines in oncology. *J Natl Compr Cancer Netw JNCCN.* 2020;18:873–898. https://doi.org/10.6004/jnccn.2020.0031.
12. Posner MR, Hershock DM, Blajman CR, et al. Cisplatin and fluorouracil alone or with docetaxel in head and neck cancer. *N Engl J Med.* 2007;357:1705–1715. https://doi.org/10.1056/NEJMoa070956.
13. Lacas B, Carmel A, Landais C, et al. Meta-analysis of chemotherapy in head and neck cancer (MACH-NC): an update on 107 randomized trials and 19,805 patients, on behalf of MACH-NC Group. *Radiother Oncol J Eur Soc Ther Radiol Oncol.* 2021;156:281–293. https://doi.org/10.1016/j.radonc.2021.01.013.
14. Cohen EEW, LaMonte SJ, Erb NL, et al. American cancer society head and neck cancer survivorship care guideline. *CA Cancer J Clin.* 2016;66:203–239. https://doi.org/10.3322/caac.21343.
15. Twigg JA, Anderson JM, Humphris G, Nixon I, Rogers SN, Kanatas A. Best practice in reducing the suicide risk in head and neck cancer patients: a structured review. *Br J Oral Maxillofac Surg.* 2020;58:e6–e15. https://doi.org/10.1016/j.bjoms.2020.06.035.
16. Licitra L, Keilholz U, Tahara M, et al. Evaluation of the benefit and use of multidisciplinary teams in the treatment of head and neck cancer. *Oral Oncol.* 2016;59:73–79. https://doi.org/10.1016/j.oraloncology.2016.06.002.

17. Chopra D, Shinn E, Teo I, et al. A cognitive behavioral therapy-based intervention to address body image in patients with facial cancers: results from a randomized controlled trial. *Palliat Support Care*. 2023:1−8. https://doi.org/10.1017/S1478951523000305.

18. Taberna M, Gil Moncayo F, Jané-Salas E, et al. The multidisciplinary team (MDT) approach and quality of care. *Front Oncol*. 2020;10:85. https://doi.org/10.3389/fonc.2020.00085.

19. Kalman NS, Zhao SS, Anscher MS, Urdaneta AI. Current status of targeted radioprotection and radiation injury mitigation and treatment agents: a critical review of the literature. *Int J Radiat Oncol Biol Phys*. 2017;98:662−682. https://doi.org/10.1016/j.ijrobp.2017.02.211.

20. Zhao W, Robbins MEC. Inflammation and chronic oxidative stress in radiation-induced late normal tissue injury: therapeutic implications. *Curr Med Chem*. 2009;16:130−143. https://doi.org/10.2174/092986709787002790.

21. Jones D. ICRU report 50—prescribing, recording and reporting photon beam therapy. *Med Phys*. 1994;21:833−834. https://doi.org/10.1118/1.597396.

22. Hodapp N. The ICRU Report 83: prescribing, recording and reporting photon-beam intensity-modulated radiation therapy (IMRT). *Strahlenther Onkol Organ Dtsch Rontgengesellschaft Al*. 2012;188:97−99. https://doi.org/10.1007/s00066-011-0015-x.

23. Bentzen SM, Constine LS, Deasy JO, et al. Quantitative analyses of normal tissue effects in the clinic (QUANTEC): an introduction to the scientific issues. *Int J Radiat Oncol Biol Phys*. 2010;76:S3−S9. https://doi.org/10.1016/j.ijrobp.2009.09.040.

24. Brouwer CL, Steenbakkers RJHM, Bourhis J, et al. CT-based delineation of organs at risk in the head and neck region: DAHANCA, EORTC, GORTEC, HKNPCSG, NCIC CTG, NCRI, NRG Oncology and TROG consensus guidelines. *Radiother Oncol J Eur Soc Ther Radiol Oncol*. 2015;117:83−90. https://doi.org/10.1016/j.radonc.2015.07.041.

25. Daly-Schveitzer N, Juliéron M, Tao YG, Moussier A, Bourhis J. Intensity-modulated radiation therapy (IMRT): toward a new standard for radiation therapy of head and neck cancer? *Eur Ann Otorhinolaryngol Head Neck Dis*. 2011;128:241−247. https://doi.org/10.1016/j.anorl.2011.04.001.

26. King SN, Dunlap NE, Tennant PA, Pitts T. Pathophysiology of radiation-induced dysphagia in head and neck cancer. *Dysphagia*. 2016;31:339−351. https://doi.org/10.1007/s00455-016-9710-1.

27. Nutting C, Finneran L, Roe J, et al. Dysphagia-optimised intensity-modulated radiotherapy versus standard intensity-modulated radiotherapy in patients with head and neck cancer (DARS): a phase 3, multicentre, randomised, controlled trial. *Lancet Oncol*. 2023;24:868−880. https://doi.org/10.1016/S1470-2045(23)00265-6.

28. Dirix P, Nuyts S, Van den Bogaert W. Radiation-induced xerostomia in patients with head and neck cancer: a literature review. *Cancer*. 2006;107:2525−2534. https://doi.org/10.1002/cncr.22302.

29. Eisbruch A, Rhodus N, Rosenthal D, et al. How should we measure and report radiotherapy-induced xerostomia? *Semin Radiat Oncol*. 2003;13:226−234. https://doi.org/10.1016/S1053-4296(03)00033-X.

30. Nutting CM, Morden JP, Harrington KJ, et al. Parotid-sparing intensity modulated versus conventional radiotherapy in head and neck cancer (PARSPORT): a phase 3 multicentre randomised controlled trial. *Lancet Oncol*. 2011;12:127−136. https://doi.org/10.1016/S1470-2045(10)70290-4.

31. Kutuk T, McAllister NC, Rzepczynski AE, et al. Submandibular gland transfer for the prevention of radiation-induced xerostomia in oropharyngeal cancer: dosimetric impact

in the intensity modulated radiotherapy era. *Head Neck*. 2022;44:1213–1222. https://doi.org/10.1002/hed.27021.

32. Moreno AC, Frank SJ, Garden AS, et al. Intensity modulated proton therapy (IMPT)—the future of IMRT for head and neck cancer. *Oral Oncol*. 2019;88:66–74. https://doi.org/10.1016/j.oraloncology.2018.11.015.

33. Gribb JP, Wheelock JH, Park ES. Human papilloma virus (HPV) and the current state of oropharyngeal cancer prevention and treatment. *Del J Public Health*. 2023;9:26–28. https://doi.org/10.32481/djph.2023.04.008.

34. Ang KK, Harris J, Wheeler R, et al. Human papillomavirus and survival of patients with oropharyngeal cancer. *N Engl J Med*. 2010;363:24–35. https://doi.org/10.1056/NEJMoa0912217.

35. Marur S, Li S, Cmelak AJ, et al. E1308: phase II trial of induction chemotherapy followed by reduced-dose radiation and weekly cetuximab in patients with HPV-associated resectable squamous cell carcinoma of the oropharynx—ECOG-ACRIN cancer research group. *J Clin Oncol Off J Am Soc Clin Oncol*. 2017;35:490–497. https://doi.org/10.1200/JCO.2016.68.3300.

36. Yom SS, Torres-Saavedra P, Caudell JJ, et al. Reduced-dose radiation therapy for HPV-associated oropharyngeal carcinoma (NRG oncology HN002). *J Clin Oncol*. 2021;39:956–965. https://doi.org/10.1200/JCO.20.03128.

37. Carnaby-Mann G, Crary MA, Schmalfuss I, Amdur R. "Pharyngocise": randomized controlled trial of preventative exercises to maintain muscle structure and swallowing function during head-and-neck chemoradiotherapy. *Int J Radiat Oncol Biol Phys*. 2012;83:210–219. https://doi.org/10.1016/j.ijrobp.2011.06.1954.

Treatment modalities, surgical principles, and rehabilitation considerations in head and neck cancer

Hani Samarah, BS, BS [1], Meghan B. Crawley, MD [1,2], Geoffrey D. Young, MD, PhD, FACS [1,2]

[1]*Florida International University, Herbert Wertheim College of Medicine, Miami, FL, United States;* [2]*Miami Cancer Institute, Baptist Health South Florida, Miami, FL, United States*

Introduction

In 1905, George Crile published a landmark paper presenting an astonishing 3-year survival rate of 75% in patients who underwent block resection of head and neck tumors (HNTs) compared with only 19% in those who did not.[1] Crile's work was based on his insight that tumors of the head and neck typically do not metastasize to distant sites and primarily drain through the neck's lymphatic pathways. Within this paradigm, this makes HNTs potentially curable through resection of the primary tumor and its associated lymph nodes. The surgical principles pioneered by Crile were later reinforced in 1951 by Dr. Hayes Martin and colleagues in a paper titled, "Neck dissection." This work solidified Crile's legacy by emphasizing strict adherence to the principles of block dissection in head and neck surgery.[2] Although nonsurgical treatments such as chemotherapy and radiation therapy have emerged, surgical resection remains an important standard of care for the vast majority of head and neck cancers (HNCs) and will likely remain an important treatment modality.[3]

Cancers of the head and neck region rank as the seventh most common cancer worldwide[4] and typically refer to soft tissue neoplasms that arise from the oral cavity, pharynx, larynx, nasal cavity, the paranasal sinuses, and the salivary glands (Fig. 4.1). Malignancies of the head and neck present a unique challenge to treat due to complex anatomy and physiology. Vital anatomic structures in proximity and the need to consider both functional and esthetic factors require a multidisciplinary approach to the diagnoses, treatment, and rehabilitation of patients afflicted with HNC.[5] This chapter will focus on the surgical treatment principles of HNC and the considerations of rehabilitation.

Head and Neck Cancer Rehabilitation. https://doi.org/10.1016/B978-0-443-11806-7.00015-1
Copyright © 2025 Elsevier Inc. All rights reserved, including those for text and data mining, AI training, and similar technologies.

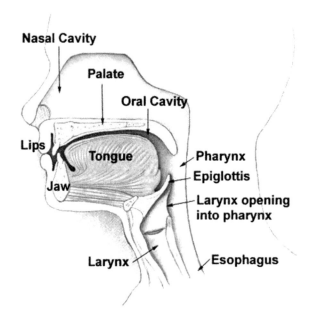

FIGURE 4.1

Head and neck overview illustrating the major soft tissues of the head and neck. This image is a work of the Centers for Disease Control and Prevention, part of the United States Department of Health and Human Services, taken or made as part of an employee's official duties. As a work of the US federal government, the image is in the public domain.[6]

Treatment modalities in head and neck cancer: Surgery, radiation therapy, and chemotherapy

Interdisciplinary approach to treatment

An interdisciplinary evaluation is often required to develop an appropriate treatment plan for patients with HNC. A comprehensive HNC team involves surgeons, medical oncologists, radiation oncologists, dentists, speech/swallowing pathologists, dietitians, psychosocial oncology specialists, prosthodontists, and rehabilitation therapists, among others. Research by Wuthrick et al. (2015) emphasizes the importance of directing patients with advanced HNC to high-volume centers for optimal survival results. The study shows that individuals treated at historically low-volume centers had inferior outcomes compared with those treated at historically high-volume centers.[7] This emphasizes the necessity for extensive expertise spanning various disciplines and the provision of high-quality radiation therapy in the comprehensive care of these patients.[8] Notably these results were reinforced in 2023, when evaluating the impact of hospital volume on overall mortality in a surgical group of head and neck squamous cell carcinoma (HNSCC) patients, finding that higher-volume facilities were associated with significantly improved patient survival, supporting the regionalization of care to high-volume head and neck centers with comprehensive facilities and supportive services to optimize outcomes.[9]

The treatment guidelines for HNSCC are dictated by the stage of the disease, considering tumor site, functional outcomes, patient-specific factors, and treatment modalities. HNCs are staged using the eighth edition of the Tumor, Node, Metastasis (TNM) classification system, developed by the American Joint Committee on Cancer (AJCC) and the Union for International Cancer Control (UICC). However, TNM staging changes depending on the anatomic location of the primary tumor.[9] The revisions for HNC staging went into effect on January 1, 2018, and will now be uniform between the AJCC and UICC.[10] Guidelines are outlined based on the site and stage of HNC, offering specific suggestions for pretreatment assessment and therapeutic approaches. In cases of localized (early stage) disease, surgery is the preferred approach due to better cure rates and lower toxicity. For intermediate staged disease, a multimodality approach is favored, incorporating radiation therapy and chemotherapy. In advanced cases or metastatic disease, palliative systemic therapy, immunotherapy, and supportive care are primary considerations. Further, patients with locoregionally recurrent disease may benefit from salvage surgery or reirradiation. Lastly, palliative radiation therapy can alleviate symptoms in cases involving metastatic disease.

Preoperative evaluation

A thorough preoperative evaluation is important for HNC patients undergoing ablative and reconstructive surgery. A preoperative evaluation may include fiberoptic evaluation of swallowing (FEES) or a modified barium swallow study, which may identify preexisting deficits. Depending on the patient's age or the pathology, they may exhibit varying degrees of swallowing impairment. These studies establish a baseline, especially crucial for older individuals who may face deficits in functions such as swallowing and speaking due to age-related factors. By thoroughly assessing the patient's current functional status, the surgical and medical teams can develop a personalized rehabilitation plan and set realistic expectations for postoperative recovery, ultimately enhancing the overall quality of care and patient outcomes.

Radiation therapy in head and neck cancer

While surgery typically forms the foundation for a patients treatment, evidence suggests that adjuvant radiation therapy (RT) or chemotherapy may provide an increased survival or decreased recurrence benefit.[11–15] Moreover, adjuvant therapies are typically recommended following surgery for patients with positive resection margins, lymphovascular or perineural invasion, extranodal extension, or pathologically positive lymph nodes.[16] Alternatively, in patients with borderline resectable or functionally unresectable disease, neoadjuvant therapy is sometimes utilized as the initial therapy, with the aim to shrink the tumor, facilitating subsequent surgical resection.[17] However, more investigations are necessary to evaluate survival advantage, and long-term toxicity of this approach.[18–20] Despite the technological advancements enhancing oncological outcomes, RT in the head and neck region still poses challenges due to a high rate of acute and late side effects, along with significant loco-regional recurrence within 3 years for high-risk patients.[21] To optimize the cost/benefit ratio of RT, efforts in recent decades have focused on personalized treatment plans considering both technological progress in photon-based RT, such as three-dimensional conformal RT and intensity-modulated RT, as well as emerging approaches such as heavy particle RT.[22]

Chemotherapy in head and neck cancer

Combining chemotherapy and radiation (chemoradiation) has shown to be more effective in controlling locoregional disease and improving disease-free survival for patients at high risk of recurrent HNC cancer compared with adjuvant radiation therapy alone.[23,24] The effectiveness of this approach is particularly significant for patients with positive surgical margins and/or extranodal extension.[25] Regimens in adjuvant chemoradiation for cancers of the head and neck include platinum-based chemotherapy, such as cisplatin for eligible patients.[26] Further, clinical trials are exploring other potential options such as cetuximab[27] and docetaxel to further refine and optimize the adjuvant treatment strategies for HNC.

Surgical management of head and neck cancer

The surgical treatment modalities for HNC typically involve comprehensive tumor excision along with resection of the surrounding margins. Evidence suggests that positive margins are associated with poorer prognosis and often require adjuvant postoperative radiation therapy and/or chemotherapy.[28,29] Tumor resection is often performed through a transcervical approach and may necessitate lip-split mandibulotomy or mandibulectomy.[30] The clinical decision between classical open cancer resection and minimally invasive resection hinges on the tumors location, tumor anatomy, and characteristics. For instance, tumors that have invaded surrounding structures and involve locoregional lymph nodes will likely require open neck dissection. Traditional transcervical surgical methods for the neck involving neck dissection typically utilize a U-shaped or Y-shaped incision.[31] However, a classic open surgical approach may result in undesirable esthetic outcomes.[32] Recent advancements in robotic-assisted HNC surgery have optimized appearance-related outcomes without compromising surgical completeness and oncological results.[33]

Approximately 40% of patients afflicted with HNC present with cervical lymph node metastasis.[34] Further, the most critical prognostic factor in HNC is the status of the lymph nodes, as their involvement significantly reduces overall survival by approximately 50%.[30] Fig. 4.2 illustrates the anatomy and nomenclature of the

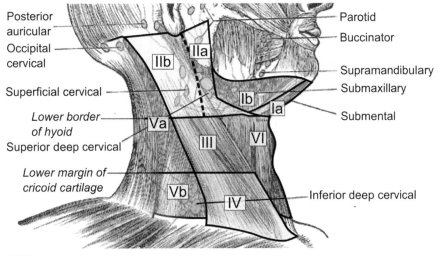

Posterior auricular
Occipital
cervical
Superficial cervical
Lower border of hyoid
Superior deep cervical
Lower margin of cricoid cartilage

IIb
IIa
Ib
Ia
Va
III
VI
Vb
IV

Parotid
Buccinator
Supramandibulary
Submaxillary
Submental
Inferior deep cervical

FIGURE 4.2

The classification of superficial cervical lymph nodes and their corresponding lymph node levels was originally delineated by the Memorial Sloan-Kettering Cancer Center in New York, NY. Subsequently, it was further refined and detailed by the Committee. Image made available under the Creative Commons CCO 1.0 Universal Public Domain Dedication.[36]

current lymph node levels of the head and neck. Therefore, cervical lymphadenectomy is a vital procedure to decrease disease burden achieved through one of the classifications of radical neck dissections (RNDs) described in the following. The RND involves the comprehensive removal of cervical lymph node groups on one side of the neck, ranging from the mandible's lower border to the clavicle and extending from the sternohyoid muscle's lateral border to the medial aspect of the contralateral anterior belly of the digastric muscle, and further to the anterior border of the trapezius. Levels I—V are included in this procedure. Three significant non-lymphatic structures are also removed in RNDs: the internal jugular vein, the sternocleidomastoid muscle, and the spinal accessory nerve.[35] The modified radical neck dissection (MRND) has emerged as a more common approach, involving the removal of cervical lymph nodes from levels I to V without removing either the spinal accessory nerve, the internal jugular vein, or the sternocleidomastoid muscle.[30] Next, the selective neck dissection (SND) involves the preservation of one of the lymph node groups typically excised during an RND or MRND. Finally, an extended neck dissection involves the removal of additional lymphatic and nonlymphatic structures not included in the other dissections described before (Table 4.1).

Depending on the presence of clinical or radiographic lymphadenopathy, neck dissection can be either therapeutic or elective. Elective neck dissection aims to rule out cancer metastasis, potentially eliminating the need for adjuvant therapy after surgery.[35,37—40] Cervical lymph nodes are stratified into seven group levels, enabling

Table 4.1 Comparison and classification of neck dissections.

	Radical neck dissection (RND)	Modified radical neck dissection (MRND)	Selective neck dissection (SND)	Extended neck dissection
Lymphatic structures	Levels I–V	Levels I–V	Preservation of one or more lymph nodes in levels I–V	Levels I–V and additional lymph nodes in the neck not routinely removed in other dissections
Nonlymphatic structures	Internal jugular vein, sternocleidomastoid muscle, spinal accessory nerve, other nonlymphatic structures	Preservation of internal jugular vein, sternocleidomastoid muscle, spinal accessory nerve	None	Excising nonlymphatic structures not typically removed in a radical neck dissection, such as the carotid artery, hypoglossal nerve, or overlying skin

a structured approach for removal (Fig. 4.2). Currently, RND is less common, as MRND and SND are more frequently employed supported by curative evidence while preserving nonlymphatic structures.[30]

Minimally invasive surgeries developed in the past few decades saw the development of minimally invasive surgical techniques, such as transoral laser microsurgery (TLM) and transoral robotic surgery (TORS). Depending on the neoplasm and its location, these techniques allow good access to tumors without an external epidermal excision. These techniques are especially useful for lesions of the mouth, pharynx, and larynx. These advancements have paved the way for improved functional and esthetic outcomes in HNC management for patients who may not undergo classical open surgery.[41]

Types of surgery and postoperative deficits

Head and neck cancer treatment involves a range of surgical procedures, each with specific purposes and potential outcomes. Ablative surgery, which entails the removal of tumors or affected tissues, is a fundamental component of cancer management. Ablative surgery and reconstructive surgery are essential to addressing tumors of the head and neck. Ablative surgery involves the removal of tumors or affected tissues, aiming to eliminate cancerous growth and prevent its spread. Reconstructive surgery focuses on restoring form and function after ablation, utilizing techniques to rebuild and repair the affected area. The interplay between these two approaches is pivotal in achieving comprehensive treatment outcomes that encompass both cancer eradication and the restoration of patients' quality of life. In the text that follows, we explore the various surgical types and their associated postoperative deficits, emphasizing the importance of rehabilitation in the recovery process.

Postoperative deficits

Ablative surgery involves tumor resection with clear margins, which may involve the intentional or unintentional sacrifice of major vascular, neurologic, and soft tissue structures. This can result in cranial nerve deficits, dysphagia, dysphonia, and lymphedema. Refer to Table 4.2 for specific postoperative deficits and associated procedures.

Facial nerve injuries

Iatrogenic facial nerve injuries most frequently occur during surgeries involving the parotid and submandibular salivary glands. Although these injuries often lead to cosmetic concerns, they may necessitate rehabilitation. The likelihood of facial nerve dysfunction is contingent upon surgical technique, tumor size, and the tumor lobes' depth.[42–44] The incidence of postoperative facial weakness is relatively uncommon and is diminishing due to the adoption of less invasive methods.[45] Reported

Table 4.2 Postoperative deficits and associated procedures.

Deficit	Type of surgery
Facial nerve	Salivary gland surgery Neck dissections
Vagus nerve	Carotid surgery Neck dissections Cervical spine procedures
Recurrent laryngeal nerve	Thyroidectomy
Accessory nerve	Neck dissections
Hypoglossal nerve	Carotid surgery Surgeries involving the base of tongue (including TORS) Neck dissections
Dysphagia	TORS Oral cavity surgery Laryngeal surgery Hypopharyngeal surgery
Dysphonia	Laryngeal surgery Tongue surgery Thyroidectomy
Lymphedema	Neck dissections

rates of facial nerve injury, at least 12 months postparotid gland surgery, range from 0.6%[43] to 6.8%.[46] Moreover, neck dissections involving submandibular area's level 1 tissues (as depicted in Fig. 4.2) can result in facial nerve injuries, with reported rates as high as 16%–23%.[47]

Vagal nerve and recurrent laryngeal nerve injuries

Given its relation to the great vessels, the vagus nerve is considered at risk during most major neck procedures. However, injury rates of the vagus proper are low.[48] The most common vagus nerve-related deficit usually results from iatrogenic injury of the recurrent laryngeal nerve (RLN).[49] Studies report rates of RLN compromise, during thyroidectomy, as high as 11%.[50] However, the rates of RLN injury are lower (2.5%)[51] in the hands of an experienced thyroid surgeon who performs more than 50 thyroid procedures annually.[52] The RLN can also be injured in cervical spinal surgery[53,54] and is significantly higher in patients undergoing cervical spinal surgery who have had previous neck surgery[55] or radiation.[56] Unilateral injury to the RLN often results in dysphonia and possibly dysphagia, whereas bilateral RLN injury often results in airway compromise requiring tracheostomy.

Accessory nerve injuries

The accessory nerve, also known as the spinal accessory nerve or cranial nerve XI, is frequently encountered during neck dissection surgery. Preservation of this nerve from iatrogenic injury is crucial to avoid debilitating sequelae, such as "shoulder syndrome," which can be challenging due to variations in its anatomic course.[57] The accessory nerve is the most commonly compromised cranial nerve in neck dissections[58] Compromise to the accessory nerve can lead to trapezial dysfunction, which will require aggressive physical therapy for rehabilitation.

Hypoglossal nerve injuries

The hypoglossal nerve, identified as cranial nerve XII, governs tongue movement, contributing significantly to speech and swallowing. Surgical procedures such as carotid endarterectomy,[59] neck dissection,[60] and tongue base surgeries including TORS[61] carry the risk of hypoglossal nerve injury. Such injuries give rise to dysphagia and dysphonia, impacting the patient's overall quality of life. Postoperative occupational therapy or other interventions may be necessary to manage these complications.

Dysphagia

Dysphagia is a common side effect of head and neck surgery. It can result from cranial nerve injury as described before. In addition, surgery in the oral cavity, pharynx, and larynx can all lead to soft tissue deficits that can cause dysphagia. The degree of dysphagia varies, and early intervention by a speech language pathologist is generally encouraged for best outcomes.[62-64] However, more research is necessary to optimize the timing, intensity, and duration of therapy for the best results.[65,66] Severe dysphagia that is unresponsive to aggressive swallow therapy or results in aspiration may require placement of a feeding tube.

Dysphonia

As previously discussed, dysphonia can manifest as a result of injury to the RLN or cranial nerve XII. Additionally, pathologic or iatrogenic soft tissue defects in the oral cavity can also cause dysphonia.[67,68] Laryngeal and hypopharyngeal surgeries frequently give rise to dysphonia, although minimally invasive techniques such as TLM and robotic surgery can mitigate this risk by preserving critical laryngeal structures.[69,70] However, for early glottic carcinomas, it is noteworthy that postsurgical dysphonia may exceed that observed after radiation therapy,[71] leading to the preference for radiation therapy as the primary treatment modality for most early-stage glottic tumors.

Laryngeal procedures, whether open or minimally invasive, often result in dysphonia. This is not surprising given the intricacies of larynx and its role in voice production. However, medical advancements have offered various techniques and options to address postsurgical voice issues and improve the quality of life for patients. Partial laryngectomies were developed as a surgical approach to preserve certain components of the larynx while removing the cancerous tissue. This approach is intended to preserve a certain degree of vocal quality for patients. However, it is important to note that even with partial laryngectomies, achieving the best possible voice outcomes often requires aggressive speech therapy and rehabilitation.[72]

In contrast, total laryngectomy involves the complete removal of the larynx, resulting in complete dysphonia. The field of HNS and rehabilitation offers innovative options to help patients regain their ability to communicate. These include esophageal speech, electrolarynx, AI generated speech and tracheoesophageal puncture (TEP).[73] Esophageal speech is a technique where patients learn to force air into the esophagus and then expel it to create sound. This method can be effective for some individuals, although it may require dedicated practice and training with a speech therapist.[74] An electrolarynx, a handheld device applied to the neck or skin, allows users to generate speech. While it does not fully mimic the natural voice, it provides an efficient communication method.[75] Advances in technology have led to the development of artificial intelligence (AI) systems that can generate speech based on user input. These systems can be programmed to mimic the patient's natural voice, allowing for more personalized and natural communication. TEP is a surgical procedure that establishes a small stoma in the tracheoesophageal wall, facilitating the passage of air from the lungs to the esophagus. This enables patients to generate speech by redirecting air through the new fistula. Quality of life assessments and evaluation of efficacy have shown that TEP with vocal prosthesis is a favorable approach to voice restoration posttotal laryngectomy.[76–79]

The choice of voice rehabilitation method often depends on the patient's individual preferences, physical capabilities, and goals for communication. Each option has its unique advantages and limitations, and a thorough evaluation by a speech–language pathologist and collaboration with a multidisciplinary team can help determine the most suitable approach for each patient's specific needs. Ultimately, the goal is to empower individuals who have undergone laryngectomy surgery to regain their ability to communicate effectively and maintain their quality of life.

Lymphedema following head and neck surgery

Disruptions to the lymphatic drainage system during neck surgery can lead to lymphedema. Lymphedema may manifest as facial swelling, which can be visually prominent and concerning for patients, known as external lymphedema. Alternately, patients may experience internal lymphedema, which will manifest as swelling of the mucosa associated with the aerodigestive tract. Lymphedema can occur in cases where there is injury to the internal jugular vein, an important blood vessel for lymphatic and venous drainage.[80] Like various other treatment-related side effects in HNC cases, head and neck lymphedema (HNL) can profoundly affect a patient's quality of life. HNL's effects extend beyond cosmetic concerns; extensive lymphedema in the facial, oral, and neck regions can lead to significant functional challenges in speaking, reading, writing, hearing, eating, and breathing.[81] The incidence of lymphedema is notably higher after bilateral neck procedures compared with unilateral ones.[82] Further, concomitant radiotherapy has been shown to be a factor in the development of cervicofacial lymphedema.[83,84] Data suggest that lymphedema affecting the head, neck, and face requires distinct therapies compared with lymphedema therapy in other anatomic sites.[85] Treatment for cervicofacial lymphedema consists of complete decongestive therapy (CDT). CDT typically involves manual lymphatic drainage (MLD), compression therapy, head and neck exercises, skin and hygiene care, and lifestyle modifications.[80] Importantly, data support the efficacy of these therapeutic interventions.[85]

Reconstruction in head and neck surgery following ablative surgery

Regional and microvascular reconstruction plays a crucial role in the treatment of HNCs following ablative surgery. After the removal of tumors or affected tissues, the reconstruction of both soft and bony defects is essential for restoring both form and function to the head and neck region.[86] This complex process involves the use of various surgical techniques to rebuild and repair the affected areas. In the following text, we will discuss regional and microvascular reconstruction, including the types of defects encountered and the importance of rehabilitation for patients undergoing these surgeries.

Soft tissue and bone defects

Following ablative surgery for HNCs, patients often experience significant soft tissue and bony defects. Soft tissue defects involve the loss of skin, muscle, and mucosa, leading to functional and esthetic challenges. On the other hand, bone defects refer to the removal critical structures such as the jaw or facial bones, which can impact a patient's ability to speak, chew, and maintain facial symmetry. These defects vary in size and complexity depending on the extent of the cancer and the surgical procedure performed. Effective reconstruction techniques are essential to address these defects and improve the patient's quality of life.[86]

Pedicled and microvascular flap reconstruction

Reconstruction following ablative surgery for HNCs typically involves pedicled flap reconstruction and microvascular flap reconstruction. Pedicled flaps entail the transfer of tissue from a nearby donor site with an intact blood supply, often utilizing a pedicle or stalk to maintain blood flow. This approach is suitable for smaller defects or instances where microvascular surgery is not feasible due to patient-specific factors.[87]

Conversely, microvascular flap reconstruction is a more intricate procedure that involves transplanting tissue, including skin, muscle, and bone, from a distant donor site to the affected area. This method demands microsurgical expertise to restore blood circulation at the recipient site, offering greater versatility for addressing complex defects.[87] Microvascular flap reconstruction is typically the preferred choice for larger and more challenging cases. In the realm of head and neck reconstruction, both pedicled and microvascular flap techniques play crucial roles in restoring function and optimizing cosmesis for patients with soft and bony defects resulting from ablative surgery.[87] Several types of microvascular free-tissue flaps play a crucial role in reconstructive surgery to address the specific reconstructive needs in various anatomical areas. Specific application of each flap type can vary depending on individual patient factors and anatomical considerations. Table 4.3 provides an overview

Table 4.3 Overview of select microvascular free-tissue flaps used in clinical applications and their clinical applications.

Flap type	Clinical applications
Scapular free flap	This approach is commonly used in maxillofacial and mandibular reconstruction, particularly for complex defects involving multiple subsites.[88]
Anterolateral thigh (ALT) free flap	Used in a variety of soft tissue applications, including tongue, cutaneous, pharyngeal, orbital, skull-base defects.[89]
Radial forearm free flap	Effective for soft and bony defects including mandible, orbit, maxillary, and skull base defects. Especially used in tongue and floor of mouth reconstruction.[90]
Fibular free flap	Utilized in bony reconstruction including mandibular and midface reconstruction.[91]
Pectoralis major myocutaneous flap	Commonly used as a primary and salvage soft tissue reconstructive option.

of select microvascular free-tissue flaps used in clinical applications, along with typical use cases.

Rehabilitation after reconstruction surgery

Rehabilitation is critical to the recovery process after head and neck reconstruction surgery. Patients often experience a range of functional deficits following surgery, including dysphagia, dysphonia, and alteration in neck and shoulder mobility. These deficits are not only due to the ablative portion of the case but also due to iatrogenic alteration of the form and function secondary to reconstruction. The reconstructed tissue is typically bulkier than the native tissue, which can displace the alignment and mechanics of the remaining tissue. It is important to recognize the effect of the reconstruction to help patients develop strategies to compensate. The goal of rehabilitation is to optimize these functions and enhance the patient's overall quality of life.

An important function to evaluate before and after surgery is the patient's ability to swallow. Consequences of dysphagia include malnutrition, aspiration pneumonia, weight loss, and choking. As discussed previously, speech therapists assess the patient's ability to swallow before and after surgery. We are able to identify the phase (oral, pharyngeal, or esophageal) of swallowing dysfunction with FEES or a modified barium swallow. They provide techniques to aid the patient in swallowing safely in addition to providing food consistency recommendations. Further, nutritional support is essential to ensure that patients receive proper nourishment, especially if dysphagia affects the types of food or drink, they can consume.

The duration and intensity of rehabilitation can vary based on the extent of the surgical resection and reconstruction and the patient's individual needs. It is a collaborative effort between the medical team and the patient to achieve the best possible outcomes and restore normalcy to their daily lives.

Typical recipient site functional changes following microvascular flap reconstruction

Following free tissue flap surgery, patients may experience a range of recipient site functional changes within the head and neck depending on what tissue was transferred, where it was transferred to, and other patient factors. Functional changes following surgery may include dysphagia, dysphonia, changes in facial esthetics and mobility, and sensory deficits. As discussed earlier, the reconstructed tissue often has more bulk than the native tissue, potentially leading to the displacement of alignment and mechanics in the surrounding tissue. Preoperative and postoperative evaluation of a patient's phonation, mastication, and deglutition can highlight what the functional changes are following surgery.

When developing a rehabilitation plan, special attention should be given to the type of tissue used, and where the tissue was specifically transferred to. For instance, tissue transferred to the floor of the oral cavity may lead to different functional outcomes than patients who receive free-flap reconstruction of the tongue. Hence, it is essential to assess the patient's swallowing efficacy to evaluate functional changes in the oral preparatory, oral, pharyngeal, or esophageal phases using a modified barium swallow or FEES to tailor appropriate rehabilitation strategies. Analogous approaches should be used when approaching the rehabilitation of a patients speech, mastication, and other functional changes of the head, neck, and face.

Common anatomic and physiologic deficits at donor sites and rehabilitation considerations

Free-flap surgery can lead to specific anatomic and physiologic deficits at the donor sites. These deficits may include scarring, functional limitations, and sensory changes. To address these issues, donor site rehabilitation is essential to enhance the patient's overall recovery experience. Table 4.4 summarizes the common deficits encountered at donor sites and the required rehabilitation.

Anterolateral thigh flap

The anterolateral thigh (ALT) flap is a versatile microvascular free-tissue flap widely employed in reconstruction of soft tissue defects, used for its bulk and ample amount of tissue.[89] At the donor site in the thigh, patients may encounter functional limitations in the perioperative period, such as muscle weakness and discomfort. Collins and colleagues (2012) reviewed 42 articles encompassing 2324 ALT flaps for donor site complications.[94] Lateral thigh paresthesia emerged as the most common complication, while severe complications such as compartment syndrome and muscle necrosis were rare. Twenty-four percent of patients experienced lateral thigh paresthesia, 4.8% experienced musculoskeletal dysfunction, 4.8% were afflicted with hypertrophic scarring or wound dehiscence, and 3.3% complained of donor site pain.[94] Physical therapy focuses on maintaining strength and overall leg range of motion (ROM) and stability. Simultaneously, occupational therapists address activities of daily living (ADLs) that might be affected by the donor site discomfort, developing strategies to adapt and perform these tasks effectively.[89] By employing

Table 4.4 Common deficits encountered at donor sites following select microvascular free-flap surgery and rehabilitation considerations.

Type of flap surgery	Common deficit	Required rehabilitation
Scapular free flap	Scarring, decreased strength, sensory deficit	Physical therapy, scar management, mobility exercises[89]
Anterolateral thigh (ALT) free flap	Scarring/wound healing complications and sensory deficits, decreased range of motion of the wrist	Scar management, range of motion exercises[90]
Radial forearm free flap	Altered shoulder mobility and strength	Physical therapy, range of motion exercises, strength training[88]
Fibular free flap	Ankle instability, decreased ankle range of motion, wound healing complications[92]	Physical therapy, gait training, strength training[91]
Pectoralis major myocutaneous flap	Chest wall discomfort, decreased strength, and range of motion of the arm	Physical therapy, breathing exercises, pain management[93]

both PT and OT early in the course of recovery, this can ensure that the patient does not further decompensate.

Radial/ulnar forearm free flap

The radial forearm free flap (RFFF) involves tissue harvested from the patient's volar forearm, including skin, fascia, and blood vessels. The RFFF is known for its thin, pliable tissue, making it suitable for head and neck reconstructions, particularly in cases involving the floor of mouth, palate, and tongue. The RFFF has distinct rehabilitation considerations at the donor site.[95] Typically, a split thickness skin graft is used to close the donor site, which can lead to contraction of the wound site and limit the wrist ROM. Additionally, early in the postoperative period, surgeons will limit the amount of motion that patients should engage in to prevent skin graft loss.

While the RFFF is widely utilized, it is noteworthy for its considerable donor site–related issues. Early complications frequently involve challenges such as wound breakdown and the loss of skin grafts, which subsequently lead to delayed wound healing and the exposure of tendons.[96] Studies conducted in the past have shown that in the long term, these complications can result in diminished mobility in the wrist, weakened wrist or hand function, sensory impairments, persistent pain, reduced hand dexterity, and cosmetic abnormalities, as indicated by both objective measurements and subjective evaluations.

Patients may experience restriction in wrist mobility and grip strength. Therefore, a comprehensive rehabilitation plan is essential to address these concerns. Physical therapists play a crucial role in helping patients regain wrist ROM and strength through targeted exercises and interventions. Occupational therapists focus on adapting daily activities to accommodate potential grip strength changes and help patients maintain independence in tasks that require fine motor skills involving the hand and wrist.[90] It is imperative for patients to participate in occupation and physical therapy exercise following forearm free flap harvest to prevent permanent ROM and functional deficits. If patients do not exercise the wrist following the surgery, the wrist will lose most of its ROM, severely limiting the use of the hand and wrist.

Scapula free flap

The osteocutaneous scapula free flap reconstruction offers both soft tissue and bone for complex head and neck reconstruction. It involves taking tissue from the scapular region, including skin, muscle, and bone, to address defects involving both bone and soft tissues. This flap can be particularly useful for reconstructing the jaw when there is a large soft tissue defect, as it provides both structural support along with ample tissue coverage.[88]

The scapular free flap is often chosen for its minimal impact on the donor site. Several studies have indicated that the morbidity associated with the donor site after scapular free flap harvesting is relatively mild.[97] However, only a handful of studies have shown objective methods to evaluate upper limb morbidity following scapular free flap surgery.[98] Various studies consistently support the idea that scapular free flap harvesting leads to low donor site morbidity, even when involving the extensive removal of both soft and hard tissues, allowing patients to regain functionality and maintain their quality of life.[97-100] Further, patients should be able to return to activities of daily living with minimal limitations within 12 months.[97-100]

Fibular free flap

The fibular free flap is a microvascular reconstruction technique that utilizes tissue from the patient's lower leg, including the fibula bone, skin, and muscle. This flap is often employed for mandibular reconstruction, as the fibula's long, straight bone can be fashioned to replace missing segments of the jaw—offering excellent functional and esthetic outcomes.[91]

After surgery, patients may experience various donor-site deficits that can affect their ankle stability, ROM (ROM), extension, flexion, and big toe plantar flexion. Ling and colleagues (2012) conducted a systematic review of donor site deficits following free fibula flap surgery.[92] Donor-site morbidities following surgery can vary in severity, but they are generally considered minor and often transient.[88]

An evaluation of 42 relevant articles found that approximately 5.8% of patients experienced ankle instability as a late donor-site morbidity.[92] Ankle instability can result from the removal of a portion of the fibula, which plays a role in stabilizing the ankle joint. This instability can affect a patient's ability to maintain balance and stability while walking or engaging in physical activities. Further, the review reported that about 11.5% of patients had limited ROM in their ankles as a late donor-site morbidity.[92] Limited ankle ROM can restrict the foot's movement and may lead to difficulties in performing tasks that require flexibility in the ankle joint. Reduced muscle strength was noted in approximately 4.0% of patients as another late donor-site morbidity.[92] Muscle weakness may occur due to the removal of a portion of the flexor hallucis longus muscle, which can impact a patient's ability to generate force during activities involving the ankle and foot. Lastly, a weakness in dorsiflexion of the great toe was observed in approximately 3.6% of patients.[92] This deficit can affect the patient's ability to flex the big toe properly, potentially impacting their gait and overall mobility.

It is essential to note that these donor-site deficits, while documented, were generally considered manageable, and many patients remained satisfied with their functional and esthetic outcomes. Surgeons can mitigate these issues through careful surgical techniques. Further, postoperative care and early rehabilitation can optimize the patient's recovery and minimize long-term morbidity.

Pectoralis major myocutaneous flap

The pectoralis major myocutaneous flap is a pedicled flap reconstruction technique. It involves transferring tissue from the patient's chest wall, including skin, muscle, and blood vessels, to the head and neck region. This flap is commonly used for reconstruction following surgery involving the throat and neck, providing reliable coverage and support.[93] After surgery, patients may encounter various donor-site deficits, such as stiffness and limited ROM.[101]

Specifically, reports have indicated that patients may experience a decrease in shoulder abduction following surgery.[101]

In female patients, PMMC flap in head and neck reconstruction poses unique challenges, primarily due to the potential for significant breast deformity resulting from the primary closure of the flap's donor site.[102] Typically, patients will exhibit medial displacement of the nipple—areola complex following flap reconstruction.[102] When alternatives to the PMMC flap are not viable, novel approaches to donor site closure are being developed to improve the donor sites form and enhance the reliability of this flap. A study, published by Mehta et al. (2016), showed that when employing modified PMMC techniques, all 47 of their patients achieved good breast contour and esthetic positioning of the nipple—areola complex.[102]

Finally, following surgery physical therapy is a fundamental component of the rehabilitation process, focusing on restoring ROM in the shoulder joint and enhancing the strength of the pectoral muscles. Patients typically undergo targeted exercises and therapies to regain functional use of the affected shoulder. Occupational therapists may also be involved in assisting patients in adapting to daily activities that may require adjustments due to chest wall mobility changes.[103]

Conclusion
Goals of rehabilitation and expected outcomes

Rehabilitation following HNC surgery is integral to improving patients' postoperative experiences. Its primary objectives encompass enhancing functional outcomes and overall quality of life. Rehabilitation programs are tailored to individual patient needs, focusing on specific areas of concern. Speech therapists work diligently to improve swallowing function and enhance speech clarity, addressing common post-surgery issues such as dysphagia and dysphonia. Physical therapists play a pivotal role in restoring neck and shoulder mobility, ensuring patients regain a full ROM and function.

Moreover, rehabilitation aims to facilitate a smooth transition back to daily activities and routines. Occupational therapists assist patients in adapting to any changes resulting from surgery, ensuring they regain independence in activities such as eating, speaking, and maintaining personal hygiene. Additionally, dietitians are vital in providing nutritional support, especially when dysphagia affects patients' ability to consume food and liquids.

Expected outcomes of rehabilitation include restored swallowing function, improved speech clarity, normalized neck and shoulder mobility, and the ability to perform daily activities independently. The duration and intensity of rehabilitation are determined by the extent of surgery and individual patient requirements. Ultimately, the collaborative effort between healthcare providers and patients in the rehabilitation process is geared toward enhancing function and overall quality of life.

References

1. Crile GW. On the surgical treatment of cancer of the head and neck. *Trans South Surg Gynecol Assoc*. 1905;18:109−127.
2. Martin H, Del Valle B, Ehrlich H, Cahan WG. Neck dissection. *Cancer*. 1951;4: 441−499. https://doi.org/10.1002/1097-0142(195105)4:3<441::aid-cncr2820040303>3.0.co;2-o.
3. Stepnick D, Gilpin D. Head and neck cancer: an overview. *Semin Plast Surg*. 2010;24: 107−116. https://doi.org/10.1055/s-0030-1255328.
4. Mehanna H, Paleri V, West CM, Nutting C. Head and neck cancer−Part 1: epidemiology, presentation, and prevention. *Br Med J*. 2010;341:c4684. https://doi.org/10.1136/bmj.c4684.
5. Wheless SA, McKinney KA, Zanation AM. A prospective study of the clinical impact of a multidisciplinary head and neck tumor board. *Otolaryngol Head Neck Surg*. 2010;143: 650−654. https://doi.org/10.1016/j.otohns.2010.07.020.
6. Contributors, W.C. *Head Neck*. Wikimedia Commons; 2023.

7. Wuthrick EJ, Zhang Q, Machtay M, et al. Institutional clinical trial accrual volume and survival of patients with head and neck cancer. *J Clin Oncol.* 2015;33:156–164. https://doi.org/10.1200/jco.2014.56.5218.

8. Corry J, Peters LJ, Rischin D. Impact of center size and experience on outcomes in head and neck cancer. *J Clin Oncol.* 2015;33:138–140. https://doi.org/10.1200/jco.2014.58.2239.

9. Rygalski CJ, Huttinger ZM, Zhao S, et al. High surgical volume is associated with improved survival in head and neck cancer. *Oral Oncol.* 2023;138:106333. https://doi.org/10.1016/j.oraloncology.2023.106333.

10. Shah JP. Staging for head and neck cancer: purpose, process and progress. *Indian J Surg Oncol.* 2018;9:116–120. https://doi.org/10.1007/s13193-018-0723-0.

11. Kokal WA, Neifeld JP, Eisert D, et al. Postoperative radiation as adjuvant treatment for carcinoma of the oral cavity, larynx, and pharynx: preliminary report of a prospective randomized trial. *J Surg Oncol.* 1988;38:71–76. https://doi.org/10.1002/jso.2930380202.

12. Mishra RC, Singh DN, Mishra TK. Post-operative radiotherapy in carcinoma of buccal mucosa, a prospective randomized trial. *Eur J Surg Oncol.* 1996;22:502–504. https://doi.org/10.1016/s0748-7983(96)92969-8.

13. Lavaf A, Genden EM, Cesaretti JA, Packer S, Kao J. Adjuvant radiotherapy improves overall survival for patients with lymph node-positive head and neck squamous cell carcinoma. *Cancer.* 2008;112:535–543. https://doi.org/10.1002/cncr.23206.

14. Huang DT, Johnson CR, Schmidt-Ullrich R, Grimes M. Postoperative radiotherapy in head and neck carcinoma with extracapsular lymph node extension and/or positive resection margins: a comparative study. *Int J Radiat Oncol Biol Phys.* 1992;23:737–742. https://doi.org/10.1016/0360-3016(92)90646-y.

15. Lundahl RE, Foote RL, Bonner JA, et al. Combined neck dissection and postoperative radiation therapy in the management of the high-risk neck: a matched-pair analysis. *Int J Radiat Oncol Biol Phys.* 1998;40:529–534. https://doi.org/10.1016/s0360-3016(97)00817-1.

16. Koyfman SA, Ismaila N, Crook D, et al. Management of the neck in squamous cell carcinoma of the oral cavity and oropharynx: ASCO clinical practice guideline. *J Clin Oncol.* 2019;37:1753–1774. https://doi.org/10.1200/jco.18.01921.

17. Kiong KL, Lin FY, Yao C, et al. Impact of neoadjuvant chemotherapy on perioperative morbidity after major surgery for head and neck cancer. *Cancer.* 2020;126:4304–4314. https://doi.org/10.1002/cncr.33103.

18. Licitra L, Grandi C, Guzzo M, et al. Primary chemotherapy in resectable oral cavity squamous cell cancer: a randomized controlled trial. *J Clin Oncol.* 2003;21:327–333. https://doi.org/10.1200/jco.2003.06.146.

19. Zhong LP, Zhang CP, Ren GX, et al. Randomized phase III trial of induction chemotherapy with docetaxel, cisplatin, and fluorouracil followed by surgery versus upfront surgery in locally advanced resectable oral squamous cell carcinoma. *J Clin Oncol.* 2013;31:744–751. https://doi.org/10.1200/jco.2012.43.8820.

20. Chaukar D, Prabash K, Rane P, et al. Prospective phase II open-label randomized controlled trial to compare mandibular preservation in upfront surgery with neoadjuvant chemotherapy followed by surgery in operable oral cavity cancer. *J Clin Oncol.* 2022;40:272–281. https://doi.org/10.1200/jco.21.00179.

21. Alterio D, Marvaso G, Ferrari A, Volpe S, Orecchia R, Jereczek-Fossa BA. Modern radiotherapy for head and neck cancer. *Semin Oncol.* 2019;46:233–245. https://doi.org/10.1053/j.seminoncol.2019.07.002.

22. Caudell JJ, Torres-Roca JF, Gillies RJ, et al. The future of personalised radiotherapy for head and neck cancer. *Lancet Oncol.* 2017;18:e266−e273. https://doi.org/10.1016/s1470-2045(17)30252-8.

23. Bernier J, Domenge C, Ozsahin M, et al. Postoperative irradiation with or without concomitant chemotherapy for locally advanced head and neck cancer. *N Engl J Med.* 2004;350:1945−1952. https://doi.org/10.1056/NEJMoa032641.

24. Cooper JS, Pajak TF, Forastiere AA, et al. Postoperative concurrent radiotherapy and chemotherapy for high-risk squamous-cell carcinoma of the head and neck. *N Engl J Med.* 2004;350:1937−1944. https://doi.org/10.1056/NEJMoa032646.

25. Bernier J, Cooper JS, Pajak TF, et al. Defining risk levels in locally advanced head and neck cancers: a comparative analysis of concurrent postoperative radiation plus chemotherapy trials of the EORTC (#22931) and RTOG (# 9501). *Head Neck.* 2005;27:843−850. https://doi.org/10.1002/hed.20279.

26. Szturz P, Wouters K, Kiyota N, et al. Weekly low-dose versus three-weekly high-dose cisplatin for concurrent chemoradiation in locoregionally advanced non-nasopharyngeal head and neck cancer: a systematic review and meta-analysis of aggregate data. *Oncol.* 2017;22:1056−1066. https://doi.org/10.1634/theoncologist.2017-0015.

27. Harari PM, Harris J, Kies MS, et al. Postoperative chemoradiotherapy and cetuximab for high-risk squamous cell carcinoma of the head and neck: radiation Therapy Oncology Group RTOG-0234. *J Clin Oncol.* 2014;32:2486−2495. https://doi.org/10.1200/jco.2013.53.9163.

28. Bradley PJ, MacLennan K, Brakenhoff RH, Leemans CR. Status of primary tumour surgical margins in squamous head and neck cancer: prognostic implications. *Curr Opin Otolaryngol Head Neck Surg.* 2007;15:74−81. https://doi.org/10.1097/MOO.0b013e328058670f.

29. Zanoni DK, Migliacci JC, Xu B, et al. A proposal to redefine close surgical margins in squamous cell carcinoma of the oral tongue. *JAMA Otolaryngol Head Neck Surg.* 2017;143:555−560. https://doi.org/10.1001/jamaoto.2016.4238.

30. Holmes JD. Neck dissection: nomenclature, classification, and technique. *Oral Maxillofac Surg Clin North Am.* 2008;20:459−475. https://doi.org/10.1016/j.coms.2008.02.005.

31. Roy S, Shetty V, Sherigar V, Hegde P, Prasad R. Evaluation of four incisions used for radical neck dissection- A comparative study. *Asian Pac J Cancer Prev.* 2019;20:575−580. https://doi.org/10.31557/apjcp.2019.20.2.575.

32. Rumsey N, Clarke A, White P. Exploring the psychosocial concerns of outpatients with disfiguring conditions. *J Wound Care.* 2003;12:247−252. https://doi.org/10.12968/jowc.2003.12.7.26515.

33. Möckelmann N, Lörincz BB, Knecht R. Robotic-assisted selective and modified radical neck dissection in head and neck cancer patients. *Int J Surg.* 2016;25:24−30. https://doi.org/10.1016/j.ijsu.2015.11.022.

34. Mendenhall WM, Million RR, Cassisi NJ. Elective neck irradiation in squamous-cell carcinoma of the head and neck. *Head Neck Surg.* 1980;3:15−20. https://doi.org/10.1002/hed.2890030105.

35. Robbins KT, Clayman G, Levine PA, et al. Neck dissection classification update: revisions proposed by the American Head and Neck society and the American academy of LOtolaryngology-Head and Neck Surgery. *Arch Otolaryngol Head Neck Surg.* 2002;128:751−758. https://doi.org/10.1001/archotol.128.7.751.

36. Contributors, W.C. *Cervical Lymph Nodes and Levels*. Wikimedia Commons; 2022.
37. Calearo CV, Teatini G. Functional neck dissection. Anatomical grounds, surgical technique, clinical observations. *Ann Otol Rhinol Laryngol*. 1983;92:215−222. https://doi.org/10.1177/000348948309200301.
38. Bocca E. Supraglottic laryngectomy and functional neck dissection. *J Laryngol Otol*. 1966;80:831−838. https://doi.org/10.1017/s0022215100066032.
39. Gavilán J, Gavilán C, Herranz J. Functional neck dissection: three decades of controversy. *Ann Otol Rhinol Laryngol*. 1992;101:339−341. https://doi.org/10.1177/000348949210100409.
40. Medina JE. A rational classification of neck dissections. *Otolaryngol Head Neck Surg*. 1989;100:169−176. https://doi.org/10.1177/019459988910000301.
41. Wahle B, Zevallos J. Transoral robotic surgery and de-escalation of cancer treatment. *Otolaryngol Clin North Am*. 2020;53:981−994. https://doi.org/10.1016/j.otc.2020.07.009.
42. Mashrah MA, Al-Sharani HM, Al-Aroomi MA, Abdelrehem A, Aldhohrah T, Wang L. Surgical interventions for management of benign parotid tumors: systematic review and network meta-analysis. *Head Neck*. 2021;43:3631−3645. https://doi.org/10.1002/hed.26813.
43. Kadletz L, Grasl S, Grasl MC, Perisanidis C, Erovic BM. Extracapsular dissection versus superficial parotidectomy in benign parotid gland tumors: the Vienna Medical School experience. *Head Neck*. 2017;39:356−360. https://doi.org/10.1002/hed.24598.
44. Ruohoalho J, Mäkitie AA, Aro K, et al. Complications after surgery for benign parotid gland neoplasms: a prospective cohort study. *Head Neck*. 2017;39:170−176. https://doi.org/10.1002/hed.24496.
45. Jin H, Kim BY, Kim H, et al. Incidence of postoperative facial weakness in parotid tumor surgery: a tumor subsite analysis of 794 parotidectomies. *BMC Surg*. 2019;19:199. https://doi.org/10.1186/s12893-019-0666-6.
46. Hernando M, Echarri RM, Taha M, Martin-Fragueiro L, Hernando A, Mayor GP. Surgical complications of submandibular gland excision. *Acta Otorrinolaringol Esp*. 2012;63:42−46. https://doi.org/10.1016/j.otorri.2011.08.001.
47. Sharma N, George NA, Sebastian P. Neurovascular complications after neck dissection: a prospective analysis at a tertiary care centre in South India. *Indian J Surg Oncol*. 2020;11:746−751. https://doi.org/10.1007/s13193-020-01229-w.
48. Larsen MH, Lorenzen MM, Bakholdt V, Sørensen JA. The prevalence of nerve injuries following neck dissections-a systematic review and meta-analysis. *Dan Med J*. 2020;67:A08190464.
49. Kern KA. Medicolegal analysis of errors in diagnosis and treatment of surgical endocrine disease. *Surgery*. 1993;114:1167−1173. discussion 1173−1164.
50. Dralle H, Sekulla C, Lorenz K, Brauckhoff M, Machens A. Intraoperative monitoring of the recurrent laryngeal nerve in thyroid surgery. *World J Surg*. 2008;32:1358−1366. https://doi.org/10.1007/s00268-008-9483-2.
51. Boudourakis LD, Wang TS, Roman SA, Desai R, Sosa JA. Evolution of the surgeon-volume, patient-outcome relationship. *Ann Surg*. 2009;250:159−165. https://doi.org/10.1097/SLA.0b013e3181a77cb3.
52. Lorenz K, Raffaeli M, Barczyński M, Lorente-Poch L, Sancho J. Volume, outcomes, and quality standards in thyroid surgery: an evidence-based analysis-European Society of Endocrine Surgeons (ESES) positional statement. *Langenbeck's Arch Surg*. 2020;405:401−425. https://doi.org/10.1007/s00423-020-01907-x.

53. Erwood MS, Hadley MN, Gordon AS, Carroll WR, Agee BS, Walters BC. Recurrent laryngeal nerve injury following reoperative anterior cervical discectomy and fusion: a meta-analysis. *J Neurosurg.* 2016;25:198−204. https://doi.org/10.3171/2015.9.SPINE15187.

54. Molteni G, Greco MG, Guarino P. Complications of cervical spine surgery. In: Boriani S, Presutti L, Gasbarrini A, Mattioli F, eds. *Atlas of Craniocervical Junction and Cervical Spine Surgery.* Springer International Publishing; 2017:217−227. https://doi.org/10.1007/978-3-319-42737-9_13.

55. Oh LJ, Dibas M, Ghozy S, Mobbs R, Phan K, Faulkner H. Recurrent laryngeal nerve injury following single- and multiple-level anterior cervical discectomy and fusion: a meta-analysis. *J Spine Surg.* 2020;6:541−548.

56. Jaruchinda P, Jindavijak S, Singhavarach N. Radiation-related vocal fold palsy in patients with head and neck carcinoma. *J Med Assoc Thai.* 2012;95:S23−S28.

57. Shah F, Qamar SN, Jaffer M, Crosbie R. Dual spinal accessory nerve: an anatomical anomaly during neck dissection. *BMJ Case Rep.* 2023;16:e249866. https://doi.org/10.1136/bcr-2022-249866.

58. Tatla T, Kanagalingam J, Majithia A, Clarke PM. Upper neck spinal accessory nerve identification during neck dissection. *J Laryngol Otol.* 2005;119:906−908. https://doi.org/10.1258/002221505774783511.

59. Kakisis JD, Antonopoulos CN, Mantas G, Moulakakis KG, Sfyroeras G, Geroulakos G. Cranial nerve injury after carotid endarterectomy: incidence, risk factors, and time trends. *Eur J Vasc Endovasc Surg.* 2017;53:320−335. https://doi.org/10.1016/j.ejvs.2016.12.026.

60. Prim MP, De Diego JI, Verdaguer JM, Sastre N, Rabanal I. Neurological complications following functional neck dissection. *Eur Arch Otorhinolaryngol Head Neck.* 2006;263:473−476. https://doi.org/10.1007/s00405-005-1028-9.

61. Chia SH, Gross ND, Richmon JD. Surgeon experience and complications with transoral robotic surgery (TORS). *Otolaryngology-Head Neck Surg (Tokyo).* 2013;149:885−892.

62. Sullivan CA, Jaklitsch MT, Haddad R, et al. Endoscopic management of hypopharyngeal stenosis after organ sparing therapy for head and neck cancer. *Laryngoscope.* 2004;114:1924−1931.

63. Lee WT, Akst LM, Adelstein DJ, et al. Risk factors for hypopharyngeal/upper esophageal stricture formation after concurrent chemoradiation. *Head Neck.* 2006;28:808−812.

64. Denk D-M, Swoboda HW, Schima W, Eibenberger K. Prognostic factors for swallowing rehabilitation following head and neck cancer surgery. *Acta Otolaryngol.* 1997;117:769−774.

65. Waters TM, Logemann JA, Pauloski BR, et al. Beyond efficacy and effectiveness: conducting economic analyses during clinical trials. *Dysphagia.* 2004;19:109−119.

66. Pauloski BR. Rehabilitation of dysphagia following head and neck cancer. *Phys Med Rehabil Clin.* 2008;19:889−928. https://doi.org/10.1016/j.pmr.2008.05.010. x.

67. Lehes L, Numa J, Sõber L, Padrik M, Kasenõmm P, Jagomägi T. The effect of velopharyngeal insufficiency on voice quality in Estonian Children with Cleft Palate. *Clin Linguist Phon.* 2021;35:393−404. https://doi.org/10.1080/02699206.2020.1780323.

68. Przerwa E. [Voice emission and the tongue]. *Ann Acad Med Stetin.* 2006;52(Suppl 3):31−35.

69. Wang CC, Lin WJ, Liu YC, et al. Transoral robotic surgery for pharyngeal and laryngeal cancers-A prospective medium-term study. *J Clin Med.* 2021;10. https://doi.org/10.3390/jcm10050967.

70. Hamzany Y, Shoffel-Havakuk H, Devons-Sberro S, Shteinberg S, Yaniv D, Mizrachi A. Single stage transoral laser microsurgery for early glottic cancer. *Front Oncol.* 2018;8: 298.

71. Park JJ, Won S. Voice outcomes after transoral laser microsurgery or radiotherapy in early glottic cancer: factors to consider. *Clin Exp Otorhinolaryngol.* 2019;12: 233−234. https://doi.org/10.21053/ceo.2019.00787.

72. Dawson C, Pracy P, Patterson J, Paleri V. Rehabilitation following open partial laryngeal surgery: key issues and recommendations from the UK evidence based meeting on laryngeal cancer. *J Laryngol Otol.* 2019;133:177−182. https://doi.org/10.1017/s0022215119000483.

73. Maniaci A, Lechien JR, Caruso S, et al. Voice-related quality of life after total laryngectomy: systematic review and meta-analysis. *J Voice.* 2021. https://doi.org/10.1016/j.jvoice.2021.09.040.

74. Martin H. Esophageal speech. *Ann Otol Rhinol Laryngol.* 1950;59:687−689. https://doi.org/10.1177/000348945005900309.

75. Kaye R, Tang CG, Sinclair CF. The electrolarynx: voice restoration after total laryngectomy. *Med Devices (Auckl).* 2017;10:133−140. https://doi.org/10.2147/mder.S133225.

76. Maniaci A, La Mantia I, Mayo-Yáñez M, et al. Vocal rehabilitation and quality of life after total laryngectomy: state-of-the-art and systematic review. *Prosthesis.* 2023;5: 587−601.

77. Allegra E, La Mantia I, Bianco MR, et al. Verbal performance of total laryngectomized patients rehabilitated with esophageal speech and tracheoesophageal speech: impacts on patient quality of life. *Psychol Res Behav Manag.* 2019:675−681.

78. Cocuzza S, Maniaci A, Grillo C, et al. Voice-related quality of life in post-laryngectomy rehabilitation: tracheoesophageal Fistula's wellness. *Int J Environ Res Publ Health.* 2020;17:4605.

79. Saltürk Z, Arslanoğlu A, Özdemir E, et al. How do voice restoration methods affect the psychological status of patients after total laryngectomy. *HNO.* 2016;64:163−168.

80. Smith BG, Lewin JS. Lymphedema management in head and neck cancer. *Curr Opin Otolaryngol Head Neck Surg.* 2010;18:153−158. https://doi.org/10.1097/MOO.0b013e32833aac21.

81. Lewin JS, Hutcheson KA, Barringer DA, Smith BG. Preliminary experience with head and neck lymphedema and swallowing function in patients treated for head and neck cancer. Perspectives on Swallowing and Swallowing Disorders. *Dysphagia.* 2010;19: 45−52.

82. Ahn C, Sindelar WF. Bilateral radical neck dissection: report of results in 55 patients. *J Surg Oncol.* 1989;40:252−255. https://doi.org/10.1002/jso.2930400410.

83. Queija DDS, Dedivitis RA, Arakawa-Sugueno L, et al. Cervicofacial and pharyngolaryngeal lymphedema and deglutition after head and neck cancer treatment. *Dysphagia.* 2020;35:479−491. https://doi.org/10.1007/s00455-019-10053-6.

84. Kim D, Nam J, Kim W, et al. Radiotherapy dose−volume parameters predict facial lymphedema after concurrent chemoradiation for nasopharyngeal carcinoma. *Radiat Oncol.* 2021;16:172. https://doi.org/10.1186/s13014-021-01901-7.

85. Smith BG, Hutcheson KA, Little LG, et al. Lymphedema outcomes in patients with head and neck cancer. *Otolaryngol Head Neck Surg.* 2015;152:284−291. https://doi.org/10.1177/0194599814558402.

86. Kushida-Contreras BH, Manrique OJ, Gaxiola-García MA. Head and neck reconstruction of the vessel-depleted neck: a systematic review of the literature. *Ann Surg Oncol.* 2021;28:2882−2895. https://doi.org/10.1245/s10434-021-09590-y.

87. Gabrysz-Forget F, Tabet P, Rahal A, Bissada E, Christopoulos A, Ayad T. Free versus pedicled flaps for reconstruction of head and neck cancer defects: a systematic review. *J Otolaryngol Head Neck Surg.* 2019;48:13. https://doi.org/10.1186/s40463-019-0334-y.

88. Kearns M, Ermogenous P, Myers S, Ghanem AM. Osteocutaneous flaps for head and neck reconstruction: a focused evaluation of donor site morbidity and patient reported outcome measures in different reconstruction options. *Arch Plast Surg.* 2018;45:495−503. https://doi.org/10.5999/aps.2017.01592.

89. Bai S, Zhang ZQ, Wang ZQ, et al. Comprehensive assessment of the donor-site of the anterolateral thigh flap: a prospective study in 33 patients. *Head Neck.* 2018;40:1356−1365. https://doi.org/10.1002/hed.25109.

90. Liu J, Liu F, Fang Q, Feng J. Long-term donor site morbidity after radial forearm flap elevation for tongue reconstruction: prospective observational study. *Head Neck.* 2021;43:467−472. https://doi.org/10.1002/hed.26506.

91. Jenkins GW, Kennedy MP, Ellabban I, Adams JR, Sellstrom D. Functional outcomes following mandibulectomy and fibular free-flap reconstruction. *Br J Oral Maxillofac Surg.* 2023;61:158−164. https://doi.org/10.1016/j.bjoms.2022.11.287.

92. Ling XF, Peng X. What is the price to pay for a free fibula flap? A systematic review of donor-site morbidity following free fibula flap surgery. *Plast Reconstr Surg.* 2012;129:657−674. https://doi.org/10.1097/PRS.0b013e3182402d9a.

93. Shindo ML, Costantino PD, Friedman CD, Pelzer HJ, Sisson GA,S, Bressler FJ. The pectoralis major myofascial flap for intraoral and pharyngeal reconstruction. *Arch Otolaryngol Head Neck Surg.* 1992;118:707−711. https://doi.org/10.1001/archotol.1992.01880070037007.

94. Collins J, Ayeni O, Thoma A. A systematic review of anterolateral thigh flap donor site morbidity. *Can J Plast Surg.* 2012;20:17−23. https://doi.org/10.1177/229255031202000103.

95. Barret JP, Roodenburg JL. Functional rehabilitation in advanced intraoral cancer. *Int J Surg Oncol (N Y).* 2017;2:e10. https://doi.org/10.1097/ij9.0000000000000010.

96. Timmons MJ, Missotten FE, Poole MD, Davies DM. Complications of radial forearm flap donor sites. *Br J Plast Surg.* 1986;39:176−178. https://doi.org/10.1016/0007-1226(86)90078-0.

97. Wallner J, Rieder M, Schwaiger M, Remschmidt B, Zemann W, Pau M. Donor site morbidity and quality of life after microvascular head and neck reconstruction with a chimeric, thoracodorsal, perforator-scapular flap based on the angular artery (TDAP-Scap-aa flap). *J Clin Med.* 2022;11. https://doi.org/10.3390/jcm11164876.

98. Ferri A, Perlangeli G, Bianchi B, Zito F, Sesenna E, Ferrari S. Maxillary reconstruction with scapular tip chimeric free flap. *Microsurgery.* 2021;41:207−215. https://doi.org/10.1002/micr.30700.

99. Bot SD, Terwee CB, van der Windt DA, Bouter LM, Dekker J, de Vet HC. Clinimetric evaluation of shoulder disability questionnaires: a systematic review of the literature. *Ann Rheum Dis.* 2004;63:335−341. https://doi.org/10.1136/ard.2003.007724.

100. Kennedy CA. *The DASH and QuickDASH Outcome Measure User's Manual.* (Institute for Work & Health); 2011.

101. Refos JW, Witte BI, de Goede CJ, de Bree R. Shoulder morbidity after pectoralis major flap reconstruction. *Head Neck*. 2016;38:1221−1228. https://doi.org/10.1002/hed.24404.
102. Mehta S, Agrawal J, Pradhan T, et al. Preservation of aesthetics of breast in pectoralis major myocutaneous flap donor site in females. *J Maxillofac Oral Surg*. 2016;15: 268−271. https://doi.org/10.1007/s12663-015-0820-3.
103. Manske RC, Prohaska D. Pectoralis major tendon repair post surgical rehabilitation. *N Am J Sports Phys Ther*. 2007;2:22−33.

Head and neck cancer rehabilitation across the continuum of care

5

Jack B. Fu, MD [1], **Carsyn Cunningham, MA** [2], **Price Lucks, MS** [2]

[1]*Department of Palliative, Rehabilitation & Integrative Medicine, University of Texas MD Anderson Cancer Center, Houston, TX, United States;* [2]*Department of Head & Neck Surgery, University of Texas MD Anderson Cancer Center, Houston, TX, United States*

Introduction

Head and neck cancer (HNC) rehabilitation's continuum of care can be categorized within the framework of Dietz's four stages of cancer rehabilitation: preventative, restorative, supportive, and palliative.[1] Rehabilitation professionals can treat H&N cancer patients from prehabilitation before surgery, during the postsurgical acute care stay, postacute inpatient rehabilitation, during survivorship care, and at the end of life.

Prehabilitation/preventative phase

Prehabilitation before head and neck surgery can prepare the patient for the challenges of surgery and postsurgical recovery. General physical conditioning prehabilitation focusing on conditioning and nutrition may be useful to build overall strength (and muscle mass), optimize nutrition, and through patient education.[2] Many head and neck cancer patients may not be in optimal health prior to surgery due to older age, alcohol abuse, tobacco use, cachexia, and sedentary lifestyle.[3] A general conditioning prehabilitation program can include moderate intensity aerobic exercise and strengthening exercises. In addition, nutrition optimization through an emphasis on protein intake (through food or nutritional formulas) is emphasized.[4] Patients compliant with a prehabilitation exercise program can demonstrate significant improvements in mobility and prevention of pulmonary morbidity.[5]

Pretreatment speech language pathology care

A presurgical speech language pathology (SLP) consult is a best practice, and National Comprehensive Cancer Network (NCCN) recommended standard prior to surgery for oral cavity, pharyngeal, or laryngeal tumors.[6] Regardless of the type of

Copyright © 2025 Elsevier Inc. All rights reserved, including those for text and data mining, AI training, and similar technologies.
63

treatment anticipated, best practice begins with a thorough baseline evaluation including a detailed cranial nerve exam, motor speech evaluation, clinical swallowing evaluation, and many times an instrumental evaluation of swallowing.[7] Instrumental swallowing evaluations include the fiberoptic endoscopic evaluation of swallowing (FEES) or the modified barium swallow study (MBS) that both afford visualization of the anatomy and physiology of swallowing and the safety and efficiency of swallowing.[6] The SLP consult includes a detailed review of anatomy and physiology of communication, swallowing, and breathing. The patient is educated on anticipated acute/subacute changes including short- and long-term rehabilitation needs, and any relevant prehabilitation strategies. For patients with baseline impairment, it is appropriate to initiate optimization therapy prior to surgery where time and capacity allow. For example, if a patient has a history of head and neck radiotherapy and is now planned to receive a mandibulectomy for osteoradionecrosis, they likely have some degree of baseline dysphagia prior to surgery, which will be exacerbated by surgery plus disuse muscle atrophy that occurs during a mandatory NPO period for surgical healing.[8] This presents an opportunity to attempt to optimize current swallow status with exercise or training to habituate compensatory swallow strategies in hopes of attenuating both acute functional impairment and improving long-term functional outcomes.

Proactive dysphagia therapy is one of the most common forms of prehabilitation in HNC, which has been studied and implemented for more than two decades.[9] Prehabilitation is predicated by a comprehensive baseline swallowing evaluation including instrumentation such that therapy can be scaled appropriately to the functional status of the individual. A swallowing prehabilitation therapy session with the SLP should include education on acute radiation effects and risk for long-term edema and fibrosis that may impact eating and swallowing. This education generates patient buy-in, helps the patient to understand why they must intentionally work on swallowing, when many of the patients do not have baseline dysphagia, and empowers patients to have ownership in their own functional outcomes. The overarching goal of prehabilitative swallowing therapy is to engage pharyngeal swallowing musculature at least to baseline capacity to prevent disuse muscle atrophy related to treatment toxicities.[10] Individualized goals are set to promote maximal swallowing activity before and during treatment including addressing any baseline dysphagia with compensatory swallowing strategies (to maintain safe/efficient swallows during radiation therapy), initiation of a home program of jaw and pharyngeal swallowing exercises,[11] and a hierarchical approach to ensuring the patients are eating the densest foods possible to get maximal muscle engagement during radiation to prevent muscle atrophy.[10] As side effects from radiation progress, it is often necessary to adjust this program to the individualized need of each patient.[10,12,13] Though traditionally proactive swallowing therapy has been delivered in person, a small cohort received telehealth visits for proactive swallowing training and education and reported that this method of delivery did not impact their learning when compared with in-person sessions.[14]

Restorative phase
Postsurgical hospitalization

Functional decline after H&N cancer surgery, particularly in older patients, has been demonstrated.[15] During the postsurgical acute care stay, physical and occupational therapy may be required to assist with mobility and deconditioning particularly if the patient experienced a complicated postsurgical course (e.g., infections, wound dehiscence, intensive care units stays).

Patients who have suffered deconditioning and cancer-related fatigue due to a complicated postoperative course may not be able to discharge home safely. Physical medicine and rehabilitation may be required to help with postacute inpatient rehabilitation triage if the patient is unable to safely discharge to their home setting. Perhaps due in part to the Medicare 60% rule, H&N cancer patients account for only about 1% of all cancer patients admitted to American acute inpatient rehabilitation facilities.[16] Prehead and neck surgery risk factors for requiring postacute inpatient rehab such as a skilled nursing facility or acute inpatient rehabilitation include increased age, lower body mass index, and comorbidities.[17] Postoperative rehabilitation considerations include the need for tube feedings and plastic surgery flap precautions. Flap precautions often consist of restrictions at the resection and graft harvest site with respect range of motion and weight bearing. The need for enteral nutritional support both during the postsurgical hospitalization and long term is quite common to allow for healing and/or dysphagia. Nutritionist assistance in selecting a nutritional formula, rate, and free water hydration is usually required. Enteral feeding intolerance can occur with tube feed initiation and can include diarrhea, nausea, vomiting, and abdominal discomfort and may require feeding adjustments.

Postsurgical communication and swallowing impairment may occur acutely or chronically, most commonly in patients undergoing surgery to the oral cavity, pharynx, or larynx. The functional impairment varies based on surgical site, defect volume, and reconstruction. For instance, dysarthria and voicing changes often occur in oral cavity resection patients due to area of lesion, frequent and possibly adynamic reconstruction, and typically transient tracheostomy,[18,19] whereas after total laryngectomy, patients have many different functional changes they must adjust to including stoma breathing, establishment of alaryngeal communication, and changes to swallowing.[20]

Acute/perioperative SLP care

For patients treated with oral cavity resection, the SLP in the inpatient environment provides basic dysarthria strategies to begin mobilizing any residual native lingual tissue and promote early neuromuscular reeducation to adapt to postoperative reconstruction and swelling. Surgical procedures with reconstruction often require the patient to undergo a temporary tracheotomy for airway management in anticipation of postoperative edema. The SLP will assess readiness for a speaking valve that may aid in secretion management, airway protection during swallowing, sense of smell and taste, and voice and speech production.[21] Importantly, fitting of a speaking valve is also a critical step in the decannulation process. Pending surgical clearance, swallow specific exercises (e.g., effortful saliva swallows, supraglottic swallow) may be trained while the patient waits for their postoperative objective swallowing evaluation, as it is important to keep the swallowing mechanism engaged given anticipated muscle atrophy from disuse during the mandatory NPO period for healing that typically lasts several weeks postoperatively. The SLP often performs a modified barium swallow study 2−8 weeks after surgery with oral and/or pharyngeal reconstruction to assess readiness for oral intake. The postoperative MBS in this clinical population serves to jointly assess postsurgical healing ("rule out leak") and swallowing function, with timing dependent on the extent of surgery, initial healing, and radiation history. In other cases, typically without reconstruction, a clinical swallowing evaluation or bedside FEES once cleared by medical team may be sufficient to resume safe and efficient oral intake. Another critical role of the inpatient SLP is postoperative laryngectomy care. Management includes guiding the patient to initiate an alternate form of communication, most commonly the electrolarynx, training the patient and caregivers on stoma management, and reinitiation of oral intake with swallowing assessment via MBS depending on reconstructive history. It is always important to reassure the patient that life continues after surgery.

Inpatient SLP care of the HN patient in nonsurgical populations is often focused on swallowing or airway management in patients hospitalized with acute tumor or treatment-related toxicity. A retrospective review found that 35% of head and neck cancer patients undergoing treatment were hospitalized after suffering some form of treatment-related toxicity.[22] Acute toxicities can include mucositis, dysphagia, aspiration, and dermatitis.[23] A recent analysis showed that out of 376 patients, 15% had at least one hospital admission during treatment due to dehydration, mucositis, fever, and nausea/vomiting.[24] The goal of maximizing swallowing outcomes during radiation continues while a patient is admitted with continued focus on eating and exercising swallowing musculature. The SLP care starts with swallow assessment, often in the form of bedside swallowing evaluation or FEES. MBS is more rarely used during acute treatment hospitalizations unless signs and symptoms point to cervical esophageal dysfunction (e.g., obstructive dysphagia symptoms concerning for stricture). The SLP provides strategies to facilitate safe/efficient swallowing by educating the patient on personalized compensatory strategies, and the need to plan pain management around mealtime, avoid spicy/acidic foods to reduce pain, and implement good oral hygiene to prevent any future infection. These practices involve a multidisciplinary team (nutrition, oncology, nursing, etc.) to help reduce the distress associated with head and neck cancer.

Supportive phase

Depending on the location, the 5-year relative survival rate for all stages of head and neck cancers is between 52% and 91%.[25] As cancer treatment falls into the background for many, maximizing quality of life for HNC survivors becomes important. Musculoskeletal, pain, and dysphagia are common impairments. The prevalence of dysphagia within the first 2 years of head and neck radiation therapy (RT) is estimated to be around 44%.[26-29]

Physical function and physiatric interventions: H&N cancer patients experience a significant decline in functional status at 1 year postsurgery.[30] The importance of maintaining exercise postsurgery cannot be emphasized enough. It will help maintain functional independence, improve cancer related symptoms, and may reduce the risk of cancer progression or recurrence.[31]

Physiatric survivorship care is largely provided on an outpatient basis. Physiatrists can assist H&N cancer survivors through exercise and lifestyle education, disability assistance,[32] and prescribing therapies.

In addition, head and neck cancer survivors may experience spasms of the neck and shoulders that may be treated with botulinum toxin injections. Patients can experience a number of complications associated with botulinum toxin injections including pain, infection, and bleeding (as with any injectable treatment). Changes in swallowing after botulinum toxin injection are relatively common (reported to be 9% by Stubblefield et al.).[33] Because most posttreatment head and neck cancer patients already have compromised swallowing (after surgery and radiation), patients are at a higher risk for experiencing noticeable changes in swallowing (compared with a noncancer patient cervical dystonia botulinum toxin patient). Swallowing changes are usually mild and may be due to temporary further weakening of swallowing musculature or exacerbation of their baseline xerostomia. Botulinum toxin has been used to treat oversalivation, and many of the salivary glands (including the parotid and submandibular gland) are in the region of frequently injected musculature. Rimabotulinum toxin is federal drug administration approved to treat chronic sialorrhea. Trismus is another condition that may benefit from botulinum toxin chemodenervation particularly if there is masseter pain and/or spasms.[34] There is also some evidence that suggests botulinum toxin chemodenervation of the salivary glands may improve first bite syndrome symptoms.[35]

Myofascial pain that can be a direct result of neck and shoulder dysfunction due to changes in the biomechanics and balance of musculature due to weakness and or scar tissue can occur. Massage (including myofascial release), trigger point injections, and rehabilitation geared toward trying to reestablishing proper musculoskeletal mechanics as much as possible may be helpful.

Neuropathic pain in the face and scalp can occur in about 14% of H&N cancer survivors often due to trigeminal and/or occipital neuralgia.[36] Nerve blocks of the trigeminal nerve (can be technically difficult and may require fluoroscopic guidance) and occipital nerve blocks can provide significant relief.[37] In addition, the use of oral medications such as gabapentin, pregabalin, and duloxetine may also be of benefit.

Carotid artery radiation late effects can lead to carotid artery stenosis and carotid baroreceptor dysfunction and orthostatic hypotension. 34% of H&N cancer patients after radiation therapy develop >50% carotid artery stenosis within 8 years postradiation.[38] Carotid artery stenosis screening is a standard of H&N survivorship care. In addition, orthostatic hypotension can occur in about two-thirds of H&N survivors and may limit functional independence due in part to baroreceptor and/or neurologic injury.[39] The use of compression stockings, abdominal binders, limiting volume-depleting or blood pressure–lowering medications (such as benign prostatic hypertrophy medications), encouraging oral fluids, and blood pressure–increasing medications such as fludrocortisone and midodrine may be needed.

Posttreatment/survivorship SLP care

Posttreatment, speech pathologists manage dysphagia,[40] dysarthria,[41] dysphonia, lymphedema,[42] and trismus with evidence-based exercise and behavioral therapy protocols. A systematic review by Heijnen et al. (2016) further describes the functional impacts on oral intake, speech, voice, and tissue integrity following oncologic interventions.[43] Outpatient SLP care includes therapies to maintain and optimize function for patient suffering chronic functional disability, and management of late functional changes many years or decades after cure (particularly late radiation-associated dysphagia, late-RAD).[10]

Outpatient SLP rehabilitation in the surgical population is ideally a seamless transition from the acute postsurgical rehabilitation started as part of the inpatient postoperative care. Surgical patients who were not yet ready for swallowing evaluation while admitted due to ongoing healing or reconstruction may return as outpatients for swallowing evaluation and diet initiation. Surgical patients requiring some form of reconstruction may undergo a rule-out-leak MBS study. A systematic protocol is recommended to limit radiation exposure to the patient and assess an array of diet textures.[44] Dynamic Imaging Grade of Swallowing Toxicity (DIGEST) is among a set of validated measurement tools for MBS and FEES. DIGEST measures pharyngeal residue and the safety (penetration/aspiration) of the swallow in the HNC population.[45] This tool allows the clinician to quantify the safety of the patient's swallow and compare it to previous studies to assess clinical presentation, in a nomenclature that aligns to the CTCAE toxicity grading framework familiar to oncologists. Following instrumental assessment, specific interventions and exercises are assigned to the patient to compensate for any physiological changes that may have impacted the safety of the swallow and/or prepare for any anticipated adjuvant treatment. Personalized therapy can be guided by performing an instrumental assessment matched to patient-reported outcome measures and other functional scales in standard fashion before and after therapy.

Postlaryngectomy patients often require lifelong SLP rehabilitation if they speak with a tracheoesophageal puncture (TEP).[46] All patients treated with a total laryngectomy require outpatient SLP care after discharge until they are independent with stoma care, stomal attachments transitioned as possible and stabilized (Lary-Tube vs. peristomal or LaryButton), swallowing the maximal tolerated diet, and have a form of alaryngeal communication. Outpatient SLP therapy for communication early after laryngectomy includes continuation of electrolarynx training, initiation of tracheoesophageal (TE) voicing, and teaching of voice prosthesis self-care in the case of primary tracheoesophageal puncture (TEP). Esophageal speech may also be an option but is rare in modern practice with popularity and better access to TEP. For patients who do not have a TEP at the time of total laryngectomy, the SLP will participate in evaluation for secondary TEP months or sometimes years after the total laryngectomy, should the patient desire this as a communication option. The SLP will evaluate TEP candidacy including insufflation testing,[47] and often a modified barium swallow that can give insight into functional potential and need for any optimization of (neo)pharyngoesophageal function prior to secondary puncture including botulinum toxin,[48] or esophageal dilation[49] to optimize TE voice.[47] Patients must be counseled on the lifelong commitment of TEP management and potential risk for complications.[50,51]

Unfortunately, side effects from radiation do not end at the conclusion of treatment. Acute toxicities can take months to dissipate, and prolonged restrictions during this recovery period may further promote chronic dysphagia by compounding normal tissue injury from radiation with muscle disuse atrophy. Proactive surveillance and rehabilitation of dysphagia have been advocated after radiation.[52] One example is the radiation swallowing pathway implemented at MD Anderson, which includes routine swallowing evaluation (MBS completed about 3–6 months postradiation) to detect patients needing more intensive, personalized therapies in concert with training on a brief lifelong home exercise program targeting maintenance of swallowing function. Once acute toxicities have resolved, there is lifelong risk for new or progressive functional impairment in speech and swallowing due to late radiation effects, including radiation fibrosis and neuropathy.[53–55] For these reasons, serial evaluation continued into long-term survivorship is advocated using instrumental means such as MBS or FEES.[54] Intervention for dysphagia, lymphedema, trismus, and dysarthria follows where relevant. One model for intensive personalized therapy for chronic or late swallowing impairment is the MD Anderson Boot Camp Swallowing Therapy Program that couples an optimization phase with a variety of personalized therapy options followed by intensive daily therapy following the McNeil Dysphagia Therapy Protocol.[56] While gains are possible in most cases, they are almost always limited as the effects of radiation fibrosis are irreversible. At times, the goal of treatment shifts from one of significant improvement to one of slowing down the often-progressive nature of radiation-associated dysphagia.[8,54] While the impact of radiation on swallowing may be inevitable, survivorship clinics seek to support long-term goals of patients with a variety of rehabilitation and other professionals and allots an opportunity to make treating and coping with changes from radiation more manageable.[54]

Conclusion

Head and neck survivors can experience significant impairments that require rehabilitation before treatment (prehabilitation), during postsurgical hospitalizations and radiation (restorative), and after completion of oncologic treatment survivorship care (supportive). Rehabilitation interventions are crucial to improve functional independence and quality of life throughout the continuum of care.

References

1. Dietz JH. Adaptive rehabilitation of the cancer patient. *Curr Probl Cancer*. November 1980;5(5):1−56.
2. Boright L, Doherty DJ, Wilson CM, Arena SK, Ramirez C. Development and feasibility of a prehabilitation protocol for patients diagnosed with head and neck cancer. *Cureus*. August 20, 2020;12(8):e9898.
3. Twomey R, Culos-Reed SN, Dort JC. Exercise prehabilitation-supporting recovery from major head and neck cancer surgery. *JAMA Otolaryngol Head Neck Surg*. August 1, 2020;146(8):689−690.
4. Cantwell LA, Fahy E, Walters ER, Patterson JM. Nutritional prehabilitation in head and neck cancer: a systematic review. *Support Care Cancer*. November 2022;30(11): 8831−8843.
5. Moore J, Scoggins CR, Philips P, et al. Implementation of prehabilitation for major abdominal surgery and head and neck surgery: a simplified seven-day protocol. *J Gastrointest Surg*. August 2021;25(8):2076−2082.
6. Pfister DG, Spencer S, Adelstein D, et al. NCCN clinical practice guidelines in oncology: head and neck cancers. *J Natl Compr Cancer Netw*. 2020;18(7):873−898.
7. Kuhn MA, Gillespie MB, Ishman SL, et al. Expert consensus statement: management of dyspahagia in head and neck cancer patients. *Otolaryngol Head Neck Surg*. 2023;168(4).
8. Strojan P, Hutcheson KA, Eisbruch A, et al. Treatment of late sequelae after radiotherapy for head and neck cancer. *Cancer Treat Rev*. 2017;59:79−92.
9. Loewen I, Jeffery CC, Rieger J, Constantinescu G. Prehabilitation in head and neck cancer patients: a literature review. *J Otolaryngol Head Neck Surg*. 2021;50(2).
10. Hutcheson KA, Bhayani MK, Beadle BM, et al. Eat and exercise during radiotherapy or chemoradiotherapy for pharyngeal cancers: use it or lose it. *JAMA Otolaryngol Head and Neck Surg*. 2013;139(11):1127−1134.
11. Greco E, Simic T, Ringash J, Tomlinson G, Inamoto Y, Martino R. Dysphagia treatment for patients with head and neck cancer undergoing radiation therapy: a meta-analysis review. *Int J Radiat Oncol Biol Phys*. 2018;101(2):421−444.
12. Barbon CEA, Peterson CB, Moreno AC, et al. Adhering to eating and exercise status during radiotherapy for oropharyngeal cancer for prevention and mitigation of radiotherapy-associated dysphagia. *JAMA Otolaryngol Head and Neck Surg*. 2022;148(10):956−964.
13. Langmore S, Krisciunas GP, Miloro KV, Evans SR, Cheng DM. Does PEG use cause dysphagia in head and neck cancer patients? *Dysphagia*. 2012;27(2):251−259.
14. Khan MM, Manduchi B, Rodriguez V, et al. Exploring patient experiences with a telehealth approach for the PRO-ACTIVE trial intervention in head and neck cancer patients. *BMC Health Serv Res*. 2022;22(1).
15. Fancy T, Huang AT, Kass JI, et al. Complications, mortality, and functional decline in patients 80 years or older undergoing major head and neck ablation and reconstruction. *JAMA Otolaryngol Head Neck Surg*. December 1, 2019;145(12): 1150−1157.

16. Mix JM, Granger CV, LaMonte MJ, et al. Characterization of cancer patients in inpatient rehabilitation facilities: a retrospective cohort study. *Arch Phys Med Rehabil*. May 2017; 98(5):971−980.

17. Freeman MH, Shinn JR, Fernando SJ, et al. Impact of preoperative risk factors on inpatient stay and facility discharge after free flap reconstruction. *Otolaryngol Head Neck Surg*. March 2022;166(3):454−460.

18. Blyth KM, McCabe P, Madill C, Ballard KJ. Speech and swallow rehabilitation following partial glossectomy: a systematic review. *Int J Speech Lang Pathol*. 2015; 17:401−410.

19. Jenkins GW, Kennedy MP, Ellabban I, Adams JR, Sellstrom D. Functional outcomes following mandibulectomy and fibular free-flap reconstruction. *Br J Oral Maxillofac Surg*. 2022;61:158−164.

20. Zenga J, Goldsmith T, Bunting G, Deschler DG. State of the art: rehabilitation of speech and swallowing after total laryngectomy. *Oral Oncol*. 2018;86:38−47.

21. Dettelbach MA, Gross RD, Mahlmann J, Eibling DE. Effect of the Passy-Muir valve on aspiration in patients with tracheostomy. *Head Neck*. 1995 July−August;17(4):297−302. https://doi.org/10.1002/hed.2880170405.

22. Ling DC, Kabolizadeh P, Heron DE, et al. Incidence of hospitalization in patients with head and neck cancer treated with intensity-modulated radiation therapy. *Head Neck*. 2015;37(12):1750−1755.

23. Muzumder S, Srikantia N, Udayashankar AH, Kainthaje PB, John Sebastian MG. Burden of acute toxicities in head-and-neck radiation therapy: a single-institutional experience. *South Asian Journal of Cancer*. 2019;08(02):120−123.

24. Patel S, Rich BJ, Schumacher L-ED, et al. Ed visits, hospital admissions and treatment breaks in head/neck cancer patients undergoing radiotherapy. *Front Oncol*. 2023;13.

25. American Cancer Society. Oral cavity and oropharyngeal cancer early detection. *Diagn Staging*. https://www.cancer.org/content/dam/CRC/PDF/Public/8765.00.pdf. Accessed 24 August 2023.

26. Hutcheson K, Nurgalieva Z, Zhao H, et al. Two-year prevalence of dysphagia and related outcomes in head and neck caner survivors: an updated SEER-medicare analysis. *Head Neck*. 2019;41(2):479−487.

27. Kamal M, Mohamed ASR, Volpe S, et al. Radiotherapy dose−volume parameters predict videofluoroscopy-detected dysphagia per DIGEST after IMRT for oropharyngeal cancer: Results of a prospective registry. *Radiother Oncol*. 2018;128(3):442−451.

28. Payakachat N, Ounpraseuth S, Suen JY. Late complications and long-term quality of life for survivors (>5 years) with history of head and neck cancer. *Head Neck*. 2012;35(6): 819−825.

29. Rock C, Grant S, Zaveri J, et al. Dose-volume correlates of the prevalence of patient-reported trismus in long-term survivorship after oropharyngeal IMRT: a cross-sectional dosimetric analysis. *Radiother Oncol*. 2020;149:142−149.

30. Bruijnen CP, de Groot LGR, Vondeling AM, et al. Functional decline after surgery in older patients with head and neck cancer. *Oral Oncol*. December 2021;123:105584.

31. Zheng A, Zhang L, Yang J, et al. Physical activity prevents tumor metastasis through modulation of immune function. *Front Pharmacol*. October 12, 2022;13:1034129.

32. Fu JB, Osborn MP, Silver JK, et al. Evaluating disability insurance assistance as a specific intervention by physiatrists at a cancer center. *Am J Phys Med Rehabil*. 2017;96(7): 523−528.

33. Stubblefield MD, Levine A, Custodio CM, Fitzpatrick T. The role of botulinum toxin type A in the radiation fibrosis syndrome: a preliminary report. *Arch Phys Med Rehabil*. March 2008;89(3):417−421.

34. Hartl DM, Cohen M, Juliéron M, Marandas P, Janot F, Bourhis J. Botulinum toxin for radiation-induced facial pain and trismus. *Otolaryngol Head Neck Surg*. April 2008; 138(4):459−463.

35. Shaikh NE, Jafary HA, Behnke JW, Turner MT. Botulinum toxin A for the treatment of first bite syndrome-a systematic review. *Gland Surg*. July 2022;11(7):1251−1263.

36. Rojo RD, Ren JL, Lipe DN, et al. Neuropathic pain prevalence and risk factors in head and neck cancer survivors. *Head Neck*. December 2022;44(12):2820−2833.

37. Mehio AK, Shah SK. Alleviating head and neck pain. *Otolaryngol Clin North Am*. February 2009;42(1):143−159.

38. Carpenter DJ, Mowery YV, Broadwater G, Rodrigues A, Wisdom AJ, Dorth JA. The risk of carotid stenosis in head and neck cancer patients after radiation therapy. *Oral Oncol*. May 2018;80:9−15.

39. Norcliffe-Kaufmann L, Palma JA. Blood pressure instability in head and neck cancer survivors. *Clin Auton Res*. August 2020;30(4):291−293.

40. Zebralla V, Wichmann G, Pirlich M, et al. Dysphagia, voice problems, and pain in head and neck cancer patients. *Eur Arch Oto-Rhino-Laryngol*. 2021;278(10):3985−3994.

41. McKinstry A, Perry A. Evaluation of speech in people with head and neck cancer: a pilot study. *Int J Lang Commun Disord*. 2003;38(1):31−46.

42. Smith BG, Lewin JS. Lymphedema management in head and neck cancer. *Curr Opin Otolaryngol Head Neck Surg*. 2010;18(3):153−158.

43. Heijnen BJ, Speyer R, Kertscher B, et al. Dysphagia, speech, voice, and trismus following radiotherapy and/or chemotherapy in patients with head and neck carcinoma: review of the literature. *BioMed Res Int*. 2016;2016:6086894.

44. Hutcheson KA, Lewin JS. Dysphagia in patients with head and neck cancer. In: Athanassios A, Ferris RL, eds. *Rosenthal. Head and Neck Cancers Evidence-Based Treatment*. New York: Demos Medical; 2018:457−478.

45. Hutcheson K. *Be Proactive! A Best Practice Guide for Treating Radiation-Associated Dysphagia*. MedBridge Blog; 2017. Retrieved April 11, 2023, from https://www.medbridgeeducation.com/blog/2017/02/be-proactive-a-best-practice-guide-for-treating-radiation-associated-dysphagia/.

46. Singer MI, Blom ED. An endoscopic technique for restoration of voice after laryngectomy. *Ann Otol Rhinol Laryngol*. 1980;89(6 Pt 1):529−533.

47. Lewin JS, Baugh RF, Baker SR. An objective method for prediction of tracheoesophagealspeech production. *JSHD J Speech Hear Disord*. 1987a;52(3):212−217.

48. Lewin JS, Bishop-Leone JK, Forman AD, Diaz Jr EM. Further experience with Botox injection for tracheoesophageal speech failure. *Head Neck*. June 2001;23(6):456−460.

49. Sweeny L, Golden JB, White HN, Magnuson JS, Carroll WR, Rosenthal EL. Incidence and outcomes of stricture formation postlaryngectomy. *Otolaryngol Head Neck Surg*. 2012;146(3):395−402.

50. Gitomer SA, Hutcheson KA, Christianson BL, et al. Influence of timing, radiation, and reconstruction on complications and speech outcomes with tracheoesophageal puncture. *Head Neck*. December 2016;38(12):1765−1771. https://doi.org/10.1002/hed.24529.

51. Hutcheson KA, Strugis EM, Lewin JS. Early risk factors for enlargement of the tracheoesophageal puncture after total laryngectomy: nodal metastasis and extent of surgery. *Arch Otolaryngol Head Neck Surg*. 2012;138(9):833−839.

52. Messing BP, Ward EC, Lazarus C, et al. Establishing a multidisciplinary head and neck clinical pathway: an implementation evaluation and audit of dysphagia-related services and outcomes. *Dysphagia*. 2018;34:89−104.

53. Aggarwal P, Zaveri J,S, Goepfert R, et al. JAMA otolaryngology: head and neck. *Surgery*. 2018;144(11):1066−1076.

54. Ebersole B, McCarroll L, Ridge JA, et al. Identification and management of late dysfunction in survivors of head and neck cancer: implementation and outcomes of an interdisciplinary quality of life (IQOL) clinic. *Head Neck*. 2021;43(7):2124−2135.

55. Hutcheson KA, Lewin JS. Functional outcomes after chemoradiotherapy of laryngeal and pharyngeal cancers. *Curr Oncol Rep*. 2012;14:158−161.

56. Malandraki GA, Hutcheson KA. Intensive therapies for dysphagia: implementation of the intensive dysphagia rehabilitation and the MD Anderson swallowing Boot Camp approaches. *Perspect ASHA Spec Interest Groups*. 2018;3(13):133−145.

Muscle wasting and frailty in head and neck cancer

6

Eric W. Villanueva, MD [1,2]**, Ryan Kelly, MD** [1,2]**, Lydia Henderson, MD** [1,2]**, Ishan Roy, MD, PhD** [1,2,3]

[1]*Shirley Ryan AbilityLab, Chicago, IL, United States;* [2]*Department of Physical Medicine and Rehabilitation, Northwestern University Feinberg School of Medicine of Medicine, Chicago, IL, United States;* [3]*Robert H. Lurie Comprehensive Cancer Center, Chicago, IL, United States*

Cachexia

Cachexia is biologically defined as a systemic muscle wasting syndrome secondary to chronic disease and is driven by a complex, multiorgan system inflammatory process and accelerated catabolic metabolism.[1] This syndrome is noted to occur in around 50% of all patients with cancer and up to 80% of those with advanced cancer.[2] Cachexia also eventually leads to progressive functional decline and disability in 50%—75% of those affected.[3] Patients with HNC are suspected to be at increased risk given anatomical location of tumors and impact on nutritional intake, with studies pointing to elevated prevalence in those diagnosed early in the course of their disease, compared with other cancers.[4] Another factor specific to HNC patients is the impact tumor location can have on taste and smell of food, leading to loss of appetite (anorexia) and exacerbation of weight loss in the setting of already-accelerated catabolic metabolism.[5]

The precise biologic mechanism of cachexia has yet to be elucidated, but proinflammatory mediators, including TNF-alpha, IL-6, and TGF-beta, are known mediators.[1] Additionally, appetite regulating factors, such as ghrelin, leptin, and GDF-15, [6—8] are also known mediators. In HNC specifically, there has not yet been a demonstrated difference in inflammatory activity in patients with or without cachexia, though there have been some data to suggest that inflammatory markers (IL-6, CRP) are higher in HNC compared with other cancers, suggesting an acute phase response is at play.[9] Cachexia, therefore, is not merely a disease of starvation or anorexia, and clinicians must remain cognizant of that fact, evaluating and treating patients with HNC with a multifaceted approach that includes, but does not solely rely on, nutritional supplementation. In fact, the consensus definition of cachexia indicates this process can occur despite adequate/ideal nutritional intake.[10]

Clearly, outcomes in terms of QoL, function, and mortality are negatively affected by a diagnosis of cachexia. Cachexia is reported as the cause of death in about 20%—30% of all cancer patients, and in HNC, 2-year survival rates drop from 57.5% to 7.5% in those with cachexia.[11,12] Before this mortality, cachexia

Head and Neck Cancer Rehabilitation. https://doi.org/10.1016/B978-0-443-11806-7.00019-9
Copyright © 2025 Elsevier Inc. All rights reserved, including those for text and data mining, AI training, and similar technologies.

also wreaks havoc on the physical function of the individual, limiting independence with activities of daily living (ADLs). Loss of muscle mass leads to impairments in overall muscle strength and limits activity tolerance including decline in proximal muscle strength, standing tolerance, and ambulation as well as cognition, all of which negatively impact QoL, treatment success, and survival.[13,14]

With this general overview in mind, it is the duty of the clinician to correctly identify and treat patients whom they believe are suffering from, or at risk of cachexia.

Diagnosis

Diagnosing cachexia can prove difficult when taking into account the existence of multiple criteria and screening measures, as well as the overlap between the similar diagnoses of sarcopenia and frailty.[15] An essential feature of cachexia is unintentional weight loss, most frequently diagnosed using the Fearon criteria. The Fearon consensus criteria is defined as "weight loss greater than 5%, or weight loss greater than 2% in individuals already showing depletion according to current body weight and height (body-mass index [BMI] $<20 \, kg/m^{(2)}$) or skeletal muscle mass (sarcopenia)."[10] Additionally, the Weight Loss Grading Scale (WLGS) addresses BMI as a modifying factor in assessment of cachexia, organizing patients into higher or lower risk categories for mortality based on weight loss and BMI and has been proposed a provisional criteria for diagnosing cachexia instead of the Fearon criteria.[16]

A strong history and physical exam are essential in the diagnosis of cachexia. Nutritional impact symptoms (NIS) such as nausea, vomiting, diarrhea, constipation, and change in taste or smell may be elicited from a thorough history, while a diligent physical exam may reveal things such as muscle atrophy, prominent in temporal or thenar regions, although these are more obvious in later disease states.[17] It is also important to screen for any reversible endocrine abnormalities (e.g., hypothyroidism, hypogonadism, and adrenal insufficiency) that may be additionally contributing to a patient's presentation. Imaging, including body impedance analysis (BIA), dual-energy X-ray absorptiometry (DEXA), and computerized tomography (CT), can also be helpful in identifying patients at risk of cachexia who may be missed by screening based on purely weight-based criteria (I.E. identifying patients with concomitant sarcopenic levels of muscle). CT specifically is useful in discriminating between muscle and fat content, and several studies have demonstrated an association between decreased muscle mass and survival, therapy tolerance, and physical function.[18,19] However, aside from the aforementioned Fearon criteria, there has not been a concerted effort in the field to merge weight loss criteria with imaging-based measurement of muscle into a combined tool that would be comprehensively useful to identify all patients at risk of muscle wasting.

Serum-based markers also have emerged as a potentially useful tool, leveraging serum inflammatory markers. C-reactive protein (CRP) is known to be commonly elevated in patients with cachexia, although its exact role in mediating the disease process remains unclear. CRP is also part of the modified Glasgow Prognostic Score, which combines it with albumin to assess cachexia severity.[20] However, CRP is not routinely collected in cancer patients in all countries,[21] limiting its utility in the real-world setting. Alternatives that utilize more commonly collected lab markers have emerged, including elevated neutrophil-to-leukocyte ratio (NLR)[22] and prognostic nutritional index (PNI),[23–25] a combination of albumin and lymphocyte count. Both of these markers have been shown to be tightly correlated with cancer outcomes in a variety of cancer populations. Serum markers may play a more significant role in cachexia assessment and diagnosis as our understanding of the pathogenesis evolves; however, as of yet, they are not easily integrated into clinical practice, similar to imaging approaches.

The importance of evaluating function when assessing for cachexia and determining treatment plan cannot be overstated. While often overlooked, function, as distinct from strength and physical activity, may be a major indicator of QoL. While strength is defined as force against resistance and physical activity as body movement by muscle expenditure, function is the ability to perform ADLs.[26,27] Often used as a proxy for one another, it is important to keep these differences in mind when assessing for cachexia. Independence with ADLs is consistently linked to increased QoL, which is a major contributor to treatment adherence and success.[28–30] A complete assessment of cachexia should, therefore, still address functional independence as it relates to ADLs.

Current patient-reported outcome assessments of function used in cachexia include the validated functional assessment of anorexia–cachexia therapy (FAACT) scale and functional assessment of cancer therapy general (FACT G) scale, which together assess QoL with relation to physical, social, emotional, and functional domains, but fail to provide details with respect to functional independent with specific tasks, making these scales less actionable.[31,32] The Short Form Health Survey (SF-36) and European Organization for the Treatment and Research of Cancer Quality of Life Questionnaire (EORTC QLQ-C30) both offer more specifics on functional independence.[33,34] In HNC specifically, the Patient-Reported Outcomes Measure Information System (PROMIS), with domains of fatigue, physical functioning, sleep disturbance, sleep-related impairment, and negative perceived cognitive function, has been shown to be a reasonable QoL measure and correlate with other HNC measures such as EORTC head and neck measures, and Voice Handicap Index (VHI-10).[35] The most detailed, but potentially burdensome, validated patient-reported outcome (PRO) scale is the Cancer Rehabilitation Evaluation Scale (CARES), which addresses not only specifics with respect to ADLs and mobility, but also sexual function.[36]

In addition to the aforementioned PROs, objective assessments of physical performance are often employed as screening tools to correlate with health, morbidity, and mortality during cachexia such as grip strength (GS), the 6-min walk test (6MWT), 30 s sit to stand (30STS), and the timed-up-and-go test (TUG).[37–39] While GS is perhaps the most widely cited in cancer cachexia, its use as an outcome to track functional independence is not recommended as it does not address specific functional change.[40,41] The others, while limited in detail about specific tasks, may be better suited to address multiple domains of functional ability. Table 6.1 illustrates current patient-reported and clinical outcome assessments of function that can be used in cachexia that covers multiple functional domains.

Many of the aforementioned measures take into account one aspect or another of the signs, symptoms, and markers for cachexia assessment, but are not comprehensive. The cachexia score (CASCO) is the only validated cachexia-specific screening tool to stage patients and is the most comprehensive, taking into account body weight loss and composition, inflammation/metabolic disturbances/immunosuppression, physical performance, anorexia, and QoL.[42] However, it is long and burdensome to administer, and thus is not often used in clinical practice.

The multitude of instruments mentioned before, each with its own limitations and complications, points to the lack of a clear, systemic approach when assessing cachexia. As a matter of practicality, it is perhaps best for the clinician to focus instead in a tiered manner. Weight-based measures, blood-based, radiological, and physical performance tests should likely be performed for screening purposes to best identify patients at risk of cachexia. Then, in those at high risk, a thorough history including NIS and functional assessments, with a graduated approach focusing firstly on ADLs followed by mobility and exercise tolerance, can be performed.[17] This can then be followed by objective assessments including a detailed neurologic and musculoskeletal exam before developing a targeted treatment plan.

Treatment

Currently, there is no standard of care or Food and Drug Administration (FDA)—approved treatment of cachexia. A multifaceted approach to treatment, in concert with the approach to aforementioned diagnosis, is recommended including nutritional optimization, pharmacologic action against NIS, and preservation/optimization of physical function.[43–46]

Though nutrition alone cannot reverse cachexia, it remains a cornerstone of cachexia treatment and is addressed in the nutrition chapter in this book. The clinician should also aim to reduce NIS to optimize nutritional intake and decrease symptom burden. Glucocorticoids and mineralocorticoids have been used mainly in the palliative, end-of-life setting for goals-of-care oriented appetite stimulation, increasing food intake, and nausea control but come at a cost of hypothalamic—pituitary—adrenal (HPA) axis suppression, delirium, osteoporosis, and proximal muscle weakness, making them less fit for a larger subset of cachexia patients.[47] Orexigenic drugs, such as dronabinol and mirtazapine, have also been used to stimulate appetite and ease nausea and early satiety in patients undergoing chemotherapy but still lack strong evidence to support their benefit.[47] Megestrol acetate (MA) is often used as an off-label appetite stimulant in cachexia. However, benefits with MA are not well demonstrated, as it may only lead to fat gain, not muscle gain, and at high doses in advanced cancers has, it paradoxically resulted in weight loss, as well as thromboembolism and edema.[48] Most recently, olanzapine, which

Table 6.1 Patient-reported and physical performance–based assessment tools of function used in cachexia that cover multiple function related domains.

Assessment tool	Type	Mobility	ADLs and iADLs	Strength	Exercise tolerance	Sexual function	QoL
FAACT + FACT G[31]	PRO						X
EORTC QLQ-C30[34]	PRO					X	X
PROMIS-Physical Function[35]	PRO	X	X		X		
CARES[36]	PRO	X	X				
6MWT[38]	Performance	X					
30STS[39]	Performance	X		X			
TUG[39]	Performance	X					

is already in use for treatment of chemotherapy-related nausea, has now been recommended by the American Society of Clinical Oncology (ASCO) as a first-line agent for treating poor appetite.[49] Anamorelin, a ghrelin receptor agonist, shows early promise with phase II and III trials demonstrating an increase in body weight and has been approved for use in Japan[50]; however, no effect has been noted with respect to physical function or long-term survival.[51] Constipation, despite being the second most common NIS (behind taste and smell alterations), is often overlooked by clinicians.[52] In one HNC study examining NIS, constipation was cited by 10% of participants as relating to reduced oral nutritional intake.[53] Multimodal, aggressive management and prevention of constipation through the use of stool softeners, promotility agents, enemas, and suppositories should not be neglected.

The role of antiinflammatories such as NSAIDs remains unclear. Some reviews point to a potential benefit in cachexia,[54] although there is not yet enough data to support this recommendation, possibly due to its known negative impacts on muscle health in the noncancer population.[55] More targeted drugs, such as the IL-6 inhibiting monoclonal antibodies clazakizumab and tocilizumab, have also shown potential benefit with respect to performance scores and symptom burden in patients with elevated IL-6 in small studies, but further investigation is needed to determine benefit in broader populations, including HNC.[56–58]

Patients with HNC are particularly susceptible to chemotherapy- and radiation-induced exacerbation of xerostomia, one of the principal detriments to QoL in this population, resulting in poor oral intake and decreased energy levels.[59] Treatment of these has largely been limited to salivary substitutes, which only provide short-term relief at best. Pharmacology approaches to treating xerostomia, including pilocarpine and amifostine, have shown mixed efficacy due to substantial side effects.[59] As a result, there has been a shift toward more preventative approaches, including gland transfers during surgery and radiation sparing techniques.[59]

When combined with the pharmacologic side effects discussed before, there exists significant risk of barriers to function and preservation of QoL, which may lead to poor treatment outcomes. These issues serve to highlight cachexia as a complex process that will not likely be solved by pharmacologic intervention alone.

While commonly used approaches in rehabilitation medicine have not yet been implemented across cancer specialties, some form of customized rehabilitation programs should be considered to prevent functional decline in cachexic patients. Exercise enhances the drive for protein synthesis and decreases insulin resistance, preventing muscle degradation.[60] While the preservation of muscle is good, the preservation of functional muscle is best. Cochrane reviews for exercise treatment have revealed exercise to be safe and decrease symptom burden, although the majority of the studies available have been small, making it difficult to determine exact exercise prescriptions for cachexia.[61] The distinction between rehabilitation, a patient and task-specific intervention focusing on ADLs and mobility, and exercise with its focus on increasing strength or endurance is often lost in clinical approaches to cachexia. Targeted muscle group resistance exercises, as opposed to aerobic training, have shown positive results for mobility and ADLs by PRO

Table 6.2 Summary of interventions for HNC patients with cachexia.[17]

Domains	Interventions
Functional autonomy	Occupational and physical therapist evaluation; evaluation for assistive devices; evaluation for caregiver services
Functional mobility	Physical or exercise therapist evaluation; evaluation for assistive devices; prescription of exercise program (resistance exercise); walking program
Social status	Social worker referral; assistance for economic or social needs; consideration for home health services; consideration for transportation aid
Nutritional status	Evaluation of nutritional intake symptoms; monitoring weight; dietitian consultation; consideration for speech–language therapist; education on diet and nutrition; elimination of medications with exacerbating side effects; consideration of pharmacologic symptom management
Cognitive status	Psychiatry and psychologic oncology referral; optimization of medications; written instructions for medication and appointments; shared information with health care proxy
Comorbidity	Coordination with primary care physician, oncology, or palliative care; review of medications; elimination

measures.[62,63] In HNC specifically, exercise-based rehabilitation programs have shown improvement in QoL.[64]

The importance of a multimodal approach when implementing cachexia patient-specific targeted therapies cannot be understated. Table 6.2 illustrates possible interventions for different domains impacted by cachexia in HNC patients. Further study is required to create a more standardized approach to cachexia-specific rehabilitation interventions, but a shift away from the perception of cachexia as a disease of malnutrition and toward its identity as a destroyer of functional independence is needed for that to happen. In the meantime, the clinician has several tools at their disposal to employ patient-specific, targeted interventions driven by stepwise analysis of the most clinically significant deficits in function.

Sarcopenia

Like cachexia, sarcopenia is a type of muscle wasting disorder. However, unlike cachexia that is mediated by chronic illness, sarcopenia is primarily associated with aging. Sarcopenia is characterized primarily by the loss of lean muscle mass and function, as well as strength. While muscle mass loss is commonly seen in cachexia, most sarcopenic individuals are not cachectic.[65] However, despite the differences between these two conditions, in reality, they can overlap and are often characterized in the literature together. For example, in the HNC population, the prevalence of malnutrition is reported to be 50%−70%.[65] Sarcopenia alone is quite common in those with HNC, but with considerable variability in the prevalence, which has been reported to be between 16% and 71%.[65] A major reason for this variability in reporting is likely inconsistent application of the accepted clinical criteria for sarcopenia.

Within the cancer population as a whole, tumor site is a known major risk factor for malnutrition, with pancreatic, GI, head and neck, and lung cancers with the highest prevalence.[66] Advanced cancer stage has also been linked to higher risk of malnutrition.[66] It is believed that a combination of reduced caloric intake, tumor burden, inflammatory status, and malabsorption all contribute to the development of malnutrition.[66] Among patients with HNC specifically, older age has consistently been identified as a risk factor for developing sarcopenia.[67,68] Both sex and BMI have contradicting data on their use as risk factors, with it reported that people with HNC and sarcopenia were more likely to be women and have higher BMIs[68] and elsewhere the opposite was found.[67]

The presence of sarcopenia has been linked to poorer outcomes in patients with HNC. For example, cisplatin toxicity is higher in those with low skeletal muscle mass and can limit dosing.[69–71] There are also higher rates of radiation toxicity (including mucositis, dysphagia, and xerostomia), more surgical complications, shorter disease-free intervals, longer postoperative hospital stays, and worse disease-specific survival and all-cause mortality in HNC patients with sarcopenia. [68–71] The detection of sarcopenia then becomes important as once a patient has been identified as having the condition, their healthcare team can risk stratify them and adjust their treatment plan as appropriate.

Diagnosis

Sarcopenia has several proposed mechanisms, including age-induced anabolic resistance, decreased physical activity, low-grade chronic inflammation, inadequate protein intake, longer term inactivity, and change in neuromuscular function.[72–75] Likely, it is a combination of several factors that contributes to the development of sarcopenia in the elderly population. In clinical medicine, this term is often applied as a general descriptor of the process that can occur in geriatric patients. Historically, sarcopenia is consistently defined as having low skeletal muscle mass,[69,70,76,77] with the most common methodology being the use of an MRI or CT scan at the C3 or L3 level to measure the cross-sectional skeletal muscle mass. It is important to note that the use of BMI alone is not considered sufficient for ruling out sarcopenia, since this can miss the loss of muscle mass despite obesity. Other methodologies for diagnosing sarcopenia have been suggested and compared to this standard, including the development of the sarcopenia index (SI), which consists of the ratio of creatinine to cystatin C.[78] The SI was shown to predict overall survival, and had a linear correlation when compared with the gold standard mentioned before, the measurement of skeletal muscle mass on MRI or CT.

Despite the strong history of diagnosing sarcopenia based solely on low muscle mass, there is an ongoing effort to begin to include physical strength criteria as well when screening for this condition. This approach takes into account the functional deficits that can occur when a patient becomes sarcopenic. The European Working Group on Sarcopenia in Older People and the Asian Working Group for Sarcopenia both released definitions that now include a focus on skeletal muscle function, particularly strength.[79–81] This distinction is important because it highlights that muscle loss causes activity intolerance and, in turn, a worsened QoL. It has been shown that QoL in aging is positively associated with performance on several functional tests, including the 400m walk, 4m walk, narrow walk, VO2 peak, stair climb, and chair stand tests[82] (Box 6.1). Key measurements of muscle strength and physical performance when diagnosing sarcopenia are now more consistently including grip strength and walking speed/distance.[79–81]

As mentioned before, previously a large majority of the literature on the diagnosis of sarcopenia in both HNC and cancer overall focused solely on the measurement of muscle mass alone. Since these studies did not examine muscle strength or function, it is unlikely that they were actually describing the current concept of sarcopenia. Rather, instead they were describing an overlap of two populations of patients: those with cancer who have true sarcopenia, or what could also be considered "primary sarcopenia," and those who have a secondary sarcopenia due to cancer. This "secondary sarcopenia" would meet criteria to be biologically defined as cachexia, since it describes a loss of muscle mass due to a disease state. Moving forward, future research should include functional measurements to only capture the population with true sarcopenia.

This shift in diagnostic criteria is apparent in emerging literature, which demonstrates a push to start including performance on functional tasks, including walking distance and grip strength.[79] This inclusion of the loss of functional muscle strength when defining and diagnosing sarcopenia also allows clinicians to shift the metrics of success when treating sarcopenia to focus on the recovery of function rather than the recovery of muscle mass alone—a distinction that often aligns with patients' priorities as well.

Box 6.1 Physical performance factors affected by sarcopenia[82]

- 400-meter walk
- 4-meter walk
- Narrow walk
- VO$_2$ peak
- Stair climb
- Chair stand
- Grip strength
- Walking speed and distance

Treatment

The treatment of sarcopenia is becoming increasingly important, especially since the aging population is rapidly expanding as people are living longer. Sarcopenia has been found to contribute to increased hospitalizations and disability, and is thought to be tied to the risk of falls and its associated comorbidities, including fractures and mortality.[2] It is therefore important for clinicians to not only identify those with sarcopenia, but also implement appropriate treatment regimens.

When determining treatment options for sarcopenia, one might assume that a higher caloric intake is better and therefore feeding tube placement should be highly considered as a treatment option since this would allow for improved, consistent nutrition. However, it has been shown that while personalized nutritional counseling is associated with higher QoL, the benefits after feeding tube placement on QoL are less consistent.[83] It is therefore important to instead focus on each patient, and tailor recommendations on how diet can be improved to each individual's needs. For this, referrals to a registered dietician might be beneficial.

However, exercise is also a key lifestyle change and might be even more important than nutrition when treating sarcopenia. One systematic review of randomized controlled trials found variable effects of nutrition alone on muscle mass, strength, and gait speed, while exercise alone was found to effectively increase gait speed and skeletal muscle mass.[80] Notably though, the benefits of individualized nutrition interventions and exercise on the recovery of function both might be potentiated if implemented together. Prior research has shown that exercise and appropriate nutrition together can improve muscle strength and function, with variable effects seen on muscle mass.[81]

When considering what type of exercise is best, resistance exercises have been suggested as first-line treatment for sarcopenia in elderly individuals. Prior studies have outlined specific regimens, with recommendations including multiple workout sessions per week with combinations of upper and lower body exercises, grouped into 1−3 sets of 6−12 repetitions for participants to cycle through with high effort expended during each set.[84]

It is worth mentioning also that while the mainstays of sarcopenia treatment focus on lifestyle interventions, there is some literature on the use of medications. However, this has not been shown to have as robust or promising a role as either nutrition or exercise. Further, there are not currently any medications approved by the FDA for the treatment of sarcopenia. One medication that has been studied is selective androgen receptor modulators, which have been shown to be effective in increasing muscle mass but not improving strength or function.[80] Additionally, growth hormone, steroids, angiotensin-converting enzyme inhibitors, β-receptor blockers, protein anabolic agents, appetite stimulants, myostatin inhibitors, and troponin activators have been studied also with variable efficacy.[85] Further research is needed to determine if there is a role for medication implementation in the treatment of sarcopenia.

As with cachexia, addressing not only the loss of lean body mass but also the loss of functionality is important to consider in sarcopenia, and a multimodal approach that includes lifestyle interventions, nutritional counseling, and dietary supplements altogether is more likely to be successful in the long run.

Frailty

The concept of frailty has become increasingly recognized as one of the most important issues in healthcare and health outcomes.[86] Approximately 11% of community dwelling adults aged 65 and older have frailty with a range of 4%−60%.[87] As the population continues to age, the burden of frailty may become even greater. As the elderly make up a significant proportion of patients diagnosed with cancer and account for approximately 80% of cancer deaths each year,[88] frailty is of particular importance in cancer. The prevalence of frailty in older adults with cancer is approximately 40%−50%, depending on the patient population and the method used to assess frailty.[89] In the HNC population, the prevalence of frailty has been reported to be 68.6% and 72% for patients referred for radiotherapy with or without chemotherapy.[90,91]

However, defining frailty can be challenging. Several definitions of frailty have been proposed, and one conceptual framework for frailty has been established. Simply put, frailty is "a state of increased vulnerability, resulting from age-associated declines in reserve and function across multiple physiologic systems, such that the ability to cope with every day or acute stressors is compromised." [92] It is a condition marked by a decline in multiple physiologic systems, often in an age-related fashion (although not exclusively), and has been described as both a predisability state and coexisting with, although decidedly distinct from, disability and chronic disease.[92,93] Both cancer itself and the therapies offered can be significant additional stressors that challenge a patient's physiologic reserve. Frailty may also be considered the result of an accumulation of age-related deficits on a spectrum from fit to frail.[94] Although frailty is typically associated with advanced age, it is important to understand that younger patients outside the geriatric population can have frailty as well. This is particularly true for patients with cancer, in whom the disease itself, and not necessarily age, may be responsible for the most significant or only declines in physiologic reserve. The concepts of frailty, sarcopenia, and cachexia are often conflated when they are distinct conditions that can exist simultaneously. In fact, frailty can be a consequence of sarcopenia or cachexia or both. Sarcopenia and cachexia are discussed further in this chapter. Similarly, in older patients with cancer, comorbidity (i.e., the burden of chronic illness), disability (i.e., the loss of function and autonomy), and frailty often coexist.[95]

The importance of frailty as a concept in cancer cannot be understated. In general, people with frailty have an increased likelihood of unmet care needs, falls and fractures, hospitalizations, lowered QoL, iatrogenic complications, and early mortality.[92,96] In the cancer population, frailty has been identified as a predictor of postoperative complications, chemotherapy intolerance, disease progression, and death.[95] Frailty may pose competing risks of morbidity and mortality independent of cancer and its treatment. Thus, the identification of frailty is important in the treatment planning phase of therapy. Efforts have been made to determine a patient's individual degree of frailty before the start of cancer therapy and to use this information to adjust the oncological treatment.[97,98] Once frailty has been identified in cancer patients, treating physicians have changed treatments[99] and have prescribed interventions for a large percentage of patients.[100]

Assessment

The fundamental goal of frailty assessment in patients with cancer is to protect them from both general and oncology-specific adverse health outcomes (Table 6.3).[101]

To this end, international and national oncologic medical societies alike (e.g., the International Society of Geriatric Oncology [SIOG] and ASCO) have developed detailed recommendations for the assessment of frailty in older adults prior to the initiation of cancer therapy.[102,103] Most societal recommendations posit that frailty assessment in patients with cancer should start with a quick screening to identify those patients who are presumably vulnerable and could benefit from a comprehensive assessment. Practical recommendations on the assessment of frailty in older patients with cancer are based on clinical studies examining whether an assessment was able to predict the occurrence or reduced the incidence of such outcomes. [102,103]

Table 6.3 General and oncology-specific adverse health outcomes related to frailty.[101]

General frailty outcomes	Oncologic-specific frailty outcomes (by treatment)
Early death Hospital admission Nursing home admission Falls Delirium Exacerbation/progression of chronic diseases Onset of acute illness Adverse drug reactions Unmet care needs	Chemotherapy • Increased drug toxicity • Unplanned treatment interruption • Premature treatment discontinuation • Drug–drug interactions • Unplanned hospitalization Radiation therapy • Increased toxicity • Unplanned treatment interruption • Premature treatment discontinuation • Unplanned hospitalization Surgery • Prolonged immobilization • Postoperative nutritional problems • Postoperative delirium or depression • Postoperative wound healing disorders • Postoperative bleeding disorders • Delayed recovery • Postoperative infection

Table 6.4 Fried Frailty Phenotype.[92]

Unintentional weight loss	10 pound weight loss in past year
Hand grip strength weakness	Grip strength in lowest 20% based on sex and body mass index
Diminished walking speed	Time it takes to walk 15 feet at normal speed
Exhaustion	Self-reported exhaustion, fatigue, and/or loss of motivation
Decreased physical activity level	Kilocalories of expenditure based on self-reported physical activities

Historically, there are two approaches to the assessment of frailty. One is the Fried Frailty Phenotype, which defines the condition as the presence of three or more of the following indicators: unintentional weight loss, hand grip strength weakness, diminished walking speed, self-reported exhaustion, and decreased physical activity level (Table 6.4).[92]

The second approach, termed the Rockwood Frailty Index, classifies frailty as the accumulation of age-related deficits.[94] Deficit items include various diseases, signs from clinical examinations, and impairments of ADLs. The index is calculated by dividing the number of deficits diagnosed by the total number of 70 predefined deficits. With the 70-item model, an index of 0.25 or more may indicate frailty. In contrast to the Fried Frailty Phenotype, the deficit-accumulation model not only determines whether frailty is present or not but also quantifies the extent of frailty in a patient in the form of the index value. However, the burden of calculating the 70-item index may be too cumbersome for routine use.[95,101] Furthermore, in the cancer context, a minority of studies have used Fried Frailty Phenotype or the Rockwood Frailty Index to identify and measure frailty in older cancer patients.[89,95]

While more than 70 screening tools exist to identify or measure frailty, and only a few of which have been validated, several have been utilized in the cancer context. SIOG and ASCO recommend initial screening for frailty in older cancer patients using the Geriatrics 8 (G8) screening tool or the Vulnerability Elders Survey-13 (VES-13).[102,103] The G8 screening tool is a self-administered survey that consists of eight items: one item for age and seven items assessing nutritional status, motor skills, psychological status, number of medications, and self-perception of health.[104] A G8 screening score ≤ 14 identities patients with possibly increased vulnerability and should prompt a more comprehensive assessment. In the largest prospective multicenter cohort study evaluating the diagnostic accuracy of screening tools in geriatric oncology, the G8 questionnaire was validated as a means of selecting patients for CGA and for prognosticating 1-year survival. On subgroup analysis of HNC patients, the G8 was found to have a sensitivity of 94.1% and specificity of 83.3% (positive predictive value of 98.5%, negative predictive value of 55.6%) for determining frailty in this cohort.[105] In HNC patients ≥ 65 years old who underwent surgery, G8 scores of 15 or less were indicative of frailty and correlated with severe postoperative complications.[106] Recently, the G8 screening tool has been validated as a screening tool to identify frail patients in HNC patients <70 years old.[107] The VES-13 is a self-administered survey that consists of 13 items: 1 item for age and 12 items assessing health, functional capacity, and physical performance.[108] Scores greater than 3 are associated with frailty. It should be noted that G8 has a high sensitivity albeit lower specificity; whereas, VES-13 has lower sensitivity but higher specificity than G8.[90,109]

For cancer patients ages ≥65–70 years who were identified as presumably vulnerable by prior frailty screening, SIOG and ASCO strongly recommend to perform the comprehensive Geriatric Assessment (GA).[102,103] The GA is considered the gold standard in identifying frailty in elderly patients. ASCO recommendations for frailty screening specifically refer to the subset of cancer patients receiving chemotherapy,[103] whereas SIOG just refers to patients aged 70 or greater.[102] GA is a multidimensional and multidisciplinary assessment to identify and manage vulnerabilities in elderly patients. According to SIOG, the domains of a GA should include physical function including instrumental activities of daily living (IADLs), ADLs, mobility, social status and support, nutrition, cognition, mood, comorbidity, and polypharmacy.[102] To decrease both assessor and respondent burden in the GA, a modified GA called the Cancer-Specific Geriatric Assessment is a brief and more focused tool that combines both self-administered and in-office assisted assessments.[110] Frailty assessed by preoperative CGA, but not chronological age, was significantly associated with major postoperative complications in patients aged ≥70 who underwent elective cancer surgery.[111] A number of retrospective and prospective, noncomparative and comparative GA studies in older patients with cancer have indicated that GA uncovers geriatric impairments, predicts treatment tolerability and feasibility, predicts (all-cause) mortality, facilitates communication about treatment goals and preferences, results in changes of oncological treatment plans, and enables targeted treatment of geriatric impairments in older cancer patients.[101]

In the interest of identifying frailty in patients, biomarkers of frailty have attempted to be identified. A comprehensive review has highlighted multiple physiologic processes associated with frailty including structural and functional brain changes; endocrine dysregulation due to changes in growth hormones, thyroid hormones, adrenocorticoids, and estradiol- and testosterone-related hormones; and dysregulation of carbohydrate metabolism, insulin signaling, and vitamin D metabolism hormones related to energy metabolism (e.g., adiponectin, leptin).[112] Similar to sarcopenia and cachexia, as defined elsewhere in this chapter, there is evidence that a state of mild chronic inflammation may serve as a biomarker of frailty. As summarized by Zampino, Ferrucci, and Semba (2020), numerous studies have reported that elevated inflammatory markers and white blood cells are associated with adverse events, age-related diseases, disability, and all-cause mortality in the elderly.

Managing frailty

Following the initial frailty assessment at the start of a cancer therapy, the overall frailty level may undergo changes during treatment and throughout a patient's further life. Over time, alterations to factors associated with frailty including social situation, physical and mental functionality, and comorbidities may occur.

Observations from studies suggest that both deterioration and improvements are possible.[113,114] However, the currently available recommendations by SIOG and ASCO on frailty assessment in older cancer patients do not advise on how to monitor this condition during or after cancer treatment.[102,103]

Once a patient has been clinically diagnosed with frailty, treatment goals center around improving the current deficits and preventing onset of new ones.[101] As the GA is the gold standard for identification of frailty, many studies have evaluated the delivery of GA-directed interventions for frailty. Four pivotal randomized-controlled trials (RCTs) have found that GA-directed management of vulnerabilities is able to reduce the risk of these patients to experience toxicity or premature discontinuation of systemic cancer treatment.[113,115–117] Table 6.5 illustrates specific

Table 6.5 Interventions targeting vulnerabilities in adults with cancer in randomized-controlled trials.[100,113,115–117]

Domains	Vulnerabilities	Interventions
Functional autonomy	Impairment of IADL Impairment of ADL	Occupational therapist and physical therapist evaluation; evaluation for assistive devices; evaluation for caregiver services
Functional mobility	Decreased gait speed Falls Weakness	Physical therapist evaluation; evaluation for assistive devices; prescription of exercise program; evaluation of iatrogenic causes (medications)
Social status	Loneliness Poverty	Social worker referral; assistance for economic or social needs; consideration for home health services; consideration for transportation aid; consideration for health care proxy
Nutritional status	Swallowing problems Digestion problems Low food or oral intake	Dietitian consultation; consideration for speech-language therapist; education on diet and nutrition
Cognitive status	Mild cognitive impairment	Psychiatry referral; optimization of medications; written instructions for medication and appointments; shared information with health care proxy
Emotional status	Depression Anxiety	Psychologist referral; spiritual services referral; local support groups; optimization of medications
Comorbidity	Coexisting chronic disease	Coordination with primary care physician, geriatrician; review of medications
Polypharmacy	High number of drugs Drug–drug interaction	Pharmacist referral; pill box; communication with primary care physician; education on polypharmacy

interventions aimed at assessed vulnerabilities by the GA as demonstrated in the aforementioned RCTs. For a large percentage of cancer patients identified with frailty, treating physicians do prescribe interventions, the most common being allied health support to address deficiencies of social support, polypharmacy, and nutrition.[100]

Much of the general literature on frailty in cancer may be applicable to the elderly HNC patient. Due to the location of tumors in the upper aerodigestive tract, patients with HNC are uniquely vulnerable to dysphagia and malnutrition due to the physical effects of tumors and subsequently to treatment effects of radiotherapy and/ or chemotherapy. In patients referred for radiotherapy with or without chemotherapy for HNC, the most commonly deficient domains assessed by the GA were those of comorbidity (77%−84.3%) and malnutrition (48.0%−49.0%).[90,91] Vulnerabilities in nutritional status are addressed elsewhere in this book.

Summary

Muscle wasting and frailty are major factors in the overall health and well-being of individuals with HNC. In addition, these conditions play a direct role in the progression of disease and response to treatment. Thus, addressing these conditions is crucial to achieving improved cancer and health outcomes. Approaches to diagnosis and assessment cachexia, sarcopenia, and frailty are still evolving and have significant overlap. While frailty focuses fundamentally on the impact of muscle wasting and deficit accumulation, cachexia and sarcopenia allude to distinct biological mechanisms that both lead to muscle loss and functional loss. Thus, clinicians should be aware of the limitations of screening approaches to identifying patients with these conditions and how they relate to both current treatment guidelines and emerging strategies more closely tied to specific biology. Nevertheless, it is clear that a multimodal approach is necessary to addressing muscle wasting and frailty, and should include comprehensive rehabilitation services, improved nutrition, medical/pharmacologic care directed at associated symptoms, psychological care, and broader social assistance.

References

1. Baracos VE, Martin L, Korc M, Guttridge DC, Fearon KCH. Cancer-associated cachexia. *Nat Rev Dis Primers*. 2018;4(1):17105. https://doi.org/10.1038/nrdp. 2017.105.
2. Morley JE, Anker SD, von Haehling S. Prevalence, incidence, and clinical impact of sarcopenia: facts, numbers, and epidemiology-update 2014. *J Cachexia Sarcopenia Muscle*. 2014;5(4):253−259. https://doi.org/10.1007/s13539-014-0161-y.
3. Naito T. Evaluation of the true endpoint of clinical trials for cancer cachexia. *Asia-Pac J Oncol Nurs*. 2019;6:227−233. https://doi.org/10.4103/apjon.apjon_68_18.

4. Jager-Wittenaar H, Dijkstra PU, Dijkstra G, et al. High prevalence of cachexia in newly diagnosed head and neck cancer patients: an exploratory study. *Nutrition*. 2017;35: 114—118. https://doi.org/10.1016/j.nut.2016.11.008.

5. Muthanandam S, Muthu J. Understanding cachexia in head and neck cancer. *Asia Pac J Oncol Nurs*. 2021;8(5):527—538. https://doi.org/10.4103/apjon.apjon-2145.

6. Garcia JM, Garcia-Touza M, Hijazi RA, et al. Active ghrelin levels and active to total ghrelin ratio in cancer-induced cachexia. *J Clin Endocrinol Metab*. 2005;90(5): 2920—2926. https://doi.org/10.1210/jc.2004-1788.

7. Patel S, Alvarez-Guaita A, Melvin A, et al. GDF15 provides an endocrine signal of nutritional stress in mice and humans. *Cell Metab*. 2019;29(3):707—718.e8. https://doi.org/10.1016/J.CMET.2018.12.016.

8. Suriben R, Chen M, Higbee J, et al. Antibody-mediated inhibition of GDF15—GFRAL activity reverses cancer cachexia in mice. *Nat Med*. 2020;26(8):1264—1270. https://doi.org/10.1038/s41591-020-0945-x.

9. Richey LM, George JR, Couch ME, et al. Defining cancer cachexia in head and neck squamous cell carcinoma. *Clin Cancer Res*. 2007;13(22 Pt 1):6561—6567. https://doi.org/10.1158/1078-0432.CCR-07-0116.

10. Fearon K, Strasser F, Anker SD, et al. Definition and classification of cancer cachexia: an international consensus. *Lancet Oncol*. 2011;12(5):489—495. https://doi.org/10.1016/S1470-2045(10)70218-7.

11. von Haehling S, Anker MS, Anker SD. Prevalence and clinical impact of cachexia in chronic illness in Europe, USA, and Japan: facts and numbers update 2016. *J Cachexia Sarcopenia Muscle*. 2016;7(5):507—509. https://doi.org/10.1002/jcsm.12167.

12. Brookes GB. Nutritional status–a prognostic indicator in head and neck cancer. *Otolaryngol Head Neck Surg*. 1985;93(1):69—74. https://doi.org/10.1177/019459988509300114.

13. Roy I, Huang K, Bhakta A, Marquez E, Spangenberg J, Jayabalan P. Relationship between cachexia and the functional progress of patients with cancer in inpatient rehabilitation. *Am J Phys Med Rehabil*. 2023;102(2):99—104. https://doi.org/10.1097/PHM.0000000000002024.

14. Schmidt SF, Rohm M, Herzig S, Berriel Diaz M. Cancer cachexia: more than skeletal muscle wasting. *Trends Cancer*. 2018;4(12):849—860. https://doi.org/10.1016/j.trecan.2018.10.001.

15. Gingrich A, Volkert D, Kiesswetter E, et al. Prevalence and overlap of sarcopenia, frailty, cachexia and malnutrition in older medical inpatients. *BMC Geriatr*. 2019; 19(1):1—10. https://doi.org/10.1186/s12877-019-1115-1.

16. Martin L, Senesse P, Gioulbasanis I, et al. Diagnostic criteria for the classification of cancer-associated weight loss. *J Clin Oncol*. 2015;33(1):90—99. https://doi.org/10.1200/JCO.2014.56.1894.

17. Fram J, Vail C, Roy I. Assessment of cancer-associated cachexia — how to approach physical function evaluation. *Curr Oncol Rep*. 2022;24(6):751—761. https://doi.org/10.1007/s11912-022-01258-4.

18. Martin L, Birdsell L, MacDonald N, et al. Cancer cachexia in the age of obesity: skeletal muscle depletion is a powerful prognostic factor, independent of body mass index. *J Clin Oncol*. 2013;31(12):1539—1547. https://doi.org/10.1200/JCO.2012.45.2722.

19. Roeland EJ, Phull H, Hagmann C, et al. FIT: functional and imaging testing for patients with metastatic cancer. *Support Care Cancer.* 2020;29(5):2771−2775. https://doi.org/10.1007/S00520-020-05730-4.

20. Silva GA da, Wiegert EVM, Calixto-Lima L, Oliveira LC. Clinical utility of the modified glasgow prognostic score to classify cachexia in patients with advanced cancer in palliative care. *Clin Nutr.* 2020;39(5):1587−1592. https://doi.org/10.1016/j.clnu.2019.07.002.

21. Dolan RD, McSorley ST, Horgan PG, Laird B, McMillan DC. The role of the systemic inflammatory response in predicting outcomes in patients with advanced inoperable cancer: systematic review and meta -analysis. *Crit Rev Oncol Hematol.* 2017;116:134−146. https://doi.org/10.1016/j.critrevonc.2017.06.002.

22. Barker T, Fulde G, Moulton B, Nadauld LD, Rhodes T. An elevated neutrophil-to-lymphocyte ratio associates with weight loss and cachexia in cancer. *Sci Rep.* 2020;10(1):7535. https://doi.org/10.1038/s41598-020-64282-z.

23. Go SI, Park S, Kang MH, Kim HG, Kim HR, Lee GW. Clinical impact of prognostic nutritional index in diffuse large B cell lymphoma. *Ann Hematol.* 2019;98(2):401−411. https://doi.org/10.1007/s00277-018-3540-1.

24. Nozoe T, Ninomiya M, Maeda T, Matsukuma A, Nakashima H, Ezaki T. Prognostic nutritional index: a tool to predict the biological aggressiveness of gastric carcinoma. *Surg Today.* 2010;40(5):440−443. https://doi.org/10.1007/S00595-009-4065-Y.

25. Ding JD, Yao K, Wang PF, Yan CX. Clinical significance of prognostic nutritional index in patients with glioblastomas. *Medicine.* 2018;97(48):e13218. https://doi.org/10.1097/MD.0000000000013218.

26. Katz S. Assessing self-maintenance: activities of daily living, mobility, and instrumental activities of daily living. *J Am Geriatr Soc.* 1983;31(12):721−727. https://doi.org/10.1111/j.1532-5415.1983.tb03391.x.

27. Lieber R. *Skeletal Muscle Structure, Function, and Plasticity the Physiological Basis of Rehabilitation.* 2010.

28. Viganó A, Bruera E, Jhangri GS, Newman SC, Fields AL, Suarez-Almazor ME. Clinical survival predictors in patients with advanced cancer. *Arch Intern Med.* 2000;160(6):861−868. https://doi.org/10.1001/archinte.160.6.861.

29. Cheville AL, Alberts SR, Rummans TA, et al. Improving adherence to cancer treatment by addressing quality of life in patients with advanced gastrointestinal cancers. *J Pain Symptom Manag.* 2015;50(3):321−327. https://doi.org/10.1016/j.jpainsymman.2015.03.005.

30. Ezzatvar Y, Ramírez-Vélez R, Sáez de Asteasu ML, et al. Physical function and all-cause mortality in older adults diagnosed with cancer: a systematic review and meta-analysis. *J Gerontol A Biol Sci Med Sci.* 2021;76(8):1447−1453. https://doi.org/10.1093/gerona/glaa305.

31. Meregaglia M, Borsoi L, Cairns J, Tarricone R. Mapping health-related quality of life scores from FACT-G, FAACT, and FACIT-F onto preference-based EQ-5D-5L utilities in non-small cell lung cancer cachexia. *Eur J Health Econ.* 2019;20(2):181−193. https://doi.org/10.1007/s10198-017-0930-6.

32. Blauwhoff-Buskermolen S, Ruijgrok C, Ostelo RW, et al. The assessment of anorexia in patients with cancer: cut-off values for the FAACT−A/CS and the VAS for appetite. *Support Care Cancer.* 2016;24(2):661−666. https://doi.org/10.1007/s00520-015-2826-2.

33. Hill RD, Mansour E, Valentijn S, Jolles J, van Boxtel M. The SF-36 as a precursory measure of adaptive functioning in normal aging: the Maastricht Aging Study. *Aging Clin Exp Res.* 2010;22(5−6):433−439. https://doi.org/10.1007/BF03324943.

34. Wheelwright SJ, Hopkinson JB, Darlington AS, et al. Development of the EORTC QLQ-CAX24, A questionnaire for cancer patients with cachexia. *J Pain Symptom Manag.* 2017;53(2):232−242. https://doi.org/10.1016/J.JPAINSYMMAN.2016.09.010.

35. Stachler RJ, Schultz LR, Nerenz D, Yaremchuk KL. PROMIS evaluation for head and neck cancer patients: a comprehensive quality-of-life outcomes assessment tool. *Laryngoscope.* 2014;124(6):1368−1376. https://doi.org/10.1002/lary.23853.

36. Schag CA, Ganz PA, Heinrich RL. Cancer rehabilitation evaluation system–short form (CARES-SF). A cancer specific rehabilitation and quality of life instrument. *Cancer.* 1991;68(6):1406−1413. https://doi.org/10.1002/1097-0142(19910915)68:6<1406::aid-cncr2820680638>3.0.co;2-2.

37. Song M, Zhang Q, Tang M, et al. Associations of low hand grip strength with 1 year mortality of cancer cachexia: a multicentre observational study. *J Cachexia Sarcopenia Muscle.* 2021. https://doi.org/10.1002/JCSM.12778.

38. Schmidt K, Vogt L, Thiel C, Jäger E, Banzer W. Validity of the six-minute walk test in cancer patients. *Int J Sports Med.* 2013;34(7):631−636. https://doi.org/10.1055/s-0032-1323746.

39. Blair CK, Harding E, Herman C, et al. Remote assessment of functional mobility and strength in older cancer survivors: protocol for a validity and reliability study. *JMIR Res Protoc.* 2020;9(9):e20834. https://doi.org/10.2196/20834.

40. Andrews JS, Gold LS, Reed MJ, et al. Appendicular lean mass, grip strength, and the development of hospital-associated activities of daily living disability among older adults in the health ABC studyLipsitz LA, ed. *J Gerontol: Series A.* 2021;XX:1−7. https://doi.org/10.1093/GERONA/GLAB332.

41. Ramage MI, Skipworth RJE. The relationship between muscle mass and function in cancer cachexia: smoke and mirrors? *Curr Opin Support Palliat Care.* 2018;12(4):439−444. https://doi.org/10.1097/SPC.0000000000000381.

42. Argilés JM, Betancourt A, Guàrdia-Olmos J, et al. Validation of the cachexia SCOre (CASCO). Staging cancer patients: the use of miniCASCO as a simplified tool. *Front Physiol.* 2017;8:92. https://doi.org/10.3389/fphys.2017.00092.

43. Fearon KCH. Cancer cachexia: developing multimodal therapy for a multidimensional problem. *Eur J Cancer.* 2008;44(8):1124−1132. https://doi.org/10.1016/j.ejca.2008.02.033.

44. Maddocks M, Hopkinson J, Conibear J, Reeves A, Shaw C, Fearon KCH. Practical multimodal care for cancer cachexia. *Curr Opin Support Palliat Care.* 2016;10(4):298−305. https://doi.org/10.1097/SPC.0000000000000241.

45. Parmar MP, Vanderbyl BL, Kanbalian M, Windholz TY, Tran AT, Jagoe RT. A multidisciplinary rehabilitation programme for cancer cachexia improves quality of life. *BMJ Support Palliat Care.* 2017;7(4):441−449. https://doi.org/10.1136/bmjspcare-2017-001382.

46. Vaughan VC, Harrison M, Dowd A, Eastman P, Martin P. Evaluation of a multidisciplinary cachexia and nutrition support service— the patient and carers perspective. *J Patient Exp.* 2021;8. https://doi.org/10.1177/2374373520981476.

47. Inui A. Cancer anorexia-cachexia syndrome: current issues in research and management. *CA Cancer J Clin.* 2002;52(2):72−91. https://doi.org/10.3322/canjclin.52.2.72.

48. Lim YL, Teoh SE, Yaow CYL, et al. A systematic review and meta-analysis of the clinical use of megestrol acetate for cancer-related anorexia/cachexia. *J Clin Med.* 2022; 11(13). https://doi.org/10.3390/jcm11133756.

49. Sandhya L, Devi Sreenivasan N, Goenka L, et al. Randomized double-blind placebo-controlled study of olanzapine for chemotherapy-related anorexia in patients with locally advanced or metastatic gastric, hepatopancreaticobiliary, and lung cancer. *J Clin Oncol.* 2023;41(14):2617−2627. https://doi.org/10.1200/JCO.22.01997.

50. Katakami N, Uchino J, Yokoyama T, et al. Anamorelin (ONO-7643) for the treatment of patients with non−small cell lung cancer and cachexia: results from a randomized, double-blind, placebo-controlled, multicenter study of Japanese patients (ONO-7643-04). *Cancer.* 2018;124(3):606−616. https://doi.org/10.1002/cncr.31128.

51. Temel JS, Abernethy AP, Currow DC, et al. Anamorelin in patients with non-small-cell lung cancer and cachexia (ROMANA 1 and ROMANA 2): results from two randomised, double-blind, phase 3 trials. *Lancet Oncol.* 2016;17(4):519−531. https://doi.org/10.1016/S1470-2045(15)00558-6.

52. Omlin A, Blum D, Wierecky J, Haile SR, Ottery FD, Strasser F. Nutrition impact symptoms in advanced cancer patients: frequency and specific interventions, a case-control study. *J Cachexia Sarcopenia Muscle.* 2013;4(1):55−61. https://doi.org/10.1007/s13539-012-0099-x.

53. Kubrak C, Olson K, Jha N, et al. Nutrition impact symptoms: key determinants of reduced dietary intake, weight loss, and reduced functional capacity of patients with head and neck cancer before treatment. *Head Neck.* 2010;32(3):290−300. https://doi.org/10.1002/hed.21174.

54. Christoffersen T. Cancer, cachexia, prostanoids, and NSAIDs. *Acta Oncol.* 2013;52(1): 3−5. https://doi.org/10.3109/0284186X.2012.750429.

55. Lilja M, Mandić M, Apró W, et al. High doses of anti-inflammatory drugs compromise muscle strength and hypertrophic adaptations to resistance training in young adults. *Acta Physiol.* 2018;222(2):e12948. https://doi.org/10.1111/APHA.12948.

56. Paval DR, Patton R, McDonald J, et al. A systematic review examining the relationship between cytokines and cachexia in incurable cancer. *J Cachexia Sarcopenia Muscle.* 2022;13(2):824−838. https://doi.org/10.1002/jcsm.12912.

57. Berti A, Boccalatte F, Sabbadini MG, Dagna L. Assessment of tocilizumab in the treatment of cancer cachexia. *J Clin Oncol.* 2013;31(23):2970. https://doi.org/10.1200/JCO.2012.48.4147.

58. Marceca GP, Londhe P, Calore F. Management of cancer cachexia: attempting to develop new pharmacological agents for new effective therapeutic options. *Front Oncol.* 2020;10:298. https://doi.org/10.3389/fonc.2020.00298.

59. Nathan CAO, Asarkar AA, Entezami P, et al. Current management of xerostomia in head and neck cancer patients. *Am J Otolaryngol.* 2023;44(4):103867. https://doi.org/10.1016/j.amjoto.2023.103867.

60. Zinna EM, Yarasheski KE. Exercise treatment to counteract protein wasting of chronic diseases. *Curr Opin Clin Nutr Metab Care.* 2003;6(1):87−93. https://doi.org/10.1097/00075197-200301000-00013.

61. Grande AJ, Silva V, Maddocks M. Exercise for cancer cachexia in adults: executive summary of a cochrane collaboration systematic review. *J Cachexia Sarcopenia Muscle.* 2015;6(3):208−211. https://doi.org/10.1002/jcsm.12055.

62. Oldervoll LM, Loge JH, Lydersen S, et al. Physical exercise for cancer patients with advanced disease: a randomized controlled trial. *Oncol.* 2011;16(11):1649−1657. https://doi.org/10.1634/theoncologist.2011-0133.

63. Cheville AL, Moynihan T, Herrin J, Loprinzi C, Kroenke K. Effect of collaborative tele-rehabilitation on functional impairment and pain among patients with advanced-stage cancer: a randomized clinical trial. *JAMA Oncol.* 2019;5(5):644. https://doi.org/10.1001/JAMAONCOL.2019.0011.

64. Samuel SR, Maiya AG, Fernandes DJ, et al. Effectiveness of exercise-based rehabilitation on functional capacity and quality of life in head and neck cancer patients receiving chemo-radiotherapy. *Support Care Cancer.* 2019;27(10):3913−3920. https://doi.org/10.1007/s00520-019-04750-z.

65. Powrózek T, Dziwota J, Małecka-Massalska T. Nutritional deficiencies in radiotherapy-treated head and neck cancer patients. *J Clin Med.* 2021;10(4):574. https://doi.org/10.3390/jcm10040574.

66. Bossi P, Delrio P, Mascheroni A, Zanetti M. The spectrum of malnutrition/cachexia/sarcopenia in oncology according to different cancer types and settings: a narrative review. *Nutrients.* 2021;13(6):1980. https://doi.org/10.3390/nu13061980.

67. Liu C, Cheng L, Ye W, Lin L. Risk factors for sarcopenia in patients with head and neck cancer. *Head Neck.* 2024;46(2):346−352. https://doi.org/10.1002/hed.27585.

68. Orzell S, Verhaaren BFJ, Grewal R, et al. Evaluation of sarcopenia in older patients undergoing head and neck cancer surgery. *Laryngoscope.* 2022;132(2):356−363. https://doi.org/10.1002/lary.29782.

69. de Bree R, van Beers MA, Schaeffers AWMA. Sarcopenia and its impact in head and neck cancer treatment. *Curr Opin Otolaryngol Head Neck Surg.* 2022;30(2):87−93. https://doi.org/10.1097/MOO.0000000000000792.

70. Jovanovic N, Chinnery T, Mattonen SA, Palma DA, Doyle PC, Theurer JA. Sarcopenia in head and neck cancer: a scoping review. *PLoS One.* 2022;17(11):e0278135. https://doi.org/10.1371/journal.pone.0278135.

71. Erul E, Guven DC, Onur MR, Yazici G, Aksoy S. Role of sarcopenia on survival and treatment-related toxicity in head and neck cancer: a narrative review of current evidence and future perspectives. *Eur Arch Oto-Rhino-Laryngol.* 2023;280(8):3541−3556. https://doi.org/10.1007/s00405-023-08014-9.

72. Kwon YN, Yoon SS. Sarcopenia: neurological point of view. *J Bone Metab.* 2017;24(2):83. https://doi.org/10.11005/jbm.2017.24.2.83.

73. Ali S, Garcia JM. Sarcopenia, cachexia and aging: diagnosis, mechanisms and therapeutic options - a mini-review. *Gerontology.* 2014;60(4):294−305. https://doi.org/10.1159/000356760.

74. Moreira-Pais A, Ferreira R, Oliveira PA, Duarte JA. Sarcopenia versus cancer cachexia: the muscle wasting continuum in healthy and diseased aging. *Biogerontology.* 2021;22(5):459−477. https://doi.org/10.1007/S10522-021-09932-Z.

75. Nishikawa H, Fukunishi S, Asai A, Yokohama K, Nishiguchi S, Higuchi K. Pathophysiology and mechanisms of primary sarcopenia (Review). *Int J Mol Med.* 2021;48(2):1−8. https://doi.org/10.3892/IJMM.2021.4989/HTML.

76. de Bree R, Meerkerk CDA, Halmos GB, et al. Measurement of sarcopenia in head and neck cancer patients and its association with frailty. *Front Oncol.* 2022;12. https://doi.org/10.3389/fonc.2022.884988.

77. Jogiat UM, Bédard ELR, Sasewich H, et al. Sarcopenia reduces overall survival in unresectable oesophageal cancer: a systematic review and meta-analysis.

J Cachexia Sarcopenia Muscle. 2022;13(6):2630−2636. https://doi.org/10.1002/jcsm.13082.

78. Zheng C, Wang E, Li JS, et al. Serum creatinine/cystatin C ratio as a screening tool for sarcopenia and prognostic indicator for patients with esophageal cancer. *BMC Geriatr.* 2022;22(1):207. https://doi.org/10.1186/s12877-022-02925-8.

79. Sayer AA, Cruz-Jentoft A. Sarcopenia definition, diagnosis and treatment: consensus is growing. *Age Ageing.* 2022;51(10). https://doi.org/10.1093/ageing/afac220.

80. Arai H, Wakabayashi H, Yoshimura Y, Yamada M, Kim H, Harada A. Chapter 4 treatment of sarcopenia. *Geriatr Gerontol Int.* 2018;18(S1):28−44. https://doi.org/10.1111/ggi.13322.

81. Chen LK, Woo J, Assantachai P, et al. Asian working group for sarcopenia: 2019 consensus update on sarcopenia diagnosis and treatment. *J Am Med Dir Assoc.* 2020;21(3):300−307.e2. https://doi.org/10.1016/j.jamda.2019.12.012.

82. Cummings SR, Newman AB, Coen PM, et al. The study of muscle, mobility and aging (SOMMA): a unique cohort study about the cellular biology of aging and age-related loss of mobility. *J Gerontol: Ser A.* 2023;78(11):2083−2093. https://doi.org/10.1093/gerona/glad052.

83. Baxi SS, Schwitzer E, Jones LW. A review of weight loss and sarcopenia in patients with head and neck cancer treated with chemoradiation. *Cancers Head Neck.* 2016;1(1):9. https://doi.org/10.1186/s41199-016-0010-0.

84. Hurst C, Robinson SM, Witham MD, et al. Resistance exercise as a treatment for sarcopenia: prescription and delivery. *Age Ageing.* 2022;51(2). https://doi.org/10.1093/ageing/afac003.

85. Cho MR, Lee S, Song SK. A review of sarcopenia pathophysiology, diagnosis, treatment and future direction. *J Korean Med Sci.* 2022;37(18). https://doi.org/10.3346/jkms.2022.37.e146.

86. Dent E, Martin FC, Bergman H, Woo J, Romero-Ortuno R, Walston JD. Management of frailty: opportunities, challenges, and future directions. *Lancet.* 2019;394(10206):1376−1386. https://doi.org/10.1016/S0140-6736(19)31785-4.

87. Collard RM, Boter H, Schoevers RA, Oude Voshaar RC. Prevalence of frailty in community-dwelling older persons: a systematic review. *J Am Geriatr Soc.* 2012;60(8):1487−1492. https://doi.org/10.1111/j.1532-5415.2012.04054.x.

88. Siegel RL, Miller KD, Jemal A. Cancer statistics, 2017. *CA Cancer J Clin.* 2017;67(1):7−30. https://doi.org/10.3322/caac.21387.

89. Handforth C, Clegg A, Young C, et al. The prevalence and outcomes of frailty in older cancer patients: a systematic review. *Ann Oncol.* 2015;26(6):1091−1101. https://doi.org/10.1093/annonc/mdu540.

90. Pottel L, Boterberg T, Pottel H, et al. Determination of an adequate screening tool for identification of vulnerable elderly head and neck cancer patients treated with radio(-chemo)therapy. *J Geriatr Oncol.* 2012;3(1):24−32. https://doi.org/10.1016/J.JGO.2011.11.006.

91. Pottel L, Lycke M, Boterberg T, et al. Serial comprehensive geriatric assessment in elderly head and neck cancer patients undergoing curative radiotherapy identifies evolution of multidimensional health problems and is indicative of quality of life. *Eur J Cancer Care.* 2014;23(3):401−412. https://doi.org/10.1111/ecc.12179.

92. Fried LP, Tangen CM, Walston J, et al. Frailty in older adults: evidence for a phenotype. *J Gerontol A Biol Sci Med Sci.* 2001;56(3):M146–M157. https://doi.org/10.1093/gerona/56.3.M146.

93. Fried LP, Ferrucci L, Darer J, Williamson JD, Anderson G. Untangling the concepts of disability, frailty, and comorbidity: implications for improved targeting and care. *J Gerontol A Biol Sci Med Sci.* 2004;59(3):M255–M263. https://doi.org/10.1093/gerona/59.3.M255.

94. Mitnitski AB, Mogilner AJ, MacKnight C, Rockwood K. The mortality rate as a function of accumulated deficits in a frailty index. *Mech Ageing Dev.* 2002;123(11): 1457–1460. https://doi.org/10.1016/S0047-6374(02)00082-9.

95. Ethun CG, Bilen MA, Jani AB, Maithel SK, Ogan K, Master VA. Frailty and cancer: implications for oncology surgery, medical oncology, and radiation oncology. *CA Cancer J Clin.* 2017;67(5):362–377. https://doi.org/10.3322/caac.21406.

96. Clegg A, Young J, Iliffe S, Rikkert MO, Rockwood K. Frailty in elderly people. *Lancet.* 2013;381(9868):752–762. https://doi.org/10.1016/S0140-6736(12)62167-9.

97. Extermann M. Integrating a geriatric evaluation in the clinical setting. *Semin Radiat Oncol.* 2012;22(4):272–276. https://doi.org/10.1016/j.semradonc.2012.05.003.

98. Balducci L, Extermann M. Management of the frail person with advanced cancer. *Crit Rev Oncol Hematol.* 2000;33(2):143–148. https://doi.org/10.1016/S1040-8428(99) 00063-3.

99. Kenis C, Bron D, Libert Y, et al. Relevance of a systematic geriatric screening and assessment in older patients with cancer: results of a prospective multicentric study. *Ann Oncol.* 2013;24(5):1306–1312. https://doi.org/10.1093/annonc/mds619.

100. Caillet P, Canoui-Poitrine F, Vouriot J, et al. Comprehensive geriatric assessment in the decision-making process in elderly patients with cancer: ELCAPA study. *J Clin Oncol.* 2011;29(27):3636–3642. https://doi.org/10.1200/JCO.2010.31.0664.

101. Goede V. Frailty and cancer: current perspectives on assessment and monitoring. *Clin Interv Aging.* 2023;18:505–521. https://doi.org/10.2147/CIA.S365494.

102. Wildiers H, Heeren P, Puts M, et al. International society of geriatric oncology consensus on geriatric assessment in older patients with cancer. *J Clin Oncol.* 2014; 32(24):2595–2603. https://doi.org/10.1200/JCO.2013.54.8347.

103. Mohile SG, Dale W, Somerfield MR, et al. Practical assessment and management of vulnerabilities in older patients receiving chemotherapy: ASCO guideline for geriatric oncology. *J Clin Oncol.* 2018;36(22):2326–2347. https://doi.org/10.1200/JCO.2018.78.8687.

104. Bellera CA, Rainfray M, Mathoulin-Pélissier S, et al. Screening older cancer patients: first evaluation of the G-8 geriatric screening tool. *Ann Oncol.* 2012;23(8):2166–2172. https://doi.org/10.1093/annonc/mdr587.

105. Soubeyran P, Bellera C, Goyard J, et al. Screening for vulnerability in older cancer patients: the ONCODAGE prospective multicenter cohort study. *PLoS One.* 2014;9(12): e115060. https://doi.org/10.1371/journal.pone.0115060.

106. Kunz V, Wichmann G, Wald T, et al. Frailty assessed with FRAIL scale and G8 questionnaire predicts severe postoperative complications in patients receiving major head and neck surgery. *J Clin Med.* 2022;11(16):4714. https://doi.org/10.3390/jcm11164714.

107. Bakas AT, Polinder-Bos HA, Streng F, et al. Frailty in non-geriatric patients with head and neck cancer. *Otolaryngol-Head Neck Surg (Tokyo).* 2023;169(5):1215–1224. https://doi.org/10.1002/ohn.388.

108. Saliba D, Elliott M, Rubenstein LZ, et al. The vulnerable elders survey: a tool for iden-tifying vulnerable older people in the community. *J Am Geriatr Soc*. 2001;49(12): 1691−1699. https://doi.org/10.1046/j.1532-5415.2001.49281.x.

109. Garcia MV, Agar MR, Soo WK, To T, Phillips JL. Screening tools for identifying older adults with cancer who may benefit from a geriatric assessment. *JAMA Oncol*. 2021; 7(4):616. https://doi.org/10.1001/jamaoncol.2020.6736.

110. Hurria A, Gupta S, Zauderer M, et al. Developing a cancer-specific geriatric assessment. *Cancer*. 2005;104(9):1998−2005. https://doi.org/10.1002/cncr.21422.

111. Han SH, Cho D, Mohammad R, et al. Use of the comprehensive geriatric assessment for the prediction of postoperative complications in elderly patients with head and neck cancer. *Head Neck*. 2022;44(3):672−680. https://doi.org/10.1002/hed.26958.

112. Wang J, Maxwell CA, Yu F. Biological processes and biomarkers related to frailty in older adults: a state-of-the-science literature review. *Biol Res Nurs*. 2019;21(1): 80−106. https://doi.org/10.1177/1099800418798047.

113. Mohile SG, Mohamed MR, Xu H, et al. Evaluation of geriatric assessment and man-agement on the toxic effects of cancer treatment (GAP70+): a cluster-randomised study. *Lancet*. 2021;398(10314):1894−1904. https://doi.org/10.1016/S0140-6736 (21)01789-X.

114. Montroni I, Ugolini G, Saur NM, et al. Quality of life in older adults after major cancer surgery: the GOSAFE international study. *JNCI: J Natl Cancer Inst*. 2022;114(7): 969−978. https://doi.org/10.1093/jnci/djac071.

115. Li D, Sun CL, Kim H, et al. Geriatric assessment−driven intervention (GAIN) on chemotherapy-related toxic effects in older adults with cancer. *JAMA Oncol*. 2021; 7(11):e214158. https://doi.org/10.1001/jamaoncol.2021.4158.

116. Soo WK, King MT, Pope A, Parente P, Dārziņš P, Davis ID. Integrated geriatric assess-ment and treatment effectiveness (INTEGERATE) in older people with cancer starting systemic anticancer treatment in Australia: a multicentre, open-label, randomised controlled trial. *Lancet Healthy Longev*. 2022;3(9):e617−e627. https://doi.org/ 10.1016/S2666-7568(22)00169-6.

117. Lund CM, Vistisen KK, Olsen AP, et al. The effect of geriatric intervention in frail older patients receiving chemotherapy for colorectal cancer: a randomised trial (GERICO). *Br J Cancer*. 2021;124(12):1949−1958. https://doi.org/10.1038/s41416-021-01367-0.

Oral complications from head and neck cancer therapy

7

Alessandro Villa, DDS, PhD, MPH [1,2] and Michele Lodolo, DDS [3]

[1]*Miami Cancer Institute, Baptist Health South Florida, Miami, FL, United States;* [2]*Herbert Wertheim College of Medicine, Florida International University (FIU), Miami, FL, United States;* [3]*University of California San Francisco (UCSF), San Francisco, CA, United States*

Introduction

Oral complications from head and neck cancer (HNC) therapy encompass a wide range of conditions, including mucositis, dry mouth, infections (viral, fungal, or bacterial), neuropathy, trismus/fibrosis, osteoradionecrosis, and oral immune-related adverse events (Fig. 7.1). These complications present unique challenges for healthcare professionals involved in the care of HNC patients. Understanding the pathophysiology, risk factors, and management strategies for these complications is of paramount importance.

Dental specialists play a crucial role in the prevention, early detection, and management of these complications. Their expertise in oral medicine/oral oncology and their understanding of the specific needs of HNC patients are essential for optimizing treatment outcomes and ensuring the well-being of HNC patients. This chapter aims to provide a comprehensive overview of the oral toxicities secondary to HNC therapy. It explores the role of various treatment modalities in the development of oral complications and emphasizes the importance of a proactive approach to oral care before, during, and after cancer treatment. The chapter also delves into the rationale for dental evaluation, the protocols involved, and the management strategies for each specific complication.[1]

The role of the dentist before and after cancer therapy
Rationale for a dental evaluation (pre) and dental protocols

The oral cavity is highly susceptible to the adverse effects of cancer therapy. In particular, patients scheduled to receive head and neck radiation therapy require special attention to their oral health, which involves timely and proper delivery of necessary dental care to avoid any future possible severe oral complications. As high-risk patient groups, they need thorough dental screening and clearance before undergoing therapy, and even after treatment, they are still vulnerable to oral

Head and Neck Cancer Rehabilitation. https://doi.org/10.1016/B978-0-443-11806-7.00009-6
Copyright © 2025 Elsevier Inc. All rights reserved, including those for text and data mining, AI training, and similar technologies.

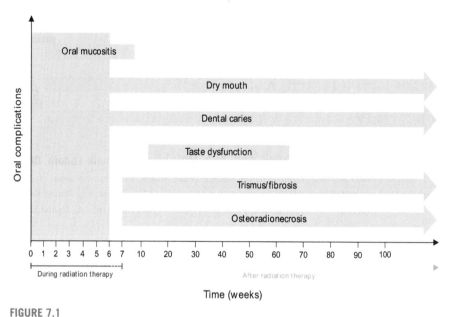

FIGURE 7.1

Onset of oral complications in patients receiving radiation therapy for head and neck cancers.

toxicities. Hence, it is crucial for oral healthcare providers to be educated and trained in delivering appropriate and effective care for this unique patient population. This section of the chapter highlights the rationale for dental evaluation before and after cancer therapy and summarizes the current dental protocols involved.

Poor oral health increases the risk of oral and systemic complications during and/or after cancer therapy. As such, a comprehensive dental and oral evaluation by a dental specialist is essential, particularly for patients awaiting head and neck radiation therapy. The primary goal of the oral and dental evaluation is to identify and eliminate any preexisting or potential dental/mucosal source of infection or intraoral trauma that could lead to complications during or following cancer therapy. Appropriate imaging studies (e.g., panoramic radiograph and, if necessary, periapical and bitewings radiographs) should be obtained, and a complete periodontal exam should be performed to identify any dental, periapical, and/or periodontal pathology. Nonrestorable teeth or partially erupted third molars with a history of recurrent pericoronitis should be extracted. Teeth with sharp and/or fractured surfaces should be smoothened or restored, as well as any ill-fitting prostheses and orthodontic appliances should be adjusted or replaced. Teeth with acute pulpal disease should be treated endodontically or extracted. In patients undergoing head and neck radiation therapy, particular attention should be given to those teeth located within the radiation field. Teeth with small dental cavities may not require immediate restoration prior to cancer treatment, especially if more conservative approaches can be adopted (e.g., aggressive topical fluoride treatment for prevention of dental caries, temporary restorations, or dental sealants). Close and good communication between the oncology and the dental team is crucial to determine the timing and extent of dental treatment required before cancer therapy. The dental and oral evaluation and treatment should be ideally performed at least 1 month before the beginning of cancer treatment to allow adequate time for healing from any invasive oral surgical procedures.

Oral hygiene and follow-up (during and post cancer treatment)

All patients should be educated about the importance of maintaining daily good oral hygiene and using prescription-strength sodium fluoride gel or toothpaste indefinitely. Patients awaiting to start cancer therapy should also receive professional dental prophylaxis and scaling (or root planning for those individuals with periodontitis). Patients should also be educated on the possible risk of acute chronic and oral complications from cancer therapy (for a complete list of oral toxicities, please refer to the following sections).

Regular dental follow-up appointments after cancer treatment should be scheduled in accordance with the patient's oncologist to identify dental, oral mucosal, and bone pathology. Oral surgical procedures that involve the manipulation of the jaw bones and gingival tissue should be avoided in patients who received head and neck radiation therapy to minimize the risk of osteoradionecrosis.[2]

Oral mucositis

Oral mucositis is one of the leading and most debilitating early toxicities of chemoradiation for HNCs that occurs due to the progressive damage and disruption of the oral mucosal integrity. Patients scheduled for head and neck radiotherapy typically receive 2 Gy of fractionated radiation daily, corresponding to 10 Gy a week, with most treatment regimens reaching a cumulative dose of 60–70 Gy. Patients usually develop mucosal erythema and mouth soreness by the end of the first week of radiation treatment. Ulceration occurs when the cumulative dose reaches 30–40 Gy, usually by the second to third week of treatment, and may persist 2–4 weeks after the completion of head and neck radiation therapy. Patients with severe oral mucositis typically present with deep ulcers often covered with a pseudomembrane of necrotic cells and bacteria (Fig. 7.2). Commonly affected oral sites are the buccal mucosa, ventral tongue, lip mucosa, floor of the mouth, and soft palate.

The pathobiology of oral mucositis is a result of a complex biological cascade characterized by five stages, which are initiated by oxidative stress, the generation of reactive oxygen species, and the activation of the innate immune response. This activation sets off a cascade of inflammatory pathways, which are further amplified by positive feedback loops. Consequently, the typical mucositis lesions

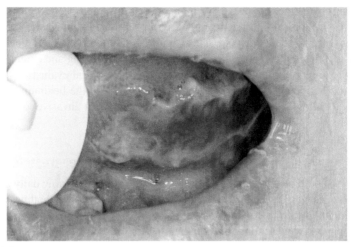

FIGURE 7.2

Mucositis. Large and shallow ulceration on the left ventrolateral tongue in a patient undergoing head and neck radiation therapy.

develop as a result of compromised epithelial integrity, and these lesions are subsequently colonized by various bacteria.[3]

Oral mucositis is often associated with significant pain that negatively affects patients' functions (e.g., chewing, swallowing, and speaking), leading to poor quality of life. Patients with severe oral mucositis may require hospitalization, parenteral nutrition, opioid use for pain management, and dose delays, reductions, or temporary discontinuation of cancer therapies, all of which can lead to poor treatment outcomes. In addition, patients with severe oral mucositis have an increased risk of local (e.g., viral, fungal, or bacterial) and systemic infections (e.g., bacteremia or sepsis).

Various scales have been suggested to evaluate and assess the severity of oral mucositis, including the National Cancer Institute Common Terminology Criteria for Adverse Events (NCI CTCAE), the World Health Organization (WHO) scale, and the Radiation Therapy Oncology Group (RTOG) scoring criteria. The WHO and NCI CTCAE scales employ criteria that consider objective characteristics such as the presence and extent of erythema and ulceration, as well as the patient's symptoms and functional capabilities, such as their ability to consume solid food or drink liquids.

Preventive and therapeutic interventions for oral mucositis have been evaluated by the Mucositis Study Group of the Multinational Association of Supportive Care in Cancer and the International Society of Oral Oncology (MASCC/ISOO). The group confirmed the importance of basic oral care and patient education to enhance oral comfort. Benzydamine hydrochloride rinses have been recommended for oral mucositis prevention in patients with HNCs undergoing a moderate-dose (<50 Gy) radiation therapy and suggested in those receiving chemoradiation.

Intraoral photobiomodulation/low-level laser therapy has shown efficacy in preventing oral mucositis secondary to head and neck radiation therapy with or without concomitant chemotherapy. Additionally, topical morphine 0.2% mouthwash has been proposed as an effective measure for pain control associated with chemoradiation-related oral mucositis. Natural agents, including honey (administrated topically and/or systemically) and oral glutamine (10−30 mg daily), have demonstrated promising results in preventing oral mucositis in patients treated with either radiotherapy and/or combined chemotherapy and radiation therapy.[4,5]

Hyposalivation and xerostomia

Hyposalivation or salivary gland hypofunction (objective reduction in the salivary flow rate) and xerostomia (subjective complaint of dry mouth) are among the most common side effects of head and neck radiation therapy.

In patients undergoing head and neck radiotherapy, hyposalivation occurs due to radiation-induced progressive damage to the acinar cells, blood vessels, and nerves of those salivary glands located within the radiation field. The extent of salivary gland damage is influenced by various factors, including the radiation dose, regimen, technique, and irradiated volume of salivary gland tissue. Permanent damage typically occurs at cumulative doses exceeding 60 Gy. Parotid glands are generally more radiosensitive than the other major salivary glands. If the cumulative radiation dose reaches 40−50 Gy, up to 75% of the parotid gland function is impaired. A 50%−60% decrease in salivary flow rate occurs in the first week of radiation therapy, and after 7 weeks, the flow rate is down to approximately 20%. Although salivary function is generally considered irreversibly impaired, partial recovery may occur 12−18 months after the completion of head and neck radiation therapy.

A diagnosis of hyposalivation is generally made when the unstimulated whole saliva (UWS) flow is ≤ 0.1 mL/min and the stimulated whole saliva (SWS) flow is $\leq 0.5-0.7$ mL/min, as measured by sialometry. Of note, hyposalivation and xerostomia do not always coexist. Xerostomia may be present due to qualitative changes in the composition of saliva in the absence of an objective reduction in the salivary flow rate.

On clinical examination, the oral mucosa of patients with hyposalivation can appear erythematous with dry secretions and depapillation of the tongue dorsum (Fig. 7.3).

Patients with hyposalivation are more prone to develop oral infections (bacterial and fungal infections), rampant dental caries, difficulties eating, swallowing, speaking, and taste dysfunction.

The MASCC/ISOO, in collaboration with the American Society of Clinical Oncology (ASCO), have formulated evidence-based guidelines for the prevention and management of salivary gland hypofunction and/or xerostomia. The panel acknowledged the efficacy of intensity-modulated radiation therapy in preventing salivary gland hypofunction and xerostomia by delivering more precise radiation

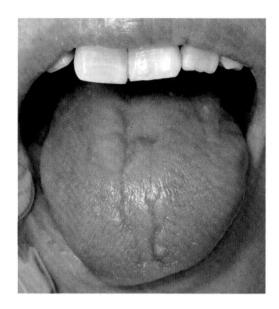

FIGURE 7.3

Atrophic tongue with complete loss of the filiform papillae in a patient with radiation-induced hyposalivation.

to the tumor while sparing surrounding normal tissues, including the salivary glands. Topical application of mucosal lubricants or saliva substitutes may be beneficial in mitigating xerostomia and salivary gland hypofunction. A strong recommendation has been made in favor of the use of oral pilocarpine or cevimeline after head and neck radiation therapy to improve xerostomia and salivary gland hypofunction in patients with a residual capacity of salivary gland tissue. However, the increase in the salivary flow induced by pilocarpine or cevimeline is often transitory. Sugar-free lozenges or chewing gum and acidic (nonerosive) sugar-free candies may be used to increase the salivary flow mechanically, but again, only in the presence of functional salivary gland tissue. While acupuncture is recommended with a lesser degree of efficacy, it is suggested for the prevention of xerostomia. Other management approaches, supported by less robust evidence, include transcutaneous electrostimulation or acupuncture-like transcutaneous electrostimulation. Furthermore, emerging strategies such as gene therapy and acinar cell replacement have exhibited promising outcomes in preventing radiation-induced damage to the salivary glands.[6,7]

Dental caries

Patients with hyposalivation are at increased risk of rampant dental caries due to the absence of crucial saliva functions, such as controlling oral pH, promoting dental remineralization, mechanical cleansing, and antimicrobial activity. Dental caries typically affects the cervical margin of the teeth and, if left untreated, can progress rapidly and potentially involve all dental surfaces.

To prevent such complications, several interventions are recommended. These include the daily and lifelong use of 1.1% neutral sodium fluoride gel with fabricated trays or brush-on applications or 1.1% sodium fluoride prescription toothpaste. Additionally, it is important to limit the consumption of cariogenic foods (high sugar content), maintain meticulous oral hygiene practices, and seek regular dental care to manage the condition effectively.[8]

Oral infections

Patients undergoing chemoradiation for HNCs face an increased risk of oral infections (i.e., viral, fungal, and bacterial). Several factors contribute to this susceptibility, such as the loss of oral mucosal integrity, dry mouth, changes in oral microbiota, and/or chemotherapy-induced immunosuppression/neutropenia. Compared with relatively healthy individuals, oral infections in cancer patients tend to exhibit a more severe clinical presentation and unpredictable progression.

Viral infections

Oral viral infections in HNC patients are primarily seen in immunocompromised individuals receiving intensive, high-dose chemotherapy regimens and typically occur due to the reactivation of Herpes Simplex Virus (HSV). Clinically, recrudescent HVS infection can present with both intraoral and extraoral lesions. Intraoral lesions appear as large, painful, shallow, irregularly shaped ulcerations that can potentially affect any surface of the oral mucosa, sometimes making them difficult to distinguish from oral mucositis. Extraoral lesions typically involve the lips and present with painful ulcerations (herpes labialis).

Treatment for oral viral infections involves hydration, nutritional support, and topical or systemic pain control. In severe cases of immunosuppression, systemic antiviral medications such as acyclovir, valacyclovir, or famciclovir may be necessary.[9]

Fungal infections

Oropharyngeal candidiasis is frequently encountered in patients undergoing HNC therapy, especially in those with hyposalivation resulting from radiation therapy. Four different clinical presentations of oral candidiasis exist and include pseudomembranous candidiasis (commonly referred to as "oral thrush"), characterized by white, thick, often removable papules resembling "cottage cheese"; erythematous candidiasis, which manifests as generalized mucosal erythema, often affecting the tongue and palate; hyperplastic candidiasis, presenting as white not removable plaques typically on the buccal commissures, tongue, and palatal mucosa; and angular cheilitis, characterized by erythema and fissures at the lip commissures. Symptoms of candidiasis range from none to burning pain, odynophagia, and dysgeusia.

The mainstay of therapy for oral candidiasis includes the use of topical antifungal medications such as clotrimazole troches or sugar-free nystatin suspension. Systemic fluconazole may be considered in case of topical treatment failure, severe immunosuppression, or as antifungal prophylaxis.[10]

Bacterial infections

Patients with poor oral hygiene undergoing chemoradiation for HNCs are at risk of developing secondary odontogenic infections. Untreated odontogenic infections may spread to surrounding soft and hard tissues, leading to severe complications, including osteomyelitis, cellulitis, cavernous sinus thrombosis, and mediastinitis.

Treatment of odontogenic infections includes the elimination of the source of infection (e.g., endodontic treatment, scaling or root planning, or extraction of affected tooth), incision and drainage in the presence of a fluctuant swelling, or empiric antibiotic therapy with large spectrum antibiotics.

Neuropathies

Neuropathy is a common and often underestimated side effect of HNC treatments (e.g., chemoradiation and surgery) that results from peripheral cranial nerve injury and typically manifests as neuropathic pain (often referred to as oral dysesthesia) and taste dysfunction. However, oral pain resembling neuropathy can also be caused by inflammation and/or ischemia resulting from the direct invasion of the HN tumor, whether primary or recurrent, into the surrounding tissues, such as the skin, muscle, or bone.

Oral dysesthesia

Oral dysesthesia can be persistent, episodic, spontaneous, or triggered by noxious and/or not-normally-evoking-pain stimuli. Oral dysesthesia is characterized by a variety of symptoms, including oral burning, tingling, numbness, and "pins and needles" sensation.

Management of oral dysesthesia is with topical anesthetics/analgesics, systemic tricyclic antidepressants (e.g., amitriptyline and nortriptyline), topical benzodiazepines (e.g., clonazepam compounded solution as a swish and spit) as well as topical or systemic γ-aminobutyric acid, or GABA analogs (e.g., gabapentin).[11]

Taste dysfunction

Taste dysfunction secondary to chemoradiation presents as hypogeusia (diminished sense of taste) or, in most cases, dysgeusia (distorted sense of taste frequently described as metallic, bitter, or unpleasant). The degree of taste impairment depends on the type of chemotherapy and/or radiation dose, the anatomical site of the cancer, and the presence of local comorbidities. Dysgeusia can be further aggravated by concomitant salivary gland hypofunction, oral candidiasis, and poor oral hygiene. In patients undergoing radiotherapy to the head and neck, taste dysfunction typically develops at 5 weeks postradiation and lasts for about 6−12 months before spontaneously resolving in most cases.

Despite the absence of an ideal treatment for dysgeusia, daily zinc supplements have shown to be beneficial in reducing taste alterations caused by chemoradiation. Other management options include topical application of GABA analogs or benzodiazepines. Taste improvement may be observed after discontinuing chemotherapy or 6−12 months after the completion of radiotherapy.[12]

Periodontitis

Periodontitis is a chronic inflammatory disease caused by multiple factors, including dysbiotic plaque biofilms and the loss of periodontal tissue support, with the presence of periodontal pockets and gingival bleeding.

Cancer treatment can potentially exacerbate preexisting periodontitis, a common condition among the general adult population. The development of periodontitis in HNC patients can be attributed to various factors, including changes in the oral microbiome, increased bacteriogenic flora, lack of saliva antimicrobial activity, and difficulties in maintaining proper oral hygiene due to common treatment toxicities such as trismus or oral mucositis. Periodontitis can result in increased tooth mobility, pain, infection, and the potential need for tooth extraction, exposing the patient to a higher risk of osteoradionecrosis. Moreover, patients with periodontal disease may develop acute periodontal infections, which can lead to bacteremia and sepsis, particularly in severely immunocompromised individuals.

Treatment of periodontal disease depends on the severity of the condition, but it generally includes professional dental prophylaxis with scaling, root planning, daily rinses with chlorhexidine mouthwash, and antibiotic therapy. Patients should be educated in maintaining lifelong daily good oral hygiene and regularly see a dental professional at least twice a year.[13]

Trismus/fibrosis

Trismus (restricted mouth opening) is a frequently encountered side effect of head and neck radiation therapy (prevalence: 30%−50%) that occurs due to the progressive damage with localized myopathy and subsequent fibrosis of the irradiated masticatory muscles (primarily masseters and pterygoids) and ligaments. Trismus can develop by the end of radiation treatment or at any time within the following 24 months, with a gradual and slowly progressive onset. Patients with trismus typically experience varying degrees of loss of function and range of mandibular motions (Fig. 7.4).

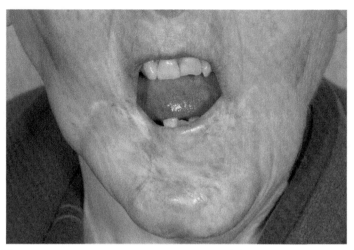

FIGURE 7.4

Trismus in a patient following surgery and radiation therapy for a right mandibular gingival squamous cell carcinoma.

A diagnosis of trismus is usually made when the measured maximum vertical opening is < 35 mm. Surgery, iatrogenic and pathologic fractures of the mandible, and odontogenic infections can potentially cause restricted mouth opening and should be considered during the process of differential diagnosis.

Trismus can significantly impair patients' ability to eat, speak, and brush their teeth, potentially leading to weight loss, malnutrition, difficulties in maintaining oral hygiene, limited access to dental treatment, and overall poor quality of life.

Early detection of trismus is crucial in minimizing the sequelae related to this complication, although a complete recovery of the mandibular range of motion is rare despite treatment.

Preventative strategies for patients undergoing radiation therapy include the fabrication of a splint to wear during radiation therapy or the use of dose-sculpting techniques such as intensity-modulated radiotherapy or image-guided radiotherapy; the first with the aim of holding adjacent healthy structures (e.g., jaw or tongue) away from the radiation field while the second of delivering more precise radiation to the tumor while sparing surrounding normal tissues.

In patients with cancers of the mandibular ramus, maxillary tuberosity, zygomatic arch, or the infratemporal fossa, prophylactic coronoidectomy and/or temporal muscle myotomy may be considered during cancer surgeries to reduce the risk of trismus. This is because temporalis fibers are particularly susceptible to developing fibrosis following surgery, radiation therapy, or immobilization. Reconstruction should be performed immediately after resection whenever feasible. Additional myotomies/scar tissue resection may be considered if other masticatory muscles are involved.

Physical therapy remains the mainstay of therapy for trismus, with a combination of active and passive mobilization exercises along with the utilization of jaw-mobilizing devices. The primary focus of active exercises is to strengthen the muscles responsible for jaw opening, while passive exercises aim to stretch the muscles involved in jaw closure. To alleviate pain and facilitate the mobilization process, analgesics or muscle relaxants may be prescribed during the initial phase of physical therapy. It is crucial to educate patients about the significance of these exercises in the treatment of trismus.

Although physical therapy remains the cornerstone of trismus treatment, additional approaches have been explored. Pentoxifylline, while showing only modest therapeutic effects on trismus, has been considered as an alternative. Furthermore, botulinum toxin injections can be utilized to alleviate pain associated with trismus, but this treatment does not seem to improve the underlying condition.[14]

Osteoradionecrosis

Osteoradionecrosis of the jaw (ORN) is a late complication of radiation therapy for HNCs, occurring in approximately 4%—37% of patients. ORN is defined as an area of exposed, nonvital bone present for more than 3—6 months in a previously irradiated field without any evidence of persisting or recurrent tumor. This definition has undergone several modifications, and there has been considerable debate regarding the criteria for mucosal breakdown and the required duration of exposure.[15,16]

Several theories have been proposed to explain the pathobiology of ORN. While the most widely acknowledged theory suggests that ORN originates from the combined effects of radiation-induced hypoxia, hypocellularity, and/or hypovascularity in the irradiated bone, a newer perspective proposes that radiation-induced fibroatrophy of the affected bone plays a pivotal role in the development of ORN along with the production of free radicals, microvascular thrombosis, and local inflammation. Regardless of the specific theory, it is widely recognized that bone exposed to radiation, especially at doses exceeding 60 Gy, exhibits increased fragility, reduced regenerative capacity, and heightened susceptibility to infections.

ORN of the jaws can occur spontaneously or, more commonly, due to procedures involving the manipulation of the bone, such as teeth extractions. The mandible is more frequently affected compared with the maxilla. In patients exposed to high-dose radiation, ORN can occur at any time after the completion of radiation therapy. Clinical signs and symptoms of ORN include ulceration or necrosis of the mucosa with exposed necrotic bone, pain, suppuration, secondary trismus, difficulties with mastication and swallowing, as well as recurrent episodes of infection (Fig. 7.5). ORN significantly impacts the quality of life of patients.

Patient scheduled to receive head and neck radiation therapy requires a thorough dental evaluation prior to treatment initiation. Hopeless teeth, especially if located within the radiation field, should be extracted to avoid future surgical procedures involving the alveolar bone during or after radiation therapy.

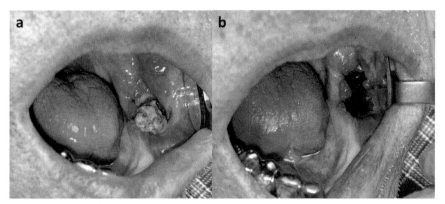

FIGURE 7.5

Osteoradionecrosis. Exposed necrotic bone of the left posterior mandible before (panel A) and after (panel B) a nonsurgical sequestrectomy.

Significant advancements have been made in the treatment of ORN with a range of surgical and nonsurgical approaches available, with controversial results. However, there is ongoing research and exploration of alternative strategies, particularly the utilization of vascularized tissue, which holds promise in improving outcomes for patients with ORN. The current treatment algorithm for ORN incorporates a combination of surgical and nonsurgical interventions. These include hyperbaric oxygen therapy, antibiotics, and the PENTOCLO protocol, involving the administration of pentoxifylline, tocopherol, and clodronate. Unfortunately, clodronate therapy, a component of the PENTOCLO protocol, is currently unavailable in the United States. Surgical debridement is usually for more severe cases, and the effectiveness of this approach can vary depending on the individual case. In recent years, there has been a growing interest in the application of vascularized tissue in the management of ORN. As research progresses, the treatment landscape for ORN is expected to further evolve.[17]

Oral immune-related adverse events

Immune checkpoint inhibitors (ICIs) have gained FDA approval for the treatment of various cancers, including certain HNCs. However, the use of ICI therapy is associated with the occurrence of systemic and oral adverse events. Oral immune-related adverse events (ir-AEs) can affect the oral mucosa and salivary glands. Clinically, oral mucosal lesions may resemble conditions such as oral lichen planus (OLP), mucous membrane pemphigoid (MMP)/bullous pemphigoid (BP), and erythema multiforme (EM). Additionally, when the salivary glands are involved, patients may develop signs and symptoms similar to those seen in Sjogren's disease, causing severe dry mouth.

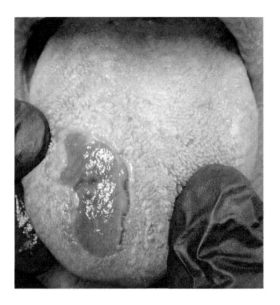

FIGURE 7.6

Oral immune-related adverse event. Large and well-defined ulceration of the right tongue dorsum in a patient taking nivolumab.

Oral ir-AEs usually develop within the initial weeks to months of treatment. OLP-like reactions are characterized by white reticular striations, erythema, and/or ulcerations mainly located on the buccal mucosa and ventral tongue (Fig. 7.6). Autoimmune blistering disorders are occasionally observed, taking the form of BP-like lesions involving the skin and rarely the oral cavity, or MMP-like lesions that typically present as desquamative gingivitis. Oral lesions resembling EM have been rarely reported in patients receiving immunotherapy. These lesions typically manifest as multiple irregularly shaped erosions and ulcers with hemorrhagic crusting of the lips. The diagnosis of these oral mucosal ir-AEs can be confirmed through histopathology and/or immunofluorescent studies, and biopsies should ideally be obtained before initiating any treatment.

Management is with topical corticosteroids, while severe cases may require systemic steroids. Patients undergoing immunotherapy may also experience Sjogren's-like signs and symptoms, such as xerostomia and hyposalivation. When evaluating a patient who has received immunotherapy and presents with dry mouth symptoms, it is crucial to consider alternative causes of xerostomia/hyposalivation, such as dehydration, polypharmacy, and anxiety. Treatment options include the use of mucosal lubricants, saliva substitutes, sugar-free lozenges, or sialogogues (e.g., pilocarpine or cevimeline), depending on the severity of the symptoms.[18]

Disfigurement from surgery and psychological/social implications

Facial disfigurement is recognized as one of the most challenging consequences of head and neck cancer (HNC) surgery for patients with large HNC. Extensive tumor resection can significantly alter facial features and profoundly impact a person's self-perception, identity, and overall well-being, potentially leading to emotional distress, anxiety, depression, or even suicidal thoughts. Additionally, visible disfigurement can subject individuals to stigma and discrimination, resulting in social exclusion. Communication challenges and functional limitations further impede social interactions and daily activities, making the situation even more difficult for those affected.

Addressing these profound implications requires a comprehensive multidisciplinary approach encompassing various support systems. Cognitive behavioral therapy and targeted interventions and tools that promote stress reduction, self-acceptance, confidence, and better participation in social interactions and intimate relationships play a crucial role. Providing education and increasing awareness can effectively combat stigma, while rehabilitation services play a significant role in aiding both physical and emotional recovery.

Support networks and patient advocacy groups also have a vital role to play, as they offer valuable connections and emotional support for individuals facing disfigurement. By fostering a compassionate and inclusive environment, it is possible to improve the well-being and quality of life for these patients, enabling them to regain confidence, rebuild relationships, and ultimately lead fulfilling lives despite the challenges they may encounter.[19]

Conclusions

HNC therapy may result in a variety of orofacial complications that significantly impact patients' quality of life and treatment outcomes. Close monitoring and appropriate management by dental specialists are crucial for patients with HNC, particularly those undergoing radiation therapy. Timely dental interventions and early identification of high-risk patients can help reduce the risk of future oral complications. Effective management of orofacial complications secondary to HNC treatment relies on the collaboration of clinicians from different teams.

References

1. National Cancer Institute. Oral Complications of Chemotherapy and Head/Neck Radiation (PDQ) Health Professional Version. https://www.cancer.gov/about-cancer/treatment/side-effects/mouth-throat/oral-complications-hp-pdq.

2. Hong CH, Napeñas JJ, Hodgson BD, et al, Dental Disease Section, Oral Care Study Group, Multi-national Association of Supportive Care in Cancer (MASCC)/International Society of Oral Oncology (ISOO). A systematic review of dental disease in patients undergoing cancer therapy. *Support Care Cancer.* August 2010;18(8):1007−1021.
3. Villa A, Sonis ST. Mucositis: pathobiology and management. *Curr Opin Oncol.* May 2015;27(3):159−164.
4. Elad S, Yarom N, Zadik Y, Kuten-Shorrer M, Sonis ST. The broadening scope of oral mucositis and oral ulcerative mucosal toxicities of anticancer therapies. *CA Cancer J Clin.* 2022;72(1):57−77.
5. Elad S, Cheng KKF, Lalla RV, et al. Mucositis guidelines leadership group of the multinational association of supportive care in cancer and international society of oral oncology (MASCC/ISOO). MASCC/ISOO clinical practice guidelines for the management of mucositis secondary to cancer therapy. *Cancer.* October 1, 2020;126(19): 4423−4431.
6. Jensen SB, Pedersen AM, Vissink A, et al, Salivary Gland Hypofunction/Xerostomia Section, Oral Care Study Group, Multinational Association of Supportive Care in Cancer (MASCC)/International Society of Oral Oncology (ISOO). A systematic review of salivary gland hypofunction and xerostomia induced by cancer therapies: prevalence, severity and impact on quality of life. *Support Care Cancer.* August 2010;18(8): 1039−1060.
7. Mercadante V, Jensen SB, Smith DK, et al. Salivary gland hypofunction and/or xerostomia induced by nonsurgical cancer therapies: ISOO/MASCC/ASCO guideline. *J Clin Oncol.* September 1, 2021;39(25):2825−2843.
8. Lu H, Zhao Q, Guo J, et al. Direct radiation-induced effects on dental hard tissue. *Radiat Oncol.* January 11, 2019;14(1):5.
9. Elad S, Ranna V, Ariyawardana A, et al, Viral Infections Section, Oral Care Study Group, Multinational Association of Supportive Care in Cancer (MASCC)/International Society of Oral Oncology (ISOO). A systematic review of oral herpetic viral infections in cancer patients: commonly used outcome measures and interventions. *Support Care Cancer.* February 2017;25(2):687−700.
10. Bensadoun RJ, Patton LL, Lalla RV, Epstein JB. Oropharyngeal candidiasis in head and neck cancer patients treated with radiation: update 2011. *Support Care Cancer.* 2011; 19(6):737−744.
11. Epstein JB, Wilkie DJ, Fischer DJ, Kim YO, Villines D. Neuropathic and nociceptive pain in head and neck cancer patients receiving radiation therapy. *Head Neck Oncol.* July 14, 2009;1:26.
12. Hovan AJ, Williams PM, Stevenson-Moore P, et al, Dysgeusia Section, Oral Care Study Group, Multinational Association of Supportive Care in Cancer (MASCC)/International Society of Oral Oncology (ISOO). A systematic review of dysgeusia induced by cancer therapies. *Support Care Cancer.* August 2010;18(8):1081−1087.
13. Al-Nawas B, Grötz KA. Prospective study of the long term change of the oral flora after radiation therapy. *Support Care Cancer.* March 2006;14(3):291−296.
14. Abboud WA, Hassin-Baer S, Alon EE, et al. Restricted mouth opening in head and neck cancer: etiology, prevention, and treatment. *JCO Oncol Pract.* October 2020;16(10): 643−653.
15. Nabil S, Samman N. Risk factors for osteoradionecrosis after head and neck radiation: a systematic review. *Oral Surg Oral Med Oral Pathol Oral Radiol.* January 2012;113(1): 54−69.

16. Nabil S, Samman N. Incidence and prevention of osteoradionecrosis after dental extraction in irradiated patients: a systematic review. *Int J Oral Maxillofac Surg*. March 2011; 40(3):229–243.
17. Sultan A, Hanna GJ, Margalit DN, et al. The use of hyperbaric oxygen for the prevention and management of osteoradionecrosis of the jaw: a Dana-Farber/Brigham and women's cancer center multidisciplinary guideline. *Oncologist*. March 2017;22(3):343–350.
18. Klein BA, Alves FA, de Santana Rodrigues VJ, et al. Oral manifestations of immune-related adverse events in cancer patients treated with immune checkpoint inhibitors. *Oral Dis*. January 2022;28(1):9–22.
19. Rhoten BA, Murphy B, Ridner SH. Body image in patients with head and neck cancer: a review of the literature. *Oral Oncol*. August 2013;49(8):753–760.

Physical therapy for head and neck cancer patients

8

Dessislava Dakova, MSPT, CLT Physical Therapist

Oncology Rehabilitation at South Miami Hospital, Miami, FL, United States

Introduction

Head and neck cancer (HNC) is the seventh most common cancer worldwide, with over 660,000 new cases and 325,000 deaths per year.[1,2] In the United States, the estimated annual burden is 65,000 new cases and 14,000 deaths, respectively. HNC is a diverse group of malignancies, which can involve the oral cavity, larynx, pharynx, tongue, nasal cavity, and the salivary glands. An exception to this category is the malignancies of the central nervous system (CNS), eye, thyroid, and the esophagus. Squamous cell carcinoma is the most prevalent HNC, accounting for about 90% of the cases.[1,2]

The incidence of HNC has been on the rise due to various factors such as socioeconomic changes, tobacco and alcohol consumption, human papillomavirus infection, and dietary consumption. The increase is global and has been seen in both the developing and developed countries,[1] with a predicted 30% annual rate increase by 2030. The most common risk factors are tobacco and alcohol use, especially smoking, and most recently, HPV infection, particularly in white males >50 years of age.[2–5] Other factors such as drinking hot liquids, diet, and Epstein–Barr virus have also been implicated. In the US and Europe, there has been a reduction in oral cancer due to a decrease in smoking and alcohol consumption. However, there has been a significant increase in oropharyngeal cancer due to HPV infection.[1,3] Southeast Asia and the Asia–Pacific regions have a very high incidence of oral cancer secondary to areca nut chewing.[1,3] Nasopharyngeal cancer (NPC), on the other hand, is more common in south China, Singapore, Vietnam and Malaysia, Northwest Canada, and Greenland, which are regions with diets rich in salt-cured fish and meat.[4] Tobacco-related HNC appears to be more prevalent in the developing countries, while HPV-related malignancies are seen more frequently in patients, particularly in men, with higher socioeconomic status. The global trend, however, is toward an increased incidence of HPV-related HNC and a decrease in the non-HPV-related cancers (in response to decreasing prevalence of smoking in North America and the Western countries).[1]

The risk of HNC increases with age, with many of the new diagnoses seen in the population >50 years, and men having two to four times higher incidences of cancer than women.[1] The majority of the HNC patients are diagnosed at stage III or IV, and the survival rates depend on the type of tumor and tumor stage at times of diagnosis.[1]

Head and Neck Cancer Rehabilitation. https://doi.org/10.1016/B978-0-443-11806-7.00008-4

Copyright © 2025 Elsevier Inc. All rights reserved, including those for text and data mining, AI training, and similar technologies.

HPV-related cancers have a much better survival rate compared with HPV-negative HNC.

HPV is one of the most common sexually transmitted infections worldwide, and HPV-related malignancies have created a global health burden.[3] HPV infection is usually asymptomatic, and women are more likely to clear the infection than men,[3] which may be a contributing factor to the higher male prevalence of HPV-related HNC. Since 1973, there has been a very significant increase in the oropharyngeal squamous cell carcinoma (OPSCC) related to HPV infection, with estimates of approximately 75% of the cases being HPV-related.[6] Currently, it is the sixth most common nonskin solid cancer among white males <65 years.[7] Approximately 90% of the patients are >50 years old with the greatest incidence found among white males aged 60−64.[7] While it affects both male and female patients, close to 75% of the patients are male as compared with 25% female. Unlike other HNC malignancies, HPV-related OPSCC presents with smaller tumors and a lower T-stage cancer, but higher lymph node tumor involvement.[7] HPV-positive HNC has better survival outcomes, and the 5-year survival rate has been estimated at 75%−80%.[8]

With increasing global incidences of HNC, reduction in the non-HPV malignancies, increasing HPV-related HNC, and improvements in diagnostics and treatment options, it is expected that there will be more HNC survivors. This calls for a responsive shift in focus to manage long-term treatment sequelae and morbidities such as speech and swallowing impairments, trismus, neuropathies, cancer-related fatigue (CRF), lymphedema, weakness, and pain.[9] Rehabilitation services (physical and occupational therapy along with speech and language pathology) play an important role in managing long term survivorship by addressing treatment related toxicities and improving overall function.[9] The goal of rehabilitation in the HNC is to be part of a multidisciplinary approach and assist in the management of the patients throughout the continuum of care, transition to survivorship, and subsequently improve their quality of life.

Treatment

Treatment of HNC may include surgical tumor resection, radiotherapy (RT), chemotherapy radiation treatment (CRT), immunotherapy, or a combination of two or more modalities. Single treatment surgery and/or radiation are the primary curative modalities, which may be used separately, or together for stage I and II disease, whereas chemotherapy is usually used in more advanced cancers. Around 80% of the patients receive RT either as the primary or adjuvant modality.[2]

Surgery

Surgical tumor resection for HNC requires careful evaluation and consideration of the expected benefits versus the risks. Potential permanent tissue, organ and vascular damage along with anticipated functional outcomes such as swallowing, breathing, and speaking is crucial in determining surgical qualification.[5] For patients with resectable tumors and acceptable organ risk, surgery is considered as the primary modality; however, for high-risk patients and those with larger tumor and nodal involvement, radiotherapy may be the preferred choice.[5]

As outlined in the Quick Reference Guide to TNM staging of Head and Neck Cancer and Neck Dissection Classification,[10] cervical dissection is classified into three main categories: radical neck dissection is considered the standard basic procedure and involves the resection of all ipsilateral cervical lymph node groups (from level I through V), the spinal accessory nerve (SAN), the internal jugular vein (IJV), and sternocleidomastoid muscle (SCM) (Figs. 8.1 and 8.2); in modified radical neck dissection, all lymph nodes (level I through V) are removed, but one or more of the other three structures (SAN, IJV, SCM) are preserved; in selective neck dissection, some lymph node groups are preserved and lymphadenectomy is based on the expected patterns of metastases from the primary tumor.[10]

The open surgical approach, however, can create significant functional and psychological morbidities. In 2009, the Food and Drug administration (FDA) approved transoral robotic surgery (TORS), a minimally invasive surgical procedure, for resection of T1-T2 malignant and benign tumors of the oral cavity, pharynx, and larynx.[11] Since then, with improvements in technology and surgical expertise, TORS has expanded to include resections of the hypopharynx, parapharyngeal space, the skull base, neck dissections, and thyroidectomy.[11] TORS is still limited, and qualifications for the procedure include medical history and existing comorbidities, tumor location and extension, patient's anatomy/surgical exposure, and surgeon experience.[11] Postoperative hemorrhage, trismus, and dental-related issues were encountered more frequently with TORS than with RT and CRT.[11]

Expected surgical side effects are pain, limited cervical ROM, soft tissue restrictions, shoulder and arm weakness, and postural changes. In the acute setting, physical therapy may be indicated for bed mobility, transfers, and early ambulation. Outpatient treatment may be warranted for cervical mobility and strengthening,

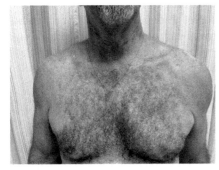 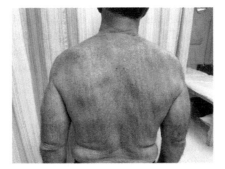

FIGURES 8.1 AND 8.2

Left shoulder muscle atrophy in patient 2 months after radical neck dissection.

soft tissue and scar tissue mobilization, upper extremities strengthening, and posture exercises.

Common functional morbidities include limited cervical extension, rotation and side bending, surgical scar pain, shoulder dysfunction related to SAN injury/resection, inability to flex and/or turn the head to the contralateral side with SCM resection, scar tissue contractures, poor food intake secondary to teeth excision, and jaw pain. Psychological distress may be related to face and neck disfigurement, chronic pain, difficulty with activities of daily living (ADLs), and limited functional independence. Rehabilitation services can be successfully used following surgery to improve pain, tissue sensitivity, cervical mobility, upper extremity function, and overall strength and endurance.

Radiation treatment

Radiation treatment (RT) is used as either the primary or adjuvant modality. RT is used to inhibit tumor cell proliferation through various molecular mechanisms[2]; however, it has significant toxicity, which may lead to severe impairments and poor quality of life. The introduction of intensity-modulated radiation therapy (IMRT), molecular imaging—guided therapy, adaptive therapy, and proton beam therapy has allowed for more precise tumor targeting and health tissue preservation and has the potential to decrease long-term toxicity.[12] Nevertheless, acute and long-term radiation-induced morbidities remain a significant burden for the cancer patient. Radiation over 50 Gr has been shown to significantly increase the risk of healthy tissue damage and neural injury. HNC patients receiving radiation treatment are at risk of developing hearing loss, changes in taste and smell function, optical neuropathies, difficulty with swallowing (dysphagia), difficulty speaking (dysphonia), radiation-induced brachial plexopathy (RIBP) leading to sensory and motor function loss, cranial nerve impairment,[2] osteoradionecrosis, and lymphedema. While some of these toxicities may be transient, many are progressive and may lead to permanent loss of function. Radiation treatment can induce both acute and late-stage symptoms. The acute symptoms such as fatigue, headache, drowsiness, and nausea are transient and usually resolve.[2] Fatigue related to RT is a component of CRF and has both physical and motivational manifestations. The late-stage symptoms such as cognitive impairment, osteoradionecrosis, lymphedema, and neuronal injury occur after several months, and may be progressive and irreversible.[2]

Radiation fibrosis

Radiation-induced fibrosis, one of the most common and devastating consequences, is a complex process of inflammation, excess production of fibroblasts,[13] ischemia, and finally fibrosis. It is unavoidable and can lead to complete sensory and motor function loss. It has a gradual onset and usually develops between 4 and 12 months after treatment.[2] The severity of fibrosis is affected by several factors and tends to be worse in older patients, larger tumors, higher radiation doses, treatment volume, additional treatments such as surgery and chemotherapy, and the patient's radiosensitivity.[13] Radiation fibrosis may lead to shoulder dysfunction, skin fibrosis and cervical musculature dystonia, and spasms.[13] Treatment includes steroid injections and rehabilitation.[13] Physical therapy can assist in improving cervical mobility and strength, minimize soft tissue restrictions, decrease edema and pain, reduce fatigue, and improve overall endurance. Trismus, also known as "lock jaw," affects the tempomandibular joint and is the result of assimilation of fibrosis in the joint and the surrounding musculature.[13] It is a devastating consequence, which interferes with the opening of the mouth, chewing, oral hygiene, nutrition, speech, and intubation.[13,14] Physical therapy and speech therapy, along with tong blade therapy and splinting devices (TheraBite, OraStretch, Dynasplint), are prescribed to improve ROM, swallowing, and strength.[13,14]

Radiation-induced brachial plexopathy

Radiation-induced brachial plexopathy (RIBP) is usually a progressive, irreversible injury to the brachial plexus caused by axonal damage, demyelination, and fibrosis of the nerve tissues.[15] It can develop at any time after the radiation treatment. Transient RIBP has also been documented and is a result of neural tissue or surrounding tissue inflammation, edema, and subsequent compression. RIBP has been documented in patients with HNC, breast cancer, lung cancer, and neoplasm of the mediastinum treated with RT.[16] The incidence of RIBP increases with age. Some patients may have higher sensitivity to RT and subsequently have an increased risk of developing RIBP.

RIBP has been estimated to affect around 22% of the patients who received RT.[2] The most common risk factors for RIBP are radiation dose, radiation technique, chemotherapy,[16] and radiation level. Radiation dose >50 Gr significantly increases the chance of neuronal injury and subsequent fibrosis.[4] The introduction of intensity-modulated radiation (IMR) allowed for more precise tumor targeting and preservation of the surrounding tissue, thus leading to less collateral damage to the adjacent healthy tissues and a lower incidence of RIBP. Chemotherapy in combination with RT seems to increase the incidence of RIBP. As for radiation level, radiation to the upper half of the cervical lymphatic drainage (levels II, III, and Va) seems to have less effect on the brachial plexus. However, radiation to the lower half of the cervical lymphatic drainage (levels IV and Vb) and especially radiation to the supraclavicular fossa seem to significantly increase the chance of RIBP.[4]

The first symptoms are usually sensory, with pain in the oral cavity, head, ipsilateral shoulder, and arm, and paresthesia (numbness, tingling, hyperesthesia) being the most frequently encountered symptom affecting nearly 50% of the patients.[2,4,15] Motor symptoms such as weakness, muscle atrophy (Fig. 8.3), diminished or absent tendon reflexes, and muscle fasciculations develop months later and may affect as

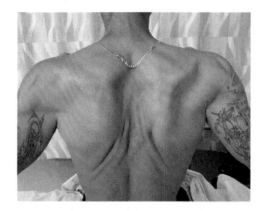

FIGURE 8.3

Right shoulder muscle wasting secondary to RIBP.

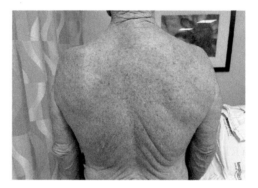

FIGURE 8.4

Left shoulder scapula winging secondary to RIBP.

many as 25% of the patients.[4,15] In HNC patients, the radiation damage affects predominantly the upper and middle trunks, predominantly in the C5 and C6 nerve root distribution.[4] Therefore, sensory and motor deficits are seen more frequently in the scapula and shoulder (Figs. 8.4–8.6). In breast cancer patients, where radiation is usually administered below the clavicle, the lower trunk of the brachial plexus is frequently injured, and the RT symptoms are seen in the hand. RIBP can be visualized on magnetic resonance imaging (MRI), whereas electromyography (EMG) and nerve conduction velocity (NCV) can be used to diagnose sensory and motor lesions.[4,16] There is no proven effective method to prevent and/or stop RIBP development, and treatment is based mostly on symptom management.[16] NSAIDs and steroids are used to decrease neuroinflammation and pain, along with opioids and gabapentin for stronger pain and paresthesia.[4,15,16] Physical therapy and occupational therapy are prescribed for cervical and shoulder ROM, pain relief, and motor function improvement. Rehabilitation focuses on gentle soft tissue and joint

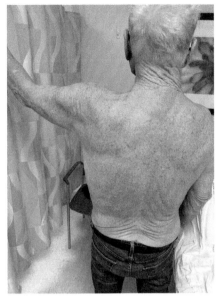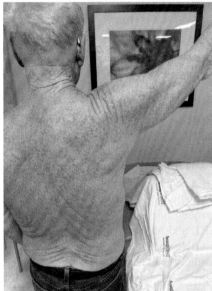

FIGURES 8.5 AND 8.6

Left shoulder muscle wasting secondary to RIBP as compared with right shoulder muscle mass.

stretching, increasing functional range of cervical extension, side bending and rotation, and shoulder mobility. Cervical and upper extremities strengthening exercises are incorporated to include gradual resistance progression along with a home exercise program education. Care is taken not to overstretch the radiated tissue, as it may lead to brachial plexus rupture.[16] For severe pain and neurovascular involvement, neurolysis is the last treatment resort and is considered an irreversible and permanent procedure.[4,16]

Drop head syndrome

Drop head syndrome (DHS) is rare, usually late-onset radiation-induced toxicity. It is characterized by weakness of the cervical extensor muscles along with fibrosis of the anterior cervical musculature and soft tissue, which results in chin-on-chest spinal deformity.[17,18] While the weakness is progressive and localized, there is no sensory involvement and paresthesia.[18] It can develop as early as 3 months after the completion of RT. DHS can lead to cervical and back pain, limited cervical ROM, dysphagia, breathing difficulties, and impaired gait.[17] It has been associated with radiation dose >50 Gy, but the etiology is not well understood.[19] Cervical bracing, either with passive brace (soft collar, Philadelphia, Miami J, Aspen Vista) or active postural brace, has been used to provide head support, reduce pain, and improve posture.[18] For mild and moderate cases, physical therapy is prescribed to improve cervical ROM, strength, posture, standing balance, and gait. Severe cases can be treated with cervical spine fusion.[17]

Lymphedema

Secondary lymphedema is a common toxicity found in many cancer patients including HNC patients. Risk factors include lymph node dissection, RT, radiation fibrosis, recurrent cancer, and additional surgeries. The addition of chemotherapy seems to increase the risk of developing lymphedema. Lymphedema is the result of impaired lymphatic drainage, which leads to the accumulation of protein-rich edema in the interstitial tissue. It develops secondary to direct tumor invasion, underlying tumor inflammation mechanism, tumor and lymph nodes dissection, RT/CRT, and fibrosis.[20−23]

HNC patients may have external, internal, or combined lymphedema. The swelling may lead to head and neck pain, stiffness, limited cervical mobility, difficulty speaking, dysphasia, hearing, vision, and respiration impairments. In extreme situations, the patient may require a tracheostomy.[20,21] In addition to the aforementioned, lymphedema carries a high psychological burden as it can cause facial and cervical disfigurement. Head and neck lymphedema is highly visible and may lead to issues with body image, self-esteem, social isolation, embarrassment, and psychological disturbance.[20,22] HNC patients seem to be particularly predisposed to depression and emotional distress due not only to the cancer treatment but also to dissatisfaction with appearance and body image.[22] The incidence of lymphedema in the HNC patients is not well established. Some studies estimate an average of 12%−75% incidence[21]; however, research by Ridner et al. found that >90% of the patients had internal, external, or combined lymphedema.[23] External lymphedema (Figs. 8.7 and 8.8) involves the soft tissue of the head and neck and can lead to tension and pain, limited cervical and shoulder ROM, and difficulty with opening the eyelids. Internal lymphedema may affect the tongue, larynx, and pharynx and can cause dysphasia, as well as difficulty with manipulating food in the mouth, respiration, and hearing. Some patients may eventually need tracheostomy and gastrostomy tube for feeding.[20]

The current treatment for HNC lymphedema involves complete decongestive therapy (CDT), physical therapy, and speech therapy.[20,21,23] CDT has four components: manual lymphatic drainage (MLD), compression therapy, exercise, and skin care. MLD is a gentle manual technique, which decongests the involved area, stimulates the mobility of the lymphatic fluid, and reroutes the lymphatic flow. Even though MLD works only on the external edema, a decrease in the external swelling triggers a reduction in the internal edema as well. Compression garments, either off the shelf or custom made, are used to exert gentle pressure and thus minimize the reaccumulation of lymphatic fluid. In HNC, they are usually worn at night, but patients with more than mild edema may need to wear them during the day as

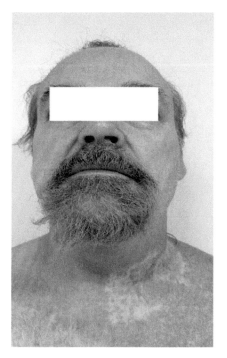

FIGURE 8.7

Head and neck external lymphedema after radiation treatment to the whole neck.

well. Exercises for the face, neck, and the upper extremities are used to improve soft tissue mobility, minimize fibrosis, improve the lymphatic flow, cervical and shoulder ROM, and posture. Patients are educated in home exercise programs and are encouraged to perform daily self-MLD, ROM, and decongestive exercises. Swallowing exercises should be done on an ongoing basis during and after RT, as they have demonstrated improved lymph flow, decrease in internal edema, prevention in constrictive fibrosis, and limited muscular atrophy.[23]

Chemotherapy

Systemic therapy is added for locoregionally and metastatic HNC management. Concomitant chemoradiotherapy (CRT) has demonstrated a survival benefit when compared with sequential treatment especially with platinum containing regiments.[24,25] HPV-positive NHC has also demonstrated sensitivity to chemoradiotherapy and better survival prognosis.[15] CRT has become a standard treatment for locoregional NHSCC.[24,25] However, it is associated with significant acute and long-term toxicities, negative impact on quality of life, and multiple, sometimes permanent functional impairments. The addition of chemotherapy to radiation seems to

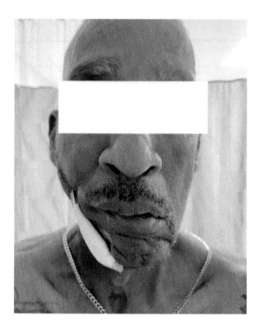

FIGURE 8.8

Lymphedema to the right side of head after tumor resection, mandibula reconstruction, and CRT.

aggravate RT complications such as xerostomia (oral dryness), fibrosis, trismus, and esophageal stenosis.[20] Chemotherapy has an accumulative effect, and regardless of the drugs used, it causes common symptoms such as CRF, peripheral neuropathy, and cognitive dysfunction.[26] These symptoms may persist for years and, unfortunately, some patients may develop permanent functional impairments. Exercise has been recommended by the American Cancer Society and Head and Neck Cancer Survivorship Care Guidelines as effective in reducing fatigue, improving balance, muscle strength, functional capacity, and quality of life.[27,28] Mild- to moderate-intensity exercises such as aerobic, flexibility, and resistance exercises have been shown to be safe and beneficial for patients who are undergoing concurrent chemoradiotherapy.[27,29,30] High-intensity exercises are not recommended as they may induce lower immune response. Exercises should follow patient-specific precautions for metastases, current, and chronic health history.

CRF may be induced by either RT and/or chemotherapy. About 60%−90% of the patients complain of fatigue while receiving treatment and 19%−38% continue to report fatigue after treatment completion.[26,29] CRF can be divided into two categories: peripheral and central. Peripheral fatigue refers to physical fatigue and lack of energy, whereas central fatigue refers to motivational fatigue.[26] CRF is disproportional to physical activity, it is not relieved by rest, and is closely associated with depression, pain, poor nutrition, sleep issues, and physical inactivity.[29,30]

Physical exercise has been shown to reduce the effects of CRF and improve fitness and quality of life.[29,30] Oncology physical therapy is recommended, and patients should be encouraged to engage in a regular exercise program.[28]

Cognitive impairment, also known as "chemobrain" or "chemofog," is another common toxicity related to chemotherapy and is reported by up to 80% of cancer patients and survivors.[26] Patients demonstrate difficulties with memory, attention, and executive function.[26,30] These cognitive problems can cause significant functional and financial burdens as patients may have trouble with activities of daily living (ADL) and may not be able to work.[30] Salerno et al. conducted a nationwide study with a cohort of 943 breast cancer patients on the relationship between chemotherapy, cognitive decline, and physical activity. The results indicated that physical activity before and during chemotherapy was associated with better cognitive function immediately and after 6 months of treatment completion.[31] Exercise is believed to be an effective behavioral intervention to improve cognitive impairment, depression, pain, anxiety, and overall function.[30]

Chemotherapy-induced peripheral neuropathy (CIPN) presents in a "glove-stocking" pattern and is reported across different chemotherapeutic agents.[26] It is characterized by pain, numbness, tingling, and temperature sensitivity, and some patients may develop skin changes in these areas. The neuropathy gradually progresses during the treatment, and some patients may be more affected than others. Once treatment is completed, the neuropathy should improve, but may persist for many months or years, and there are patients who may develop permanent neurological impairments.[28] Patients experiencing CINP may have difficulty with gross and fine motor skills such as closing hands, grasping, carrying, holding utensils and small objects, and writing. If the lower extremities are affected, the patients may experience gait and balance deficits, which may lead to falls and reduced overall mobility. In some instances, assistive devices such as a cane, walker, and wheelchair may be needed to improve the safety of transfers and gait. CIPN treatment may include pharmacology, transcutaneous nerve stimulation (TENS), acupuncture,[28] and rehabilitation services. Occupational therapy is prescribed for upper extremity desensitization, hand/fingers ROM, strengthening, and gross and fine motor skills improvement. Physical therapy is recommended for lower extremities desensitization, strengthening, endurance, balance, and gait training. Pilates, yoga, and tai chi exercises are also beneficial to improve flexibility, core strength, posture, balance, and overall strength.

Case study

The patient is a 55-year-old male who noticed left side of neck swelling in May 2021 after getting his first COVID vaccine. He attributed the edema to the vaccine and did not follow up with a physician. The mass continued to grow, and in October 2021, the patient started to experience voice changes and difficulty with turning his head. In January, he could barely speak and decided to seek medical advice. CT scan revealed a very large nodal mass in the base of the left neck extending into the inlet of the mediastinum and encasing vessels. There were enlarged lymph nodes in the left posterior cervical chain medial to the sternocleidomastoid muscle. No definitive mass was identified in the nasopharynx, oropharynx, and hypopharynx or larynx. Neck mass biopsy done in February revealed HPV-related squamous cell carcinoma (SCC). Subsequent PET scan demonstrated 8.1 × 6.8 cm FDG avid mass and metastatic disease in the left level II cervical lymph node chain. The patient was eventually diagnosed with stage T0N3M0, HPV-related, unknown primary SCC of the neck. He was treated with CRT with weekly cisplatin. The treatment started in March 2022 and was completed at the end of April 2022. The patient received cumulative cisplatin dose of 280 mg/m^2.

After the completion of treatment, the patient started to complain of significant cervical edema (Fig. 8.9), cervical pain, limited neck ROM, ringing in the ears, dry mouth, and thick saliva. He reported paresthesia (numbness and tingling) in the cervical muscles, L shoulder, hands, and feet. In addition, he also reported increased voice hoarseness and changes in high-pitch sounds. The patient was referred to physical therapy and speech therapy.

PET scan in August 2022 revealed a complete metabolic response with significant improvement in the size and resolution of abnormal FDG uptake in the cervical mass on the left side of the neck. There was no evidence of cancer recurrence and metastatic disease. In October 2022, the patient reported improved cervical edema and ROM (he was still receiving physical therapy), but continued to complain of difficulty with speaking, mouth dryness, and thick saliva. Hands and feet paresthesia had improved, and he had stopped taking gabapentin. In March 2023, the patient completed physical therapy treatment: cervical mobility has improved to normal,

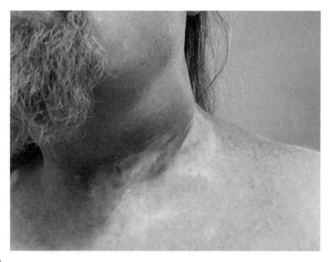

FIGURE 8.9

Cervical and left lower half of face lymphedema 2 months after completion of CRT.

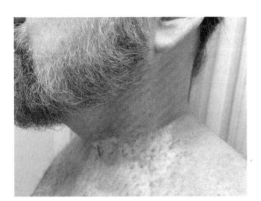
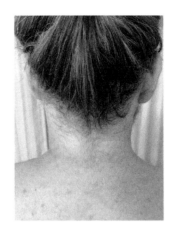

FIGURES 8.10 AND 8.11

Persistent cervical and left lower half of face lymphedema 16 months after completion of CRT.

and the pain had completely resolved. Cervical edema had improved but was still present. In August 2023, the patient was found to have left vocal cords paralysis. Speech had improved, but the patient complained that he couldn't project his voice in class—the patient is a teacher and had returned to working full time. The tinnitus was stable. The patient complained of neck tension and thickening of the skin on the left side of the neck (radiated area), along with persistent edema (Figs. 8.10 and 8.11). He was referred to continue with physical therapy (lymphedema management, cervical stretching, and strengthening) and speech therapy.

Conclusion

With a global reduction in tobacco use and increasing incidence of HPV-related HNC, there is a growing population of survivors living over 5 years, with some living a normal life span. Improved survivorship, however, allows for more treatment-related toxicities to develop, many of which lead to severe and permanent functional impairments. A multidisciplinary approach is needed to treat HNC patients from time of diagnosis to survivorship and into lifelong management of treatment-related morbidities. Physical therapy and rehabilitation services can be successfully used for the management of cervical dysfunction, CRF, chemotherapy-induced neuropathy, RIBP, weakness, and lymphedema.

References

1. Gormley M, Creaney G, Schache A, Ingarfield K, Conway D. Reviewing the epidemiology of head and neck cancer: definitions, trends, and risk factors. *Br Dent J.* 2022; 233(9):2022.
2. Azzam P, Mroueh M, Francis M, Abou Daher A, Zeidan Y. Radiation-induced neuropathies in head and neck cancer: prevention and treatment modalities. *Ecancermedicalscience.* 2020;14:1133.
3. Rahman Q, Iocca O, Kufta K, Shanti R. Global burden of head and neck cancer. *Oral Maxillofac.* 2020;32(3):367–375.
4. Cai Z, Li Y, Hu R, Rong X, Wu R, Tang Y. Radiation-induced brachial plexopathy in patients with nasopharyngeal carcinoma: a retrospective study. *Oncotarget.* 2016;7(14): 18887.
5. Powell SF, Vu L, Spanos WC, Pyeon D. The key differences between human papillomavirus-positive and −negative head and neck cancers: biological and clinical implications. *Cancers.* 2021;13:5206.
6. Thompson-Harvey A, Yetukuri M, Hansen AR, et al. Rising incidence of late-stage head and neck cancer in the United States. *Cancer J.* 2020;126(5):1090–1101.
7. Mahal BA, Catalano PJ, Haddad RI, et al. Incidence and demographic burden of HPV-associated oropharyngeal head and neck cancers in the United States. *Cancer Epidemiol.* 2019;28(10):1660–1667.
8. Perri F, Longo F, Caponigro F, et al. Management of HPV-related squamous cell carcinoma of the head and neck: pitfalls and caveat. *Cancers.* 2020;12(4):975.
9. Song JS, Vallance P, Biron V, Jeffrey CC. Epidemiological trends of head and neck cancer survivors in Alberta: towards improved understanding of the burden of disease. *J Otoraryngol Head N.* 2020;49(1):1–6.
10. Deschler DG, Moore MG, Smith RV, eds. *Quick Reference Guide to TNM Staging of Head and Neck Cancer and Neck Dissection Classification.* 4th ed. Alexandria, VA: American Academy of Otolaryngology–Head and Neck Surgery Foundation; 2014.
11. Mella MH, Chabrillac E, Dupret-Bories A, Mirallie M, Vergez S. Transoral robotic surgery for head and neck cancer: advances and residual knowledge gaps. *J Clin Med.* 2023; 12:2303.
12. Cramer J, Burtness B, Le QT, Ferris R. The changing therapeutic landscape of head and neck cancer. *Nat Rev Clin Oncol.* 2019;16:669–683.
13. Ramia P, Bodgi L, Mahmoud D, et al. Radiation-induced fibrosis in patients with head and neck cancer: a review of pathogenesis and clinical outcomes. *Clin Med Insights Oncol.* 2021;16:1–7.
14. Brook I. Late side effects of radiation treatment for head and neck cancer. *Radiat Oncol J.* 2020;38(2):84–92.
15. Delanian S, Lefaix J, Pradat P. Radiation-induced neuropathy in cancer survivors. *Radiother Oncol.* 2012;105:273–282.
16. Kibici K, Erok B, Atca AO. Radiation-induced brachial plexopathy in breast cancer and the role of surgical treatment. *Indian J Neurosurg.* 2020;9(2):99–105.
17. Verla T, Vedantam A, North R, et al. Surgical Management of postradiation, dropped head spinal deformity in patients with head and neck cancer. *World Neurosurg.* 2021; 156:e1–e8.

18. Knowlton SE, Zheng M, Diamond Y, Yakaboski M, Ruppert L. Bracing to treat dropped head syndrome in cancer patients: a retrospective review. *J Prosthet Orthot*. 2021;33(1): 20−25.

19. Inaba K, Nakamura S, Okamoto H, et al. Early-onset dropped head syndrome after radiotherapy for head and neck cancer: dose constrains for neck extensor muscles. *J Radiat*. 2016;57(2):169−173.

20. Smith BG, Lewin JS. The role of lymphedema management in head and neck cancer. *Curr Opin Otolaryngol Head Neck Surg*. 2010;18(3):153−158.

21. Jackson LK, Ridner SH, Deng J, et al. Internal lymphedema correlates with subjective and objective measures of dysphagia in head and neck cancer patients. *J Palliat Med*. 2016;19(9):949−956.

22. Deng J, Ridner SH, Murphy BA. Lymphedema in patients with head and neck cancer. *Oncol Nurs Forum*. 2011;38(1):E1−E10.

23. Ridner SH, Dietrich MS, Niermann K, Cmelak A, Mannion K, Murphy B. A prospective study of the lymphedema and fibrosis continuum in patients with head and neck cancer. *Lymphatic Res Biol*. 2016;14(4):198−205.

24. Rosenberg AJ, Vokes E. Optimizing treatment de-escalation in head and neck cancer: current and future perspectives. *Oncologist*. 2021;26(1):40−48.

25. Shibata H, Saito S, Uppaluri R. Immunotherapy for head and neck cancer: a paradigm shift from induction chemotherapy to neoadjuvant immunotherapy. *Front Oncol*. 2021; 11:727433.

26. Vichaya EG, Chiu GS, Krukowski K, et al. Mechanisms of chemotherapy-induced behavioral toxicities. *Front Neurosci*. 2015;9:131.

27. Lin K-Y, Cheng H-C, Yen C-J, et al. Effects of exercise in patients undergoing chemotherapy for head and neck cancer: a pilot randomized control trial. *Int J Environ Res Publ Health*. 2021;18:1291.

28. Goyal N, Day A, Epstein J, Goodman J, et al. Head and neck cancer survivorship consensus statement from the American Head and Neck society. *Laryngoscope Investig Otolaryngol*. 2022;7:70−92.

29. Pachman DR, Barton DL, Swetz KM, Loprinzi CL. Troublesome symptoms in cancer survivors: fatigue, insomnia, neuropathy, and pain. *J Clin Oncol*. 2012;41:7238.

30. Mustain KM, Sprod LK, Janelsins M, Peppone LJ, Mohile S. Exercise recommendations for cancer related fatigue, cognitive impairment, sleep problems, depression, pain, anxiety, and physical dysfunction: a review. *Oncol Hematol Rev*. 2013;8(2):81−88.

31. Salerno EA, Culakova E, Kleckner AS, et al. Physical activity patterns and relationships with cognitive function in patients with breast cancer before, during, and after chemotherapy in prospective, nationwide study. *J Clin Oncol*. 2021;39(29):3283−3297.

Shoulder dysfunction in head and neck cancer

9

Romer B. Orada, DO [1] and Victor F. Leite, MD [2,3]

[1]*Miami Cancer Institute, Baptist Health South Florida, Miami, FL, United States;* [2]*University of Sao Paulo, Sao Paulo, Brazil;* [3]*Hospital Israelita Albert Einstein, São Paulo, SP, Brazil*

Overview

Head and neck cancer (HNC) is one of the most common cancers and is an important cause of mortality and morbidity. According to the American Cancer Society's 2023 Cancer Statistics, HNC accounts for about 4% of all cancers in the United States.[1] In 2023, an estimated 66,920 people will be diagnosed in the United States. Worldwide, an estimated 562,328 people were diagnosed in 2020. It is estimated that 15,400 deaths will occur in the United States in 2023. In 2020, an estimated 277,597 people worldwide died from the disease.[1]

HNC has been an area of research for decades, with a particular focus on understanding the physiological and psychological effects of the disease. With increases in survivorship for patients with HNC, attention is turning to quality-of-life issues for survivors. Rehabilitation interventions are patient-specific and aim to prevent, restore, compensate, and palliate symptoms and sequelae of treatment for optimal functioning.[2]

HNC is a complex health condition that can affect a person's physical and mental health, but it can also have a tremendous impact on the patient's shoulders. Shoulder pain and dysfunction are common symptoms especially after neck dissection as a treatment.[3] This may result in muscle weakness, affect the stability of the shoulder joint resulting in pain, decreased mobility, fatigue, limited ability to perform activities of daily living, and even further complications. While it may seem like a minor issue when compared with other symptoms of HNC, its impact should not be ignored as it could lead to long-term functional impairments.

Shoulder dysfunction is one of the most observed physical side effects associated with HNC. This chapter will discuss the common causes of shoulder dysfunction in those affected by HNC, as well as treatments available, to reduce its impacts on a patient's quality of life.

Head and Neck Cancer Rehabilitation. https://doi.org/10.1016/B978-0-443-11806-7.00001-1
Copyright © 2025 Elsevier Inc. All rights reserved, including those for text and data mining, AI training, and similar technologies.

Definition and causes

HNC treatment sequelae may cause musculoskeletal impairment such as trismus, spinal accessory nerve (SAN) palsy, and radiation-induced neck fibrosis that can lead to shoulder dysfunction and disability, chronic neck pain, and postural deficits[4] and can potentially be overlooked with management of head and neck cancer patients.[5]

For some survivors, pain remains a significant problem and associated with worse quality of life.[6] The prevalence and incidence of shoulder and neck dysfunction after neck dissection varies by the type of surgery performed and how the dysfunction is measured. According to a systematic review article, the prevalence rates for shoulder pain were slightly higher after radical neck dissection (RND) (range, 10%–100%) compared with modified radical neck dissection (MRND) (range, 0%–100%) and selective neck dissection (SND) (range, 9%–25%). The incidence of reduced shoulder active range of motion depended on surgery type (range, 5%–20%), with more aggressive surgeries resulting in higher impairments. Type of neck dissection was a risk factor for shoulder pain, reduced function, and health-related quality of life.[7]

SND has become a mainstay of HNC treatment. SND helps reduce the incidence of complications associated with RND while achieving the same oncological results, especially in clinically node-negative (cN0) cases[8]; however, the most common complication with SND is shoulder syndrome from spinal accessory nerve (SAN) trauma resulting in dysfunction and shoulder disability. Extensive dissection in neck levels 2 and 5 (especially level IIb dissection) leads to SAN dysfunction.[9] Relevant SAN anatomy and its relation with neck muscles is shown in Fig. 9.1.

Even when the spinal accessory nerve is preserved, neck dissection results in a high probability of postoperative shoulder functional impairment. Data from a prospective cohort showed that about 42% of individuals were unable to abduct their shoulders by 150 degrees or more 6 months after surgery.[10] Postoperative radiation therapy was a predictor of poor shoulder function in the early postoperative period; both level V dissection and head and neck irradiation were predictors of poor shoulder function at 6 and 9 months after neck dissection.[10]

Radiation therapy involves the use of high-energy beams consisting of photons or particles such as protons, neutrons and electrons to destroy cancer cells by direct DNA or indirect tissue damage by the production of reactive oxygen species.[11] However, these packets of energy can also damage the healthy tissues surrounding the tumor site which can lead to inflammation that can evolve into a fibrotic process and eventually causing radiation fibrosis.[12] These healthy tissues may include the skin leading to dermatitis/ulceration, muscles (myopathy), ligaments (rupture), nerves/roots (radiculopathy/plexopathy/neuropathy), and other connective tissues in the shoulder region.[11] Depending on the total volume of tissue treated along with radiation dose used, over time, radiation-induced fibrosis and scarring can occur leading to pain, stiffness, and limited range of motion in the affected shoulder.

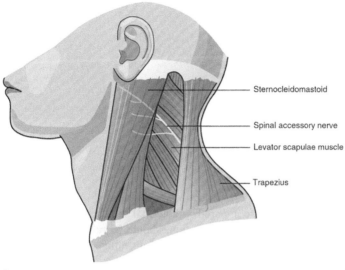

FIGURE 9.1

Anatomy of the spinal accessory nerve and its relation with neck muscles.

With permission from Rightslink #5619570612456.

Symptoms and physical findings

Shoulder dysfunction is a painful impairment that can cause a great deal of physical and emotional discomfort. Symptoms include persistent pain in the shoulder, limited range of motion, and impaired ability to raise one's arm or reach behind their back. Pain can be triggered during everyday tasks such as washing hair, reaching for an object off the top shelf at the store or even carrying groceries. Common causes of shoulder dysfunction in the HNC population are spinal accessory nerve (SAN) neuropathy, rotator cuff tears, adhesive capsulitis, bursitis, and arthritis. For the purpose of this chapter, the focus on SAN trauma is highlighted.

Signs of localized muscle atrophy may indicate a nerve injury, such as the accessory nerve or the dorsal scapular nerve.

The SAN is the main motor nerve of the trapezius and sternocleidomastoid muscles. If injured, functions such as elevation of the shoulder, rotation and tilting of the head, and flexion of the neck can be limited or even made impossible. It can lead to muscle weakness, limited range of motion (ROM), and shoulder tilt and pain, which can reduce patient functioning.[13] Although the spinal accessory nerve is preserved during most surgeries, shoulder pain and dysfunction still occur in 20%−60% of patients.[3]

Physical findings may include localized muscle atrophy, masses, and signs of radiation-induced injuries (Fig. 9.2).

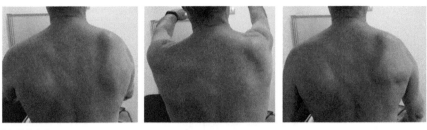

FIGURE 9.2

Physical examination in a patient with right SAN neuropathy.

With permission from Rightslink #5618780684255.

Decreased shoulder flexion, abduction, and increased pain are commonly associated with neck dissection compared with normal shoulders. Coexisting myofascial pain in the face, neck, and scapular regions should be ruled out, as they may be an important source of referred shoulder pain and disability. Other differential diagnoses include cervical spine and brachial plexus pathologies.

Abnormalities of supraspinatus tendon and subdeltoid bursa on sonography and trapezius muscle atrophy may play a key role in shoulder pain and shoulder flexion and abduction limitations.[14]

Diagnostic tests

Diagnostic tests should be guided by that hypothesis elicited during history and physical exam to ensure that the patient receives proper treatment. An experienced clinician should start with a thorough clinical exam to observe pain levels, physical deficits, and range of motion. Next, X-rays may be considered to assess for any osseous etiology, especially for those with advanced disease, or muscle asymmetry. In case a nerve injury is suspected, an electromyographic test (EMG) and nerve conduction study (NCS) should be performed.

Both MRI and US are possible tools for assessing SAN neuropathy and nerve continuity, although US performed by experienced radiologists has been reported to be superior to MRI in a small retrospective study.[15] Sonographic findings can include significant decrease in thickness and change in the echographic pattern of the trapezius muscle and loss of continuity in the SAN.[14–16]

In case a musculoskeletal disorder is suspected, a shoulder ultrasound or MRI and cervical spine MRI should be considered. In the case of shoulder pathologies, although both imaging modalities have similar accuracy for diagnosing subacromial bursitis, full- and partial-thickness rotator cuff tears,[17] MRI is superior when assessing labrum or intraarticular or bone pathologies, such as metastasis. Sonographic findings can include significant decrease in thickness of the trapezius muscle, abnormal findings of supraspinatus tendon, and subdeltoid bursa on the surgical side.[14–16] The ratio of trapezius muscle atrophy was related to shoulder pain, and subdeltoid bursa abnormalities had significant limitations on shoulder flexion and abduction.[14]

Treatment options

There are multiple treatment options for shoulder pain in head and neck cancer survivors. Treatment selection is guided by etiology and location of pain. For instance, shoulder pain caused by SAN neuropathy will be treated differently from cervical myofascial pain or rotator cuff tendinopathy. As a general principle, the treatment plan is focused on improving scapulothoracic biomechanics with range of motion and strengthening exercises (among others); providing analgesia with a combination of patient education, modalities, and medications. In select cases, orthoses can be helpful. In cases where those treatments are not sufficient, or pain is such that those treatments are not feasible, interventional procedures should be considered.

Exercises

There is moderate-certainty evidence that a supervised progressive resistance training focused in the scapular region is efficacious in improving shoulder pain and dysfunction after HNC.[3] In case neuropathic symptoms are present, nerve desensitization techniques, such as applying different textures and temperatures in a graded fashion, are recommended. In the case of shoulder pathologies not associated with cancer, rehabilitation is also recommended.[18]

Modalities

Modalities are the use of physical energies that cause physiological changes, such as ultrasound, photobiomodulation (or low-level laser therapy), or electrical stimulation.

Controlled data for the efficacy of modalities in shoulder dysfunction in the HNC population is lacking, although it is possible that photobiomodulation could be an adjunct in the treatment of HNC lymphedema,[19] which is potential etiology of shoulder pain.

Data from noncancer individuals with nonspecific shoulder pain and subacromial impingement syndrome show that pretensioned tape, ultrasound, and interferential current were found to be noneffective.[20] Despite that, several guidelines still suggest that those modalities "may be recommended" for adhesive capsulitis.[18] In the noncancer population with adhesive capsulitis, there is low quality evidence that photobiomodulation for 6 days is superior to placebo, and moderate evidence that photobiomodulation plus exercise for 8 weeks is superior to exercise alone.[21]

Acupuncture

There is low-certainty evidence that acupuncture is superior to conventional treatment for shoulder pain in the HNC population.[3] Although we do not recommend using acupuncture as a single treatment for those cases, it can definitely be an adjunct to the rehabilitation program.

Medications

Nociceptive pain due to shoulder pathology may be treated with analgesics such as a acetaminophen.[18] Several guidelines also suggest the use of NSAIDs,[18] although there is a controversial risk of this class of medication impairing tendon repair.[22] In select cases of moderate to intense pain, weak opioids could be used for a short periods of time.

Neuropathic pain can be treated with medications such as tricyclic antidepressants, serotonin norepinephrine reuptake inhibitors, gabapentinoids, and topical substances, among others.[23]

Injections

There are multiple interventional targets for treating pain in the shoulder. Choosing the most appropriate procedure depends on the etiology and topography of pain. As a general principle, one should start with procedures that are closest to the pain source, and progress to more distant ones in case there is no response. The following list is not exhaustive and includes the most common procedures we see in our practice for shoulder pain in HNC.

- Trigger-point injections or dry needling[24]
  - Myofascial pain
- Botulinum toxin injections[25]
  - Persistent myofascial pain, and peripheral neuropathy
- Subacromial bursa injection[18]
  - Shoulder tendinopathy or bursitis
- Peritendinous or intratendinous injections[18]
  - Shoulder tendinopathy
- Intraarticular[18]
  - Osteoarthritis, adhesive capsulitis, and other sources of intraarticular pain, such as osteonecrosis
- Nerve blocks
  - Neuropathic pain, bursitis, shoulder tendinopathy or intraarticular pain
- Radiofrequency
  - Cases where nerve blocks results were short-lived but effective

Surgery

In cases where a complete nerve injury occurred, as evidenced by loss of trapezius function on physical exam and NCS/EMG findings, a nerve repair surgery should be considered,[26,27] since denervated muscles will lose tonus and capacity over time. Although the optimum timing for surgical repair remains unknown, a retrospective study spanning 30 years of experience in reconstructive SAN surgery reported that the nerve injuries repaired within 3–6 months of lesion had better functional outcomes than those operated more than 8–12 months after.[28] Imaging modalities such as the United States can be useful in surgical planning, particularly assessing nerve continuity and identifying injury sites.[15,16] Lesions with nerve continuity and positive nerve action potentials can be treated with neurolysis, and for the remaining cases, end-to-end suture or interposition graft repair can be considered.[28] Nerve repair surgery can have high success rates. The abovementioned three-decades-long retrospective study showed preoperative shoulder abduction strength ≥3 in 0% of their cohort, compared with 87% 1 year postsurgery.[28]

Intraarticular shoulder pathologies that are refractory to conservative therapies could be considered for a shoulder arthroplasty.[29]

Complications of shoulder dysfunction

Shoulder dysfunction is a serious issue with long-term consequences. It can lead to loss of function, impairment, and even disability in some cases. Chronic pain caused by shoulder dysfunction can significantly reduce the quality of life of those affected and restrict their personal activities as well as their occupation. People who suffer from shoulder dysfunction often have restricted range of motion and lack strength, which in turn leads to instability in the shoulder joint, making it hard for them to perform even simple activities such as reaching up or pushing objects.

The effects of shoulder dysfunction are far-reaching and should not be ignored. In addition to physical impairment, there may be psychological implications due to ongoing pain and fatigue caused by the condition. Furthermore, individuals may not be able to work if they cannot perform necessary tasks required by their job without experiencing pain or discomfort. Many survivors exhibit late dysfunction—a survivorship clinic including surveillance by rehabilitation specialists may optimize identification of dysfunction.[30]

Conclusion

Shoulder dysfunction can be a major factor for HNC survivors as it causes pain, discomfort, and loss of mobility. Shoulder pain is frequent and can have multiple etiologies, especially in patients with high gross tumor nodal volume receiving chemoradiotherapy, long-term neck and shoulder impairment was associated with increased pain and stiffness, difficulty lifting objects, reaching overhead, and overall ability to perform work-related tasks.[31] Without proper diagnosis and treatment, quality of life can become significantly affected. Thus, it is important to identify the signs of shoulder dysfunction to provide effective treatment that takes into account the specific needs of each individual patient.

An interdisciplinary approach should be taken when dealing with such an issue since the physical and/or psychological components may need to be addressed in tandem. With accurate identification and appropriate treatment plans tailored to individual patient's needs, which usually includes exercises, oral medication and in some cases of intense and/or refractory pain, interventional pain procedures, and in rare select cases, surgical procedures, shoulder dysfunction may be alleviated, leading to improved health outcomes in head and neck cancer patients.

References

1. Siegel RL, Miller KD, Wagle NS, Jemal A. Cancer statistics, 2023. *CA A Cancer J Clin.* 2023;73(1):17−48.
2. Jamal N, Ebersole B, Erman A, Chhetri D. Maximizing functional outcomes in head and neck cancer survivors: assessment and rehabilitation. *Otolaryngol Clin.* 2017;50(4): 837−852.
3. Almeida KAM, Rocha AP, Carvas N, Pinto A. Rehabilitation interventions for shoulder dysfunction in patients with head and neck cancer: systematic review and meta-analysis. *Phys Ther.* 2020;100(11):1997−2008.
4. Ghiam MK, Mannion K, Dietrich MS, Stevens KL, Gilbert J, Murphy BA. Assessment of musculoskeletal impairment in head and neck cancer patients. *Support Care Cancer.* 2017;25(7):2085−2092.
5. Baldoman D, Vandenbrink R. Physical therapy challenges in head and neck cancer. *Cancer Treat Res.* 2018;174:209−223.
6. Cramer JD, Johnson JT, Nilsen ML. Pain in head and neck cancer survivors: prevalence, predictors, and quality-of-life impact. *Otolaryngol Head Neck Surg.* 2018;159(5): 853−858.
7. Gane EM, Michaleff ZA, Cottrell MA, et al. Prevalence, incidence, and risk factors for shoulder and neck dysfunction after neck dissection: a systematic review. *Eur J Surg Oncol.* 2017;43(7):1199−1218.
8. Garreau B, Dubreuil PA, Bondaz M, Majoufre C, Etchebarne M. The necessity of level IIb dissection for clinically negative neck oral squamous cell carcinoma. *J Stomatol Oral Maxillofac Surg.* 2020;121(6):658−660.
9. Dziegielewski PT, McNeely ML, Ashworth N, et al. 2b or not 2b? Shoulder function after level 2b neck dissection: a double-blind randomized controlled clinical trial. *Cancer.* 2020;126(7):1492−1501.
10. Imai T, Sato Y, Abe J, et al. Shoulder function after neck dissection: assessment via a shoulder-specific quality-of-life questionnaire and active shoulder abduction. *Auris Nasus Larynx.* 2021;48(1):138−147.
11. Stubblefield MD. In: *Radiation Fibrosis Syndrome.* New York: Springer Publishing Company; 2011:989−1010.

12. Hauer-Jensen M, Fink LM, Wang J. Radiation injury and the protein C pathway. *Crit Care Med*. 2004;32(5 Suppl):S325–S330.

13. Veyseller B, Aksoy F, Ozturan O, et al. Open functional neck dissection: surgical efficacy and electrophysiologic status of the neck and accessory nerve. *J Otolaryngol Head Neck Surg*. 2010;39(4):403–409.

14. Huang Y-C, Lee Y-Y, Tso H-H, et al. The sonography and physical findings on shoulder after selective neck dissection in patients with head and neck cancer: a pilot study. *BioMed Res Int*. 2019;2019:2528492.

15. Emily C, Bin L, Scott WW, et al. Ultrasound imaging of nerves in the neck. *Neurology Clin Pract*. 2020;10(5):415.

16. Shen J, Chen W, Ye X, et al. Ultrasound in the management of iatrogenic spinal accessory nerve palsy at the posterior cervical triangle area. *Muscle Nerve*. 2019;59(1):64–69.

17. Roy JS, Braën C, Leblond J, et al. Diagnostic accuracy of ultrasonography, MRI and MR arthrography in the characterisation of rotator cuff disorders: a systematic review and meta-analysis. *Br J Sports Med*. 2015;49(20):1316–1328.

18. Doiron-Cadrin P, Lafrance S, Saulnier M, et al. Shoulder rotator cuff disorders: a systematic review of clinical practice guidelines and semantic analyses of recommendations. *Arch Phys Med Rehabil*. 2020;101(7):1233–1242.

19. Robijns J, Nair RG, Lodewijckx J, et al. Photobiomodulation therapy in management of cancer therapy-induced side effects: WALT position paper 2022. *Front Oncol*. 2022;12:927685.

20. Yu H, Côté P, Shearer HM, et al. Effectiveness of passive physical modalities for shoulder pain: systematic review by the Ontario protocol for traffic injury management collaboration. *Phys Ther*. 2015;95(3):306–318.

21. Page MJ, Green S, Kramer S, Johnston RV, McBain B, Buchbinder R. Electrotherapy modalities for adhesive capsulitis (frozen shoulder). *Cochrane Database Syst Rev*. 2014;(10):Cd011324.

22. Constantinescu DS, Campbell MP, Moatshe G, Vap AR. Effects of perioperative nonsteroidal anti-inflammatory drug administration on soft tissue healing: a systematic review of clinical outcomes after sports medicine orthopaedic surgery procedures. *Orthop J Sports Med*. 2019;7(4).

23. Bates D, Schultheis BC, Hanes MC, et al. A comprehensive algorithm for management of neuropathic pain. *Pain Med*. 2019;20(Suppl 1):S2–s12.

24. Thottungal A, Kumar P, Bhaskar A. Interventions for myofascial pain syndrome in cancer pain: recent advances: why, when, where and how. *Curr Opin Support Palliat Care*. 2019;13(3):262–269.

25. Bach CA, Wagner I, Lachiver X, Baujat B, Chabolle F. Botulinum toxin in the treatment of post-radiosurgical neck contracture in head and neck cancer: a novel approach. *Eur Ann Otorhinolaryngol Head Neck Dis*. 2012;129(1):6–10.

26. Cambon-Binder A, Preure L, Dubert-Khalifa H, Marcheix PS, Belkheyar Z. Spinal accessory nerve repair using a direct nerve transfer from the upper trunk: results with 2 years follow-up. *J Hand Surg Eur*. 2018;43(6):589–595.

27. Rasulić L, Savić A, Vitošević F, et al. Iatrogenic peripheral nerve injuries-surgical treatment and outcome: 10 years' experience. *World Neurosurg*. 2017;103:841–851.

28. Park SH, Esquenazi Y, Kline DG, Kim DH. Surgical outcomes of 156 spinal accessory nerve injuries caused by lymph node biopsy procedures. *J Neurosurg Spine*. 2015;23(4):518–525.

29. American Academy of Orthopaedic Surgeons. Management of glenohumeral joint osteoarthritis. *J Am Acad Orthop Surg.* 2020;28(19):781−789.

30. Ebersole B, McCarroll L, Ridge JA, et al. Identification and management of late dysfunction in survivors of head and neck cancer: implementation and outcomes of an interdisciplinary quality of life (IQOL) clinic. *Head Neck.* 2021;43(7):2124−2135.

31. Burgin SJM, Spector ME, Pearson AT, et al. Long-term neck and shoulder function among survivors of oropharyngeal squamous cell carcinoma treated with chemoradiation as assessed with the neck dissection impairment index. *Head Neck.* 2021;43(5):1621−1628.

Head and neck cancer associated lymphedema

10

Carolina Gutiérrez, MD [1] and John C. Rasmussen, PhD [2]

[1]*Department of Physical Medicine and Rehabilitation, The University of Texas Health Science Center at Houston, Houston, TX, United States;* [2]*Brown Foundation Institute of Molecular Medicine, The University of Texas Health Science Center at Houston, Houston, TX, United States*

Cancer is a disease in which cells of the body grow out of control, negatively affecting the surrounding tissues and, if left untreated, can result in death. Cancers of the head and neck (H&N) arise from tissues associated with the oral cavity such as the tongue, gums, nose, sinuses, salivary glands, larynx, and pharynx, including nasopharynx, oropharynx, and hypopharynx, but do not include brain cancers or cancers of the eye. The majority of H&N cancers are squamous cell carcinomas. Risk factors include tobacco use, alcohol use, a combination of tobacco and alcohol, and/or infection associated with the human papillomavirus (HPV) especially type 16.[1]

H&N cancers account for about 4% of all cancers in the United States, and in 2023, an estimated 66,920 people, including 49,190 men and 17,730 women, will be diagnosed with H&N cancer with 15,400 individuals succumbing to the disease.[1] H&N cancer is three to four times more likely to occur in men than women; however, the rate of H&N cancer in women has been rising for several decades. Treatments for H&N cancer may include surgery, radiation, chemotherapy, immunotherapy, and targeted therapy.

The 5-year relative survival rate from 2013 until 2019 was 68.5%[2]; thus, large numbers of H&N cancer survivors live to experience the short- and long-term side effects of the cancer and cancer treatment including H&N lymphedema. Given that many H&N cancer patients, particularly those with HPV-associated cancers, are being diagnosed and completing treatment at younger ages, these survivors will deal with the long-term side effects of the disease and treatment, including H&N lymphedema, for decades. These side effects can include loss of critical functions, such as swallow and speech, tracheostomy, impaired range of motion, scarring of the face and neck, and lymphedema. In this chapter, we will focus on H&N lymphedema, which is manifested by chronic swelling of the tissues, and which may be underreported and underrecognized but is believed to impact more that 75%[3] of survivors.

Head and Neck Cancer Rehabilitation. https://doi.org/10.1016/B978-0-443-11806-7.00011-4
Copyright © 2025 Elsevier Inc. All rights are reserved, including those for text and data mining, AI training, and similar technologies.

Epidemiology of H&N cancer and associated lymphedema

The lymphatic system is a secondary vascular system found throughout the body that, in many ways, acts as an interstitial sewer system by taking up excess water and macromolecules, including proteins, cellular debris, and foreign contaminants, transporting the resulting fluid, or lymph, unidirectionally through a network of lymphatic vessels for immune presentation in the lymph nodes, and ultimately for delivery into the blood vasculature. When functioning properly, the lymphatics ensure fluid homeostasis, prevent the accumulation of toxic substances within the tissues, and help regulate the body's immune response.

When lymphatic drainage is disrupted, swelling may occur in the upstream tissues and, when chronic, frequently results in lymphedema, an incurable condition characterized by irreversible swelling, tissue fibrosis, skin changes, reduced wound healing, and increased incidence of infection. In addition to the health impact, these changes negatively impact the psychosocioeconomic well-being of the affected individuals. While mosquito-borne parasites account for the majority of cases of lymphedema worldwide, in developed countries, lymphedema is generally acquired as a result of cancer and/or cancer-related treatments. In some such cases, the tumors themselves grow to a size that obstruct the lymphatic vessels or nodes, thus impeding the movement of lymph through the lymphatics. However, most cancer-related cases of lymphedema result from the trauma associated with the cancer treatment itself, as lymph nodes are removed, either for staging or treatment, and/or lymphatic vessels are severely damaged during radiation treatment. When lymphedema results from trauma or insult to the lymphatics, it is often referred to as secondary lymphedema. Primary lymphedema is rare, of genetic origin, and is typically classified by time of onset including (1) congenital lymphedema, which is diagnosed at birth or within the first couple of years of life; (2) lymphedema praecox, which occurs between puberty and age 35; and (3) lymphedema tarda, which occurs after the age of 35.

Breast cancer—related lymphedema (BCRL) is perhaps the most widely recognized and studied form of secondary lymphedema in the United States, due at least impart to the relatively high incidence of breast cancer, compared with other cancers, and how visible/apparent the swelling can be when present in the hand and/or arm of the patient. Cumulatively, approximately 8% of breast cancer survivors who undergo sentinel lymph node biopsy alone and 24.9% of breast cancer survivors who undergo complete axillary node dissection develop BCRL, with more invasive procedures having higher rates of incidence.[4,5] Similar incidences of lower limb and genital lymphedema are reported in prostate[6] and gynecologic[7] cancer survivors. The reported incidence of H&N cancer-related lymphedema ranges from 12% to 90%[8] and is particularly important to diagnose and treat as chronic swelling in the proximity of critical structures can impact vital functions including respiration and swallowing. It is not clear why some cancer survivors develop lymphedema and others, who underwent similarly invasive procedures, do not, although it has been hypothesized that some individuals may have a genetic predisposition for lymphedema (for review, see Kapellas et al.[9]).

Anatomy of H&N lymphatics

As blood is pumped through the blood capillaries, water and nutrients filter through the vessel walls into the interstitial space. As the filtrate, known as interstitial fluid, washes between the cells, it picks up cellular wastes and foreign contaminates, and is subsequently taken up by the initial lymphatics. The initial lymphatics consist of loosely connected lymphatic endothelial cells that overlap, allowing water and macromolecules to enter the saclike structures but restricting their return to the interstitial space. As the initial lymphatics fill, the fluid, or lymph as it is now called, moves into the lymphatic capillaries or microvessels, which transport the lymph to larger collecting lymphatic vessels. The collecting lymphatics are made up of series of subunits called lymphangions, which are sheathed with smooth muscle cells and contract serially to pump lymph through the vessel. Each lymphangion is bounded by valves to prevent lymphatic reflux and promote the unidirectional movement of lymph. The collecting lymphatics pump lymph through lymph nodes where it is filtered and cellular wastes, abnormal cells, and foreign contaminants such as bacteria and viruses are presented for immune response. The filtered lymph is then transported through larger and deeper lymphatic vessels, including trunks and ducts, and returned to the blood vessels at the subclavian veins. The upper right quadrant of the body, including the right half of the head, drains to the right lymphatic duct and into the right subclavian vein, while the remainder of the body, including the left half of the head, drains to the thoracic duct and into the left subclavian vein. For an in-depth review of the lymphatics, their development, and role in health and disease, see Oliver et al.[10]

Despite the H&N making up a relatively small portion of the overall volume of the body, they account for approximately 300 of the body's 800 lymph nodes. Because of the sheer number of lymph nodes and the various organs and tissues in the H&N, the lymphatic pathways can be complex and involve multiple clusters of lymph nodes (for detailed descriptions, see Foldi[11]). Many of the lymph nodes are superficial, including the submental, submandibular, parotid, mastoid, occipital, and other lymph nodes, and are generally arranged in a ring shape around the lower portion of the head near the top of the neck (Fig. 10.1A). The superficial nodes receive lymph from the skin, face, and neck and drain to subsequent deep lymph nodes, which are generally arranged vertically along the neck. While the deep lymph nodes receive lymph from the superficial lymph nodes, they also provide the initial draining pathways for deeper tissues as well as for sections of more superficial organs including the eye and ear. Regardless of origin, the H&N lymphatics converge into the deep cervical lymph nodes, which in turn drain into the jugular lymphatic trunks, and ultimately into the right lymphatic or thoracic ducts.

While the specific drainage patterns of an area of the H&N can involve multiple routes, in general, each section drains down and away (left or right) from the vertical midline of the face toward the base of the neck as shown in Fig. 10.1A (arrows). For

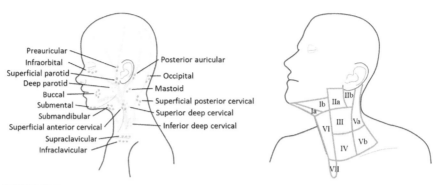

FIGURE 10.1

(A) Illustration of lymph nodes and the general lymphatic drainage patterns (*green arrows*) of the H&N. Note, this illustration is not an exhaustive representation of all the H&N lymph nodes, for a more complete description of the lymph nodes and draining pathways, see Foldi.[11]. (B) Schematic illustrating the classification levels of cervical lymph nodes frequently used for the purpose of H&N cancer staging and therapy planning.

cancer-related treatment purposes, the cervical lymph nodes are often classified by the region of the H&N in which they are found as shown in Fig. 10.1B. In this chapter, we do not consider the lymphatic drainage of the central nervous system, which has distinct, but poorly understood, features and pathways that eventually drain into the cervical lymph nodes.[12]

Pathology

Lymphedema is a common sequelae of H&N cancer treatment and is more prevalent in individuals who undergo extensive lymph node dissections in the neck followed by radiation treatment. The lymphatic trauma associated with such treatments results in the accumulation of protein-rich fluids, which triggers irreversible changes in the skin and soft tissues including skin thickening, adipose tissue deposition, and fibrosis. The immune system is also compromised, leaving the individual at increased risk of infection, particularly of cellulitis. While upregulated inflammation pathways are clearly implicated in the development and progression of lymphedema, the underlaying cellular and molecular mechanisms associated with these changes are not clearly understood. It is likely that some genetic predisposition may play a role in the development of cancer-related lymphedema. For more comprehensive reviews of what is currently known about the pathological mechanisms of lymphedema development, see Sung et al.[13] and Bernas et al.[14]

H&N cancer-associated lymphedema is particularly challenging owing to the proximity of critical structures in the H&N where even small amounts of swelling can dramatically impact the patient's ability to speak, swallow, and/or breathe and may necessitate additional life-sustaining interventions including tracheotomy and/ or the insertion of a feeding tube. The swelling in H&N lymphedema can be external, internal, or both. External swelling occurs in the superficial tissues and is the easiest to observe and diagnose.

Fig. 10.2 illustrates an example of external swelling in the face and submental region. Left untreated, external swelling may cause the eyes to swell shut, while skin changes including fibrosis and papillomatosis, increase in severity. Internal swelling occurs in the deeper tissues of the neck and may not be readily apparent from external observation. While internal swelling may be visible in the mucosa at the back of the throat, endoscopy may be necessary to measure the swelling in the deeper mucosa including the trachea, esophagus, and voice box. In addition to swelling and fibrosis, symptoms of H&N lymphedema may include heaviness,

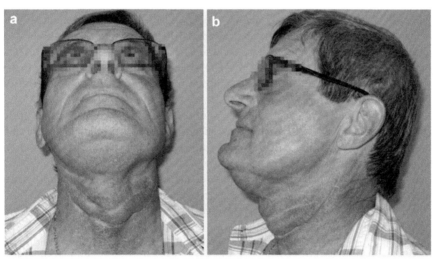

FIGURE 10.2

Example images of a patient with bilateral H&N lymphedema. Note the general puffiness the cheeks and submental areas including swollen areas in the neck above the scar line. While onset frequently occurs within the first 3 months after cancer treatment, years may pass before onset. Staging of external disease is based largely on observed tissue changes with stage 0 including patient reported symptoms such as heaviness in the neck but without any observable swelling or tissue changes. Stage 1 includes the observation of mild, reversible swelling, with (1b) or without (1a) pitting. In stage 2, the swelling becomes irreversible but without visible tissue changes. The onset of stage 3 lymphedema is marked by the development of fibrosis and other irreversible tissue changes. Staging of internal disease follows a similar progression of symptoms, but is more complicated by the difficulty of assessing internal swelling.

Reproduced from Ayestaray B, Bekara F, Andreoletti JB. π-Shaped lymphaticovenular anastomosis for head and neck lymphoedema: a preliminary study. J Plast Reconstr Aesthetic Surg 2013;66(2):201–206 (Published by Elsevier).

numbness, stiffness, tingling and/or pain in the skin or muscles of the face, head, or neck, changes in vision or hearing, and/or difficulties with breathing, swallowing, and speech.

Diagnosis
Clinical assessment and history

When evaluating a patient for H&N cancer–related lymphedema, the clinical history and physical examination play an essential role. Lymphedema frequently presents within 3 months after treatment, including surgery and/or radiation, but may present many months or years after treatment.[16]

A comprehensive clinical history including oncological medical history is essential to better understand the risk factors associated with H&N cancer–related lymphedema. The specific cancer type, anatomical location, time of diagnosis and presentation, and extent of the disease including possible neck metastasis can all factor into the presentation of lymphedema. H&N cancers frequently metastasize to the lymph nodes, and subsequent treatments of the involved nodes increase the risk of lymphedema.

Treatments for H&N cancer include surgical resection, with or without neck dissection to remove neck lymph nodes, reconstruction (local reconstruction and free flaps), chemotherapy, radiation, and targeted therapy. Neck node dissection can be unilateral or bilateral and can include (1) radical dissection where the spinal accessory nerve, sternocleidomastoid muscle, and internal jugular vein and lymph nodes from levels I to V (Fig. 10.1B) are removed or (2) modified neck dissection, which while less invasive still may involve the resection of lymph nodes from different levels (I–V) of the neck.

The risk for H&N lymphedema increases with the increased number and invasiveness of the interventions performed to control the disease in the lymph nodes. For example, the type and extent of neck dissection and radiation to the neck area may increase the risk for H&N lymphedema.[17]

Clinical history should include the cancer history and cancer treatment, and the onset of the symptoms associated with lymphedema. Lymphedema associated symptoms can include neck swelling, neck "tightness," neck heaviness, changes in voice including hoarseness, shortness of breath, and excessive submental tissue/fullness, among others. These symptoms are not specific to lymphedema but can be helpful in the lymphedema evaluation.

While obesity is a risk for lymphedema even when the lymphatic system is intact and has been identified as a risk factor for lymphedema in breast cancer,[18] it may not be a risk factor in the H&N cancer population.[3] Other risk factors include location of tumor, total dosage and duration or radiation, and number of treatment modalities (i.e., chemotherapy, surgery, and/or radiation therapy).[3] To facilitate early recognition and timely treatment, it is important to provide education to patients undergoing

H&N cancer treatment about the risk of lymphedema and symptoms that they should be aware of and report. Patient-reported outcome measures can help to identify symptoms associated with lymphedema.

Physical examination

After surgery, swelling at the H&N area is expected and is not necessarily related to lymphedema. Skin changes can be present at different times during treatment. Post-surgical incision and flaps in healing process, acute radiation dermatitis can be found and can be associated with some swelling and/or erythema. After radiation, chronic skin and tissue fibrosis can be encountered. It is important to differentiate acute and/or healing processes with signs of lymphedema. Inspection and examination will need to be repeated after surgical incision is healed and after completion of radiation.

Measurements

Unlike cases of limb lymphedema, H&N lymphedema does not have a contralateral limb that can be used for comparison purposes. In addition, facial asymmetries, whether due to enlarged lymph nodes, or cases of induration and larger masses owing to disease before cancer treatment, or posttreatment anatomical changes, related to larger resections, reconstruction, weight loss, and fibrosis, often limit the effectiveness of pre- and posttreatment facial measurements and contralateral comparisons of the bilateral face and neck as reliable methods to measure tissue changes based on volumes and to diagnose H&N cancer—related lymphedema.

MD Anderson Cancer Center developed a facial measurement technique[19] to track tissue changes in the face and neck over time. This method includes facial circumference measurements and point to point measurements including a facial composite measurement. The two facial circumferential measurements, include a (1) diagonal measurement from chin to the crown of the head and (2) submental circumference from <1 cm in front of one ear to the corresponding location in front of the contralateral ear. The point to point measurements include measurements between (1) bilateral mandibular angles, (2) bilateral tragus, as well as (3) a facial composite measurement consisting of the cumulative measurements between seven facial protuberances, as shown in Fig. 10.3, including between the (1) tragus to mental protuberance, (2) tragus to mouth angle, (3) mandibular angle to nasal wing, (4) mandibular angle to internal eye corner, (5) mandibular angle to external eye corner, (6) mental protuberance to internal eye corner, and (7) mandibular angle to mental protuberance. The method also includes a composite neck score obtained from three circumferential neck measurement at the superior, medial, and inferior neck.

While this method may provide an objective comparison between the baseline measurement and subsequent measurements, and thus may provide a numeric indication of changes in swelling over time, limitations in the precision and reliability of

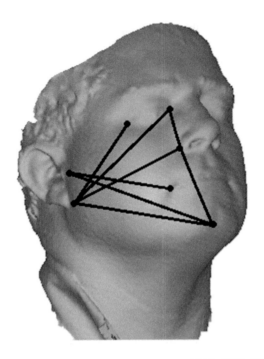

FIGURE 10.3

(A) Illustration of point-to-point measurements comprising the facial composite score as developed at MD Anderson Cancer Center.[19]

the measurements[20] limit the use of these measurements as a single test for the onset of lymphedema.

Stemmer sign

The Stemmer sign[21] is assessed by pinching the skin at the foot at the proximal phalange between the second and third toe. While it has been used as a tool to help diagnose lower extremity lymphedema, it is not useful in the diagnosis of H&N lymphedema. However, the fullness and swelling of the skin can point us toward lymphedema.

Bioimpedance

Bioimpedance spectroscopy can be used to measure body composition including fluid volume. While its use is not broadly reported in H&N lymphedema, the ALOHA trial indicates that the MoistureMeterD along with tape measurements could provide and objective measurement of H&N lymphedema.[22]

Imaging

Because the lymphatics are small and filled with clear fluid, they are difficult to directly image using standard clinical imaging techniques without the introduction of exogenous contrast agents. Lymphoscintigraphy, often considered the gold standard of lymphatic imaging and frequently cited as a diagnostic for limb lymphedema (for review, see van Heumen et al.[23]), is accomplished following the intradermal injection of a radionuclide for lymphatic uptake, enabling the visualization of lymph nodes and large lymphatic ducts and trunks. However, while this technique has been used to identify sentinel lymph nodes[24] in H&N cancers, it has not been widely adopted for the assessment of H&N lymphedema. Non–contrast-enhanced, magnetic resonance imaging (MRI) can visualize lymph nodes and large stagnant lymph trunks; however, to image smaller lymphatic vessels using MRI, a gadolinium-based contrast agent must be intradermally administered. While this technique is more established in limb lymphedema and provides opportunities to assess other tissues (for recent reviews, see Salehi et al.[25] and Miseré et al.[26]), it also has limited adoption for H&N lymphedema evaluation.

X-ray computed tomography (CT) can provide excellent images of the lymphatics, but only after surgical isolation of—and direct administration of an iodinated contrast agent into—a lymphatic vessel (for more details, see Schwartz et al.[27]), as such it is rarely used for lymphatic imaging owing to the technical expertise needed and the invasiveness of the procedure. However, CT imaging of the tissues has shown promise as a diagnostic of internal and external lymphedema following the CT Lymphedema and Fibrosis Assessment Tool (CT-LEFAT)[28] scoring systems. While still in validation, CT-LEFAT standardizes the assessment of fat stranding, epiglottic thickness, and prevertebral soft tissue thickness at specific sites to provide an objective assessment of lymphedema and fibrosis. Ultrasound may also provide excellent opportunities to assess the soft tissues and has the advantage of being noninvasive, readily available, and relatively inexpensive. Measurements such as skin-to-bone distance, the thickness of skin and subcutaneous tissues, and assessment of tissue elasticity (i.e., fibrosis) have been proposed and demonstrated but need additional validation for widespread adoption. For a more detailed review of the use of these imaging modalities in H&N lymphedema, see Fadhil and Singh.[8]

Indocyanine green (ICG) lymphography, based on near-infrared fluorescence imaging, is increasingly used to assess lymphatic function in health and disease.[29] In this technique, ICG is intradermally administered for uptake into the lymphatics. The tissues are then illuminated with an excitation light, and the resultant fluorescence signal is collected using a special camera. This technique enables the visualization of superficial lymphatic vessels and the lymph nodes. In addition, because ICG imaging involves short exposure times, active lymphatic pumping can be visualized. Healthy lymphatic vessels are well defined with active pumping. Lymphatic failure, including lymphedema, is characterized by reduced lymphatic pumping and/

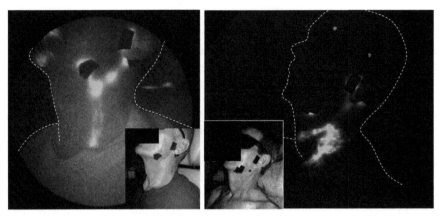

FIGURE 10.4

ICG-based near-infrared fluorescence images (with color inset) of (left) unobstructed lymphatic flow from intradermal injection sites in the jawline and near the ear (covered with black vinyl tape) and (right) dermal lymphatic backflow in the neck of a patient with lymphedema.

(left) Reproduced with permission from Rasmussen JC, Tan IC, Naqvi S, et al. Longitudinal monitoring of the head and neck lymphatics in response to surgery and radiation. Head Neck 2017;39(6):1177–1188.

or the backflow of ICG into the dermal lymphatic capillaries (see Fig. 10.4). In breast cancer–related lymphedema, dermal lymphatic backflow is visible on average 8 months prior to the onset of clinically diagnosable lymphedema, based on a 5% increase in limb volume.[30] While it is unclear if dermal lymphatic backflow will likewise precede the onset H&N lymphedema, prior studies indicate that when left untreated, dermal lymphatic backflow is persistent over months and years.[31] One study of early H&N lymphedema indicated that early physiotherapeutic intervention reduced the extent of dermal lymphatic backflow in 75% of subjects.[32] Whether dermal backflow portends the onset of H&N lymphedema and whether physiotherapy administered at the first sign of lymphatic dysfunction can prevent the onset/progression of lymphedema is currently under investigation by the authors.

Challenges diagnosing, staging, and assessing H&N lymphedema

The limb volume difference (≥5 or 10%) between the affected and contralateral limbs is frequently used as a major determinant in the diagnosis of cancer-related lymphedema in the extremities as the contralateral limb is used as a control, thus allowing the clinician to account for limb changes related to weight-loss or other phenomena that may impact bilateral limbs. In H&N cancer, the lack of a contralateral structure and occurance of asymentric treatment-related changes in the face and neck, render diagnosis by facial and neck comparisons challenging. As a result, H&N lymphedema is underrecognized and underdiagnosed resulting in poorer outcomes and lower quality of life for H&N cancer survivors.

Treatment

The first step, and maybe most important, for lymphedema treatment is recognition. Providing patients and caregivers with education about lymphedema and its treatment should be included in a prerehabilitation assessment. Education should be provided to the medical/oncology team to increase awareness about H&N lymphedema and the importance of early diagnosis and treatment. Having close monitoring and high suspicion for lymphedema especially after completion of surgery and radiation is important and can help in an early diagnosis and treatment. In addition, educating patients about lymphedema and the importance of treatment can increase their compliance and may decrease the ultimate impact of their lymphedema-associated symptoms. Early intervention has shown improved response and treatment as prevention warrants future studies.

Decongestive lymphatic therapy

The main goal of lymphedema treatment is to reduce swelling followed by maintenance to keep the swelling at a reduced level.

The decongestive lymphatic therapy (DLT) should be performed by a trained person such as physical or occupational therapist, massage therapist, speech and language pathologist, physician, and/or nurse. Most commonly therapists provide the treatment.

Decongestive lymphatic therapy has four components:

- Education and skin care to reduce the risk of infections and wounds. This includes skin inspection, the use of moisturizing agents, and wound care.
- Manual lymphatic drainage (MLD) is a very gentle and light massage technique that aims to stimulate the lymphatics and mobilize fluid from an edematous area to a nonedematous area where the lymphatic system is properly working and can take up the fluid.
- Compression bandages, including wraps, foams and padding, can be applied after MLD to assist pushing fluid from swollen areas and preventing reaccumulation in the affected area.
- Exercise: Exercise is safe and should be an essential component of lymphedema treatment during volume reduction and maintenance care. In the past, patients were advised to avoid strength training including carrying heavy objects and to avoid strenuous activities as it was thought that these activites could promote the development of lymphedema. However, multiple studies have shown that exercise, especially weight bearing/strengthening exercises,

is an essential component for lymphedema management.[33] Resistance exercises are recommended to be performed two to three times a week as part of a supervised and progressive program using the major muscle groups. Exercise helps with fluid pumping/transportation and drainage and may reduce symptoms associated with cancer and cancer treatment and thus is a key piece in survivorship and healthy lifestyle.

The maintenance phase, described also as phase 2, starts when the swelling has decreased and the patient is discharged from clinically-based therapy for home/self-based lymphedema management.

Appropriately fitted compression garments are essential to maintain the tissue volume long term. An evaluation for the appropriate garments includes proper fitting based on patient measurements of the affected area, appropriate garment pressure, ability of the patient or the caregiver to assist with donning, insurance coverage, and patient's financial status. Garments can be used for different parts of the body but can be challenging when used in the H&N area secondary to the anatomy, practical considerations such as the ability of the patients to wear a garment for prolonged amount of time, comfort, and compliance. Garments can be custom-made for the patient or generic that can be bought commercially.

The skin care and exercise should continue and should become part of the self-care routine.

Patients and caregivers can continue with self-manual lymphatic drainage.

Patient should have regular follow-up with medical team and/or therapist to monitor the lymphedema.

Pneumatic compression devices

Basic and advanced pneumatic compression devices (APCD), which simulate MLD to promote movement of fluid and stimulate lymphatic pumping, have been used for many years to treat lymphedema in the trunk and extremities.

The first APCD developed for H&N lymphedema was approved by the Food and Drug Administration (FDA) at the end of 2016. Patients using this device report improvement in swallowing and breathing, ability to perform activities of daily living, and satisfaction and comfort utilizing the pump as well as high compliance.[34]

In another study, ICG based, near-infrared fluorescence lymphatic imaging was used to assess the lymphatics before and immediately after a single APCD treatment and after 2 weeks of daily, at home use.[32] Imaging showed an increase in drainage and lymphatic uptake in all subjects after a single treatment with the APCD and, after 2 weeks, a decrease in the extent (i.e., area) of dermal backflow in six of eight subjects with complete resolution in one case (Fig. 10.5).

A recent systematic review looking at treatment intervention for H&N cancer–related lymphedema showed multiple limitations in recent studies including smaller sample size. The majority of the studies are observational with fewer randomized trials.[35] No serious adverse events associated with lymphedema treatment were

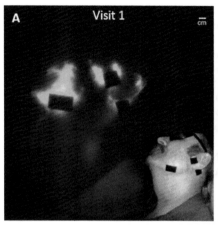
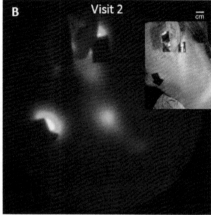

FIGURE 10.5

Resolution of abnormal dermal lymphatic backflow after 2 weeks of daily at home advanced pneumatic compression therapy in a patient with early H&N lymphedema.

Reproduced from Gutierrez C, Karni RJ, Naqvi S, et al. Head and neck lymphedema: treatment response to single and multiple sessions of advanced pneumatic compression therapy. Otolaryngol Head Neck Surg 2019;160(4): 622–626 (From STM signatory).

reported. Rehabilitation interventions including standard lymphedema therapy, the use of APCDs, and Kinesio tape can be safe and beneficial, improving the quality of life of cancer survivors.

In conclusion, H&N lymphedema can be present in a large percentage of the head and neck cancer population and can impact quality of life and function. Early identification, diagnosis and treatment of lymphedema should be an essential part of rehabilitation in head and neck cancer survivorship.

References

1. Siegel RL, Miller KD, Wagle NS, Jemal A. Cancer statistics, 2023. *CA A Cancer J Clin.* 2023;73(1):17–48.
2. Cancer of the Oral Cavity and Pharynx—Cancer Stat Facts. https://seer.cancer.gov/statfacts/html/oralcav.html.
3. Deng J, Ridner SH, Dietrich MS, et al. Prevalence of secondary lymphedema in patients with head and neck cancer. *J Pain Symptom Manag.* February 2012;43(2):244–252.
4. Naoum GE, Roberts S, Brunelle CL, et al. Quantifying the impact of axillary surgery and nodal irradiation on breast cancer-related lymphedema and local tumor control: long-term results from a prospective screening trial. *J Clin Oncol.* October 10, 2020;38(29):3430–3438.
5. Donahue PMC, MacKenzie A, Filipovic A, Koelmeyer L. Advances in the prevention and treatment of breast cancer-related lymphedema. *Breast Cancer Res Treat.* 2023;200(1):1–14.

6. Clinckaert A, Callens K, Cooreman A, et al. The prevalence of lower limb and genital lymphedema after prostate cancer treatment: a systematic review. *Cancers*. November 18, 2022;14(22):5667.

7. Dessources K, Aviki E, Leitao MM. Lower extremity lymphedema in patients with gynecologic malignancies. *Int J Gynecol Cancer*. February 2020;30(2):252−260.

8. Fadhil M, Singh R, Havas T, Jacobson I. Systematic review of head and neck lymphedema assessment. *Head Neck*. October 2022;44(10):2301−2315.

9. Kapellas N, Demiri E, Lampropoulos A, Dionyssiou D. Genetic predisposition in cancer-related lymphedema: a systematic review. *Lymphatic Res Biol*. October 2022;20(5): 478−487.

10. Oliver G, Kipnis J, Randolph GJ, Harvey NL. The lymphatic vasculature in the 21st century: novel functional roles in homeostasis and disease. *Cell*. July 23, 2020;182(2): 270−296.

11. Földi M, Földi E. *Foldi's Textbook of Lymphology for Physicians and Lymphedema Therapists*. Elsevier, Urban & Fischer Verlag; 2006.

12. Lan YL, Wang H, Chen A, Zhang J. Update on the current knowledge of lymphatic drainage system and its emerging roles in glioma management. *Immunology*. February 2023;168(2):233−247.

13. Sung C, Wang S, Hsu J, Yu R, Wong AK. Current understanding of pathological mechanisms of lymphedema. *Adv Wound Care*. July 2022;11(7):361−373.

14. Bernas M, Al-Ghadban S, Thiadens SRJ, et al. Etiology and treatment of cancer-related secondary lymphedema. *Clin Exp Metastasis*. September 30, 2023:1−24.

15. Ayestaray B, Bekara F, Andreoletti JB. π-Shaped lymphaticovenular anastomosis for head and neck lymphoedema: a preliminary study. *J Plast Reconstr Aesthetic Surg*. February 1, 2013;66(2):201−206.

16. Deng J, Ridner S, Rothman R, et al. Perceived symptom experience in head and neck cancer patients with lymphedema. *J Palliat Med*. December 2016;19(12):1267−1274.

17. Tribius S, Pazdyka H, Tennstedt P, et al. Prognostic factors for lymphedema in patients with locally advanced head and neck cancer after combined radio(chemo)therapy-results of a longitudinal study. *Oral Oncol*. July 2, 2020;109:104856.

18. Wu R, Huang X, Dong X, Zhang H, Zhuang L. Obese patients have higher risk of breast cancer-related lymphedema than overweight patients after breast cancer: a meta-analysis. *Ann Transl Med*. April 2019;7(8):172.

19. Smith BG, Lewin JS. Lymphedema management in head and neck cancer. *Curr Opin Otolaryngol Head Neck Surg*. June 2010;18(3):153−158.

20. Chotipanich A, Kongpit N. Precision and reliability of tape measurements in the assessment of head and neck lymphedema. *PLoS One*. 2020;15(5).

21. Stemmer R. A clinical symptom for the early and differential diagnosis of lymphedema. *Vasa*. 1976;5(3):261−262.

22. Purcell A, Nixon J, Fleming J, McCann A, Porceddu S. Measuring head and neck lymphedema: the "ALOHA" trial. *Head Neck*. January 2016;38(1):79−84.

23. van Heumen S, Riksen JJM, Bramer WM, van Soest G, Vasilic D. Imaging of the lymphatic vessels for surgical planning: a systematic review. *Ann Surg Oncol*. January 2023;30(1):462−479.

24. Skanjeti A, Dhomps A, Paschetta C, Tordo J, Delgado Bolton RC, Giammarile F. Lymphoscintigraphy for sentinel node mapping in head and neck cancer. *Semin Nucl Med*. January 2021;51(1):39−49.

25. Parsai Salehi B, Carson Sibley R, Friedman R, et al. MRI of lymphedema. *J Magn Reson Imag*. April 2023;57(4):977−991.
26. Miseré RML, Wolfs J, Lobbes MBI, van der Hulst RRWJ, Qiu SS. A systematic review of magnetic resonance lymphography for the evaluation of peripheral lymphedema. *J Vasc Surg Venous Lymphat Disord*. September 2020;8(5):882−892.
27. Schwartz FR, James O, Kuo PH, Witte MH, Koweek LM, Pabon-Ramos WM. Lymphatic imaging: current noninvasive and invasive techniques. *Semin Intervent Radiol*. August 2020;37(3):237−249.
28. Aulino JM, Wulff-Burchfield EM, Dietrich MS, et al. Evaluation of CT changes in the head and neck after cancer treatment: development of a measurement tool. *Lymphatic Res Biol*. February 2018;16(1):69−74.
29. Sevick-Muraca EM, Fife CE, Rasmussen JC. Imaging peripheral lymphatic dysfunction in chronic conditions. *Front Physiol*. 2023;14:1132097.
30. Aldrich MB, Rasmussen JC, DeSnyder SM, et al. Prediction of breast cancer-related lymphedema by dermal backflow detected with near-infrared fluorescence lymphatic imaging. *Breast Cancer Res Treat*. August 2022;195(1):33−41.
31. Rasmussen JC, Tan IC, Naqvi S, et al. Longitudinal monitoring of the head and neck lymphatics in response to surgery and radiation. *Head Neck*. June 2017;39(6): 1177−1188.
32. Gutierrez C, Karni RJ, Naqvi S, et al. Head and neck lymphedema: treatment response to single and multiple sessions of advanced pneumatic compression therapy. *Otolaryngol Head Neck Surg*. April 2019;160(4):622−626.
33. ACSM Blog. https://www.acsm.org/blog-detail.
34. Gutiérrez C, Mayrovitz HN, Naqvi SHS, Karni RJ. Longitudinal effects of a novel advanced pneumatic compression device on patient-reported outcomes in the management of cancer-related head and neck lymphedema: a preliminary report. *Head Neck*. August 2020;42(8):1791−1799.
35. Cheng MH, Pappalardo M, Lin C, Kuo CF, Lin CY, Chung KC. Validity of the novel Taiwan lymphoscintigraphy staging and correlation of Cheng lymphedema grading for unilateral extremity lymphedema. *Ann Surg*. 2018;268(3):513−525.

Swallowing and communication disorders in head and neck cancer

11

Casey Richardson, MA, CCC-SLP [1] **and Katherine Hutcheson, PhD** [2]

[1]*Atos Medical, Houston, TX, United States;* [2]*University of Texas MD Anderson Cancer Center, Houston, TX, United States*

Introduction

Swallowing and communication disorders are potential consequences of head and neck cancer and can significantly impact an individual's functional status and quality of life. These functional changes have a psychosocial impact, limiting social activities such as engaging in conversations, sharing meals with loved ones, and effectively communicating over the phone. Individuals with head and neck cancer are at risk for depression, with one study reporting a prevalence of 40%, and the risk of suicide is twice that of other cancers, especially in patients with primary sites in the hypopharynx or larynx.[1,2] Addressing these challenges requires a comprehensive, multidimensional approach to evaluating and treating swallowing and communication disorders.

This chapter describes the general principles of assessment of communication and swallowing disorders in individuals with head and neck cancer in addition to the normal anatomy and physiology of swallowing and voice. Within the voice section, rehabilitation post laryngectomy and tracheostomy are described.

General principles of assessment and management

Multidimensional assessment is the best practice to comprehensively assess speech, swallowing, voice, and communication. A thorough assessment of communication and swallowing disorders should encompass various vital components, including patient-reported outcomes (PROs), functional status measures as appropriate, patient and caregiver interviews, an oral mechanism exam, a motor speech profile, and a clinical or instrumental assessment of the respective system. By integrating these components, the clinician gains a holistic and global understanding of the patient. This comprehensive approach not only identifies the anatomical changes and physiologic impairments contributing to the swallowing or communication disorder but also sheds light on the broader impact of these disorders on the individual's overall quality of life. The multidisciplinary

Head and Neck Cancer Rehabilitation. https://doi.org/10.1016/B978-0-443-11806-7.00005-9
Copyright © 2025 Elsevier Inc. All rights are reserved, including those for text and data mining, AI training, and similar technologies.

team of healthcare professionals can tailor interventions and treatment that address the specific impairments that align with the patient's goals.

Patient interview

Perhaps the most essential part of the assessment is the patient interview, as the clinician can gain information about the patient's functional status, goals, and priorities. The interview is also an opportunity to build rapport and create a supportive environment throughout the individual's journey through diagnosis, treatment, and survivorship. PROs and functional measures may be administered during the patient interview and are described in more detail in the following section.

There is an increased focus in the literature on understanding the patient's journey and treating them with respect as they undergo life-changing treatment that can leave them with not only functional changes but also changes in their physical appearance. Engaging in conversation regarding prognosis of functional outcomes begins during pretreatment counseling and continues throughout the treatment and into survivorship. The conversation is an opportunity to assess the individual's understanding of their current level of function, anticipated outcomes, and readiness to engage in prehabilitation or rehabilitation program. The Serious Illness Conversation framework provides a structure for engaging in these conversations and includes setting up the conversation, assessing, sharing, exploring, and closing the conversation.[3] This guide can be used to shape the conversation with both the patient and the caregiver.

Patient-reported outcomes and functional measures

PROs assess the impact of head and neck cancer and its treatment on a patient's quality of life and well-being. These outcome measures provide valuable insights into the physical, emotional, and social aspects of the patient experience that may not be captured through clinical or instrumental assessment. The results of the PROs are crucial for delivering patient-centered care, including goal setting and tailored treatment plans. Several commonly used and validated PROs evaluate the impact of dysphagia, communication, and voice on a patient's life, and the most frequently found instruments in research and clinical practice are summarized in Table 11.1.

Functional status measures describe the patient's overall function in a specific domain. Table 11.2 describes the common measures associated with swallowing, and the National Cancer Institute's Common Toxicity Criteria for Adverse Events (CTCAE) can be used to classify a variety of toxicities, including dysphagia.

Oral mechanism exam

An oral mechanism exam (OME) is a foundational component in assessing communication and swallowing disorders and has been described in the literature since the 1970s.[13] During the examination, clinicians systematically observe, rate, and

Table 11.1 Common swallowing and communication patient-reported outcome measures.

Measure	Category	Description
MD Anderson Dysphagia Inventory (MDADI)[4]	Swallowing	20 questions that quantify physical, emotional, and functional domains of swallowing related quality of life. This tool is head and neck specific and has been validated in several languages.
University of Washington Quality of Life Questionnaire (UW-QOL)[5]	Swallowing	15 questions regarding the individual's health and quality of life over the past 7 days.
The Eating Assessment Tool-10 (EAT-10)[6]	Swallowing	10-item questionnaire of swallowing symptoms.
Sydney Swallowing Questionnaire (SSQ)[7]	Swallowing	17-question, self-report inventory, which was developed to measure the symptomatic severity of oral-pharyngeal dysphagia.
Voice Handicap Index-10 (VHI-10)[8]	Voice	10 items measuring the individual's perception of voice problems.
Voice-Related Quality of Life (V-RQOL)[9]	Voice	A 10-item questionnaire that measures the impact of voice on quality of life and has a social and physical domain.
Communicative Participation Item Bank (CPIB)[10]	Communication	A 10-item questionnaire that measures communicative participation restrictions and can be used for any etiology of communication disorder.

Table 11.2 Common swallowing and communication functional status measures.

Measure	Category	Description
Functional Oral Intake Scale (FOIS)[11]	Swallowing	Ordinal scale to categorize the patient's current level of oral intake with seven levels ranging from a total oral diet with no restriction to nothing by mouth and accounts for total or partial feeding tube dependence
Performance Status Scale for Head and Neck Cancer Patients (PSS-HN)[12]	Swallowing/ speech	Ordinal scale normalcy of diet, speech, understandability of speech, and eating in public

describe anatomical variations, symmetry, and range of motion of speech and swallowing mechanisms. Not all deviations of normal anatomy result in a functional deficit, but they should be appropriately noted.

Additionally, the clinician may observe a physical change or symptoms that warrant further evaluation by a physician. For instance, a malodorous oral cavity may indicate the need to refer to an oral oncologist to address the microbiome of the oral cavity or dehiscence of a surgical site warrants immediate referral back to the head and neck surgeon. The clinician may also note the presence of mucositis during radiation and chemotherapy that may be impacting oral intake or guarding during speech.

The OMEs should also include a cranial nerve examination, specifically assessing nerves related to speech, swallowing, and vocal function (see Table 11.3). The exam findings have implications for the disorder's diagnosis, etiology, and

Table 11.3 Cranial nerves of speech, swallowing, and voice.[20]

Number	Name	Motor function[a]	Sensory function	Suggested tasks to assess[b]
V	Trigeminal	Sensation of the face and oral cavity	Movement of the muscles of mastication	Observe during mastication; touch the individual's face
VII	Facial	Movement of muscles for facial expression/ movement	Taste (anterior two-thirds of the tongue)	Visualize symmetry; raise eyebrows, smile, pucker lips, puff cheeks with air
IX	Glossopharyngeal	Innervates muscles responsible for elevation of the larynx	Taste (posterior one-third of the tongue), gag reflex	Test gag reflex
X	Vagus	Motor innervation of the soft palate, pharynx, and larynx, including vocal folds	Gag reflex	Say "ahh" and assess soft palate; motor speech tasks to assess vocal function
XII	Hypoglossal	Motor innervation of tongue movements for speech and swallowing	No sensory function	Assess the tongue at rest

The oral motor exam provides vital information regarding the structure, function, and overall health of the mechanisms for swallowing and speech. Changes in the structures, symmetry, and range of motion may impact speech and the oral phase of swallowing or indicate risk for pharyngeal dysphagia.
[a] Functions most related to speech, swallowing, and voice are summarized in the table.
[b] Suggested tasks are those that can be seen during a physical exam. Additional tasks may be completed during a fiberoptic endoscopic examination or a modified barium swallow study to assess cranial nerve function further, e.g., observing pharyngeal shortening on videofluoroscopy, endoscopy, or manometry as a marker of IX function.

treatment. Cranial neuropathies may occur following radiation therapy. Approximately 5% of oropharyngeal cancer survivors develop hypoglossal palsy, and all of those patients develop radiation-associated dysphagia.[14] In Aggrawal et al. 2019, individuals with lower cranial neuropathy were more likely to have a feeding tube, a history of aspiration pneumonia, and a tracheostomy.[15] Additionally, a hypoglossal palsy can result in flaccid dysarthria and associated decline in speech intelligibility. Therefore, careful consideration should be given to the cranial nerves as deficits in these areas can be early indicators of late radiation-associated dysphagia and may signal the presence or onset of a decline in swallow function. This is vital information in determining the appropriate treatment paradigm, which will be discussed later in this chapter, as well as patient education regarding the prognosis of communication or swallowing disorders.

Another critical consideration is to evaluate for trismus, which is defined as an oral opening of less than or equal to 35 mm. Trismus can impact the quality of life and individual, is correlated with a more limited diet, and can impact speech.[16] Individuals with severe trismus may even become feeding tube dependent.[17] According to a systematic review by Watters et al. (2019), individuals with a primary head and neck cancer site in the oral cavity or the oropharynx are at significant risk. The prevalence of trismus in individuals with head and neck cancers is 17.3% at baseline, 44.1% at 6 months posttreatment (radiation, surgery, and/or chemotherapy), and 32.1% at 12 months posttreatment.[18] Maximum interincisal opening (MIO) can be tracked at all evaluations by using a measuring tool to achieve standardized and consistent measurement. Trismus treatment may include device-driven or manual therapies and is vital to comprehensively treat the communication and/or swallowing disorder.[19] Managing trismus may also be critical in optimizing patients for further therapeutic modalities such as bolus-driven swallowing therapy or before fabricating a prosthodontic device to aid speech or swallowing.

Motor speech evaluation

A motor speech evaluation is a fundamental component of the SLP evaluation as the presence or treatment of head and neck cancer may result in flaccid dysarthria or anatomic or structural alteration in speech (empirically referred to in the authors practice as "structural dysarthria").

Evaluation principles in summary

Head and neck cancer can result in significant functional changes and impact communication and swallowing. There are both structural changes and changes in cranial nerve function that can adversely impact swallowing and communication systems. The evaluation methods discussed in general principles are considered the fundamental building blocks of assessment ideally completed for "every patient, every time" to determine the most appropriate next steps in evaluation and treatment for each individual.

Assessment and treatment of voice disorders

Dysphonia refers to changes in voice. Dysphonia is highly prevalent in HNC with various possible sources of injury. Surgery resecting portions of the vocal fold or vocal tract can result in rough, weak, breath, or strained vocal quality or, in the case of a total laryngectomy, a complete loss of the voice or aphonia. Radiation may cause temporary or permanent changes in the voice by way of fibrotic stiffening of the laryngeal apparatus if the larynx is within the radiation field. Additionally, vocal fold paralysis may be the result of cranial neuropathy of the vagus nerve by tumor, as a delayed effect of radiation, or damage to the vagus nerve during surgery. Individuals may also have a behavioral voice disorder in addition to the structural/functional changes due to head and neck cancer treatment.

Anatomy and physiology of voice

The mechanism of voice production is a complex event that involves multiple organs, and disruption at any level can result in a voice disorder. The voice is powered by respiration, and the vocal folds are the source of phonation. The vibration of the vocal folds is filtered by the vocal tract, including the oral cavity, nasal cavity, and pharynx. The size and shape of the various cavities of the vocal tract influence the acoustic output. Vocal quality depends upon the vibratory characteristics of the vocal folds, characteristics of the vocal tract, and adequate and consistent subglottic pressure. The reader is encouraged to refer to a textbook on voice for more detailed information regarding the anatomy and physiology of voice.[21]

Evaluation

Voice evaluation includes the foundational elements discussed earlier in the chapter in addition to perceptual, vibratory, and in some cases acoustic and aerodynamic parameters of voice production. Direct visualization of the vocal tract and larynx during laryngeal videostroboscopy is essential in the head and neck cancer population. Laryngeal videostroboscopy is an office procedure that is commonly done by either a physician or a speech–language pathologist. During this endoscopic exam, a pulsed light source is used to assess vocal fold mobility and vibratory patterns of the true vocal folds. The exam provides immediate images of the presence or absence of pathology and a permanent visual record. Laryngeal videostroboscopy is often a component in diagnosing and staging laryngeal cancer and can be used in routine surveillance after treatment of head and neck cancer and documents changes in vibratory laryngeal function over time. For rehabilitation purposes, the laryngeal videostroboscopy is used to also assess for a behavioral component of the voice disorder and probe the stimulability for voice therapy techniques. The exam results, clinical observation, and patient goals drive the treatment plan for the voice disorder.

Treatment

Treatment of voice disorders in the head and neck may include behavioral voice therapy and medical management. An important consideration in treating voice disorders in the head and neck is considering the anticipated intervention outcomes and expected long-term prognosis. Suppose there is a structural change, such as after a partial laryngectomy or radiation damage. In that case, the individual's voice cannot be expected to return to its baseline function before oncologic diagnosis and treatment, but voice intervention may still improve the vocal quality.[22]

Studies indicate that voice and speech degeneration during chemoradiation improve again 1—2 months after treatment and exceed pretreatment levels after 1 year. However, voice and speech measures do not show normal values before or after treatment.[23] Additionally, a randomized control trial demonstrated that individuals with a primary larynx cancer treated with radiation improved PRO measurements following voice therapy and individuals with a supraglottic primary site had improvement in acoustic measurements of voice.[24] These studies suggest some potential improvement in voice following treatment with radiation and a role of voice for voice therapy to improve the voice quality.

Some individuals may have severe toxicities from radiation that result in a dysfunctional larynx or vocal fold paralysis due to lower cranial neuropathy. Medical management of vocal fold paralysis may include a medialization procedure such as an injection laryngoplasty or a thyroplasty to improve vocal function.[25,26] In severe cases of a dysfunctional larynx, an individual may undergo a functional total laryngectomy wherein the nonfunctional larynx is resected to improve respiratory or swallow function.[27] Understanding the underlying impairment is critical to determining the potential benefits of voice therapy and/or medical management.

Rehabilitation after tracheostomy

Voice changes can occur due to the presence of a tracheostomy. A tracheostomy is a surgical procedure that creates an opening in the trachea, most commonly between the third and fourth tracheal ring, and a tracheostomy tube is placed into that opening. The procedure's goals are to facilitate creating a patent airway below upper airway obstruction, or to facilitate weaning from a ventilator.[28] In individuals with head and neck cancer, the most common reasons for placement of a tracheostomy are significant tumor burden causing airway restriction or postoperatively due to anticipated postoperative edema. The individual may be decannulated as soon as the postoperative edema recedes, and this may occur during or after the postoperative hospital admission. In the case of significant tumor burden, the tracheostomy is often removed after surgery and/or radiation as long as there is a patent upper airway.

With a tracheostomy in place, the patient primarily inhales/exhales below the level of the vocal folds. This causes aphonia or a loss of voice. Some air can escape into the upper airway to allow voicing depending upon the degree of upper airway restriction. The speech–language pathologist's role is to assess the optimal way for the patient to achieve voice after tracheostomy. One way is through digital occlusion of the tracheostomy tube. An individual inhales and then covers the end of the tracheostomy tube to route the exhaled air through the vocal folds. While possible in the setting of partial upper airway obstruction, some individuals may not achieve voice if there is a large upper airway restriction. If the source of restriction is postoperative edema, this may change as the individual recovers from surgery as quickly as a few days allowing voicing to resume early after surgery despite the tracheostoma.

Additionally, the patient may be fit with a speaking valve. There are various speaking valves on the market, and the most commonly used device is the Passy Muir speaking valve (PMSV), a biased closed valve.[29] The valve rests in a closed position, opens on inspiration, and returns to a closed position on exhalation, routing the air through the vocal folds. There is an abundance of literature detailing the candidacy and contraindications for speaking valve placement as well as the benefits of the speaking valve, including improved swallow function, taste/smell, cough, and secretion management.[30–33] The clinician is vital in determining candidacy for a speaking valve or digital occlusion. Either of these methods for routing air through the vocal folds can cause shortness of breath or the inability to exhale fully, as a trade-off for the benefit of regaining voice.

It is generally considered best practice for the speech–language pathologist to complete a speaking valve evaluation before a swallowing evaluation. According to Marvin et al. 2021, individuals with a tracheostomy and an oropharyngeal diagnosis, including a laryngeal or oropharyngeal tumor, surgery, or infection, are at greater risk of silent aspiration. Additionally, the risk of aspiration was twice as high with an open tracheostomy versus a closed tracheostomy such as a cap or speaking valve. The risk of silent aspiration was 4.5 times greater with an open tracheostomy.[34] Thus, fitting a patient with a speaking valve or capping may help to improve airway protection against aspiration before completing an instrumental swallowing evaluation (i.e., FEES or MBSS), which will be discussed later in this chapter.

Breathing through a tracheostomy impacts the pulmonary health of the individual as there is a loss of filtration and a decline in the temperature and relative humidity of the air in the trachea/lungs, which results in excessive mucous.[35] The benefit of heat moisture exchangers (HMEs) is well described in individuals with a laryngectomy and experienced a resurgence in the perceived importance of HMEs in individuals with a tracheostomy since the onset of the COVID-19 pandemic.[36] When exhaling through an HME, the heat and moisture of the air are retained by the HME medium, which may be foam treated with a hygroscopic compound or corrugated paper. The heat and moisture are recycled when the individual inhales through the HME.[37] Research has shown significant benefits in using the HME, including reduced coughing and mucus expectoration, improved sleep, and increased patient satisfaction and compliance.[38]

In individuals with head and neck cancer, the tracheostomy tube is often temporary, but the tracheostomy can be permanent should the patient develop bilateral vocal fold paralysis, subglottic stenosis, or other treatment complications compromising the patency of the upper airway. There is evidence supporting the multidisciplinary management of the patient population with tracheostomy to both facilitate decannulation and improve communication and overall pulmonary health regardless of the duration of cannulation.[39]

Rehabilitation after total laryngectomy

During a total laryngectomy, the larynx is removed, and the upper airway is separated from the digestive tract. This results in significant functional changes, including loss of laryngeal voice, changes in swallow physiology, and altered pulmonary function, including a permanent tracheostoma. An individual may undergo a total laryngectomy for three oncologic reasons: primary, salvage, or functional. A primary laryngectomy is when an individual is diagnosed with a locally advanced primary larynx, supraglottic, hypopharyngeal, or thyroid cancer. The second type of laryngectomy is a salvage laryngectomy, which is used for recurrence of a previously treated cancer, usually in the setting of prior laryngeal radiation or chemoradiation. A functional laryngectomy is recommended when an individual has a nonfunctional larynx due to treatment, often dependent on PEG and/or tracheostomy.[40,41]

After laryngectomy, speech pathology rehabilitation targets diverse areas including pulmonary rehabilitation, swallowing assessment/treatment, and alaryngeal communication evaluation and training. Rehabilitation starts with preoperative counseling, offering an opportunity to counsel the patient and caregivers on expected anatomic and functional changes, and rehabilitation options. Shenson et al. (2017) revealed that individuals who receive preoperative counseling have a reduced length of stay postoperatively without increased readmissions.[42]

During the preoperative counseling, the speech—language pathologist begins the process of shared decision-making with the patient and multidisciplinary team about the optimal method of alaryngeal communication, including three primary options of esophageal speech, tracheoesophageal (TE) speech, and the artificial larynx. Of crucial importance is to establish the patient's desire and candidacy (beyond the scope of this chapter) for the prosthetic option of a tracheoesophageal puncture (TEP).

Tracheoesophageal speech

Tracheoesophageal (TE) speech was introduced in 1980 by Dr. Blom and Singer and is often considered the gold standard in voice restoration following a total laryngectomy as this method of alaryngeal communication has been associated with high patient satisfaction and quality of life.[43,44] Additionally, TE speech offers the closest to laryngeal voice in terms of ease of speech, fluency, and volume.[45] A TEP is a surgically created TE fistula between the esophagus and trachea, and a voice prosthesis is placed in the puncture. The voice prosthesis consists of a shaft, one-way valve to allow air passage and prevent aspiration of liquids, an esophageal flange, and a tracheal flange. The voice prosthesis is replaced on average every 2–3 months, but some voice prosthesis may remain in place for up to a year.[46] The TEP can be done primarily, at the time of the initial laryngectomy, or secondarily, any time after the initial surgery. The TE voice prosthesis may be placed at the time of surgery, primary placement, or delayed placement of the voice prosthesis.

TE voice production is an aerodynamic event that is powered by pulmonary air shunted through the tracheoesophageal puncture and voice prosthesis when the stoma is occluded manually or by a hands-free valve. The vibratory source is the pharyngoesophageal segment (PES), which is located at approximately C4–C6.[47] The sound is shaped by the articulators. Quality of TE speech is related to the vibratory qualities of the segment, and the neopharynx.[48] For example, if a patient has a narrow neopharyngeal lumen due to fibrotic radiation associated stricture or bulky reconstruction, the TE voice may sound tight or strained. The pharyngoesophageal segment (PES) that produces voicing during TE phonation can be visualized during endoscopy or fluoroscopy in the oblique and lateral views during phonation and swallowing—as critical diagnostic procedures both for TEP candidacy and TE speech failure.

TEP is associated with a high success rate in appropriately selected patients, but there are complications that may occur after the procedure.[49] Determining candidacy is critical as complications are common, but the majority of complications are treated without additional surgery.[50] Complications include premature leak through or around the voice prosthesis causing aspiration, stricture, lymphedema, pharyngocutaneous fistula, and pharyngoesophageal spasm. Additionally, the voice prosthesis requires daily maintenance to clean and manually dexterity to occlude the stoma. Candidacy is a shared decision between the patient, their loved ones, and the multidisciplinary team that balances the probability of acquiring functional speech against the probability of developing major complications associated with the TEP.

Esophageal speech

Esophageal speech predates tracheoesophageal speech and has declined in use as the TEP has become the gold standard in voice restoration.[51] Often likened to talking on a belch, to produce esophageal speech, air is volitionally propelled by the patient to the level of the PES and returned for voicing. There are three methods of propelling the air-consonant injection, lingual press, and inhalation.[52] The benefit of esophageal speech is a natural sound without risk of complications or prosthetics, but the downside is a lengthy rehabilitation and low success rates. Learning esophageal speech is typically time-consuming and requires significant patient motivation. Success rates are highly variable, ranging from 24% to 75%.[53–55] Once acquired, esophageal speech requires no ongoing maintenance and can be highly functional in select individuals. However, esophageal speech has a decreased mean length of utterance and decreased volume in comparison with TE speakers.[56] Esophageal speech is best considered in patients who are highly motivated, willing to invest significant time in learning, and want a low maintenance option after investing significant early rehabilitation efforts.

Electrolarynx

The electrolarynx or artificial larynx is an electromechanic device that moves a metal or plastic head to create vibration and serves as an external sound source. The device is placed against the neck or cheek, or via an oral adapter that is placed into the mouth. The mechanical sound is then shaped by the articulators into speech. The electrolarynx can be used immediately postoperatively offering an immediate means of communication after loss of the larynx. Some individuals may take longer to learn how to effectively use the device while other individuals before proficient in a few days following surgery.

The key factors that contribute to intelligibility with the EL are finding the correct placement on the neck, cheek, or in the mouth, overarticulation, and on/off timing. Finding the correct placement of the device is crucial and may be impacted by lymphedema, fibrosis, postsurgical incision lines, and manual dexterity. Additionally, the tone of the electrolarynx can be adjusted and impacts speaker comfort and listener acceptance.[57] Some devices offer variable pitch adjustment. Electrolarynx training often focuses on the aforementioned listed factors in addition to reducing distracting behaviors such as stoma blast (air blasts from the tracheostoma during speech).

The electrolarynx has lower risk and maintenance in comparison with TE speech in addition to a high success rate. However, the electrolarynx has an electronic sound quality and reduced intelligibility in comparison to TE speech.[56] Despite this, the electrolarynx is a reliable means of communication and is a great option for individuals at high risk for complications with a TEP or who may not want the associated short term and long-term maintenance.

Swallowing following total laryngectomy

Even though patients cannot aspirate following a total laryngectomy unless the TE voice prosthesis is leaking, individuals are at risk for dysphagia. Literature suggests that at least 50% of individuals will experience dysphagia and swallow function is impacted by closure pattern.[58-60] Individuals with a circumferential reconstruction are at more risk for a stricture than a patch flap and individuals with reconstruction are a more risk than patient with primary closure of the pharynx (no flap).[61] Additionally, those who undergo a functional total laryngectomy are at risk for requiring a long-term feeding tube as one study revealed that 18% of patients required a PEG for supplemental oral intake and 4% were completely feeding tube dependent.[41]

Swallow function is ideally assessed with a modified barium swallow study. Multiplane bolus trials in lateral, oblique, and anterior posterior views are ideal to visualize the anatomy and the pharyngoesophageal segment. High-density barium coats the neopharynx and helps the clinician assess for anatomical variation as well as function. In the oblique view, phonatory tasks including counting and maximum phonation assist in assessing the pharyngoesophageal segment.

Pulmonary health following total laryngectomy

The separation of the lower and upper airways causes significant changes in pulmonary function, including the loss of filtration, humidification, and warming of the inhaled air. When breathing through an open stoma, by the time the air reaches the lung, there is a relative humidity of approximately 50%, a level at which cilia stop functioning.[62] This results in a buildup of thick mucus and can lead to mucous plugs and frequent coughing that adversely impacts the quality of life. Since the 1990s, literature has shown the importance of wearing an HME to improve pulmonary health, reduce mucous production, and reduce coughing.[63]

The HME is attached over the stoma by a peristomal adhesive or an intraluminal device such as a laryngectomy tube or a laryngectomy button. The attachment has two main goals, which are to house the HME and provide an airtight seal to allow total air shunting into the voice prosthesis for TE voice restoration. There is not a one-size-fits-all solution due to variation in peristomal topography, stomal morphology, and patient preference.[64,65] The ideal stoma size is between 12 and 19 mm, and a stoma smaller than 12 mm may cause respiratory issues while a stoma larger than 19 mm may be impossible to occlude for speech. Individuals with stomal stenosis require an intraluminal device to maintain airway patency; some may alternate between a peristomal and intraluminal attachment depending upon severity of stomal stenosis and how quickly the stoma shrinks.

Swallowing

Dysphagia negatively impacts quality of life following head and neck cancer treatment and can also deteriorate an individual's health due to aspiration pneumonia and/or malnutrition.[66,67] These complications can occur during treatment as well as long into survivorship.[68,69] Recognizing the magnitude of the problem of radiation-associated dysphagia, there is an emphasis over recent decades on clinical trials to reduce the risk of dysphagia in individuals undergoing radiotherapy.[70–72]

All phases of swallowing including oral preparatory, oral, pharyngeal, and esophageal phases can be impacted depending upon the location of the cancer and the treatment modality. Speech–language pathologists most often focus on the evaluation and treatment of oropharyngeal dysphagia as the oropharyngeal swallow may be improved with dysphagia therapy and/or compensatory strategies.[73–77] The esophageal phase may also be impacted and can be screened during evaluation. The esophageal phase is generally managed by a gastroenterologist and may require medical management such as esophageal dilation.[78] Due to the significant effects that radiation associated dysphagia can have on an individual's functional status, quality of life, and health, there is a robust body of literature that focuses on identifying the problem, risk factors, and how to potentially mitigate those risks, as well as how to treat radiation associated dysphagia.[79–83]

Overview of normal anatomy and physiology of swallowing

Swallowing is a complex and coordinated sensorimotor event that involves five cranial nerves and over two dozen paired muscles. Swallow function is controlled by the central pattern generator in the medulla, and the oropharyngeal swallow is a patterned response, not a reflex. Motor or sensory impairment of cranial nerves, impairment of muscle function, and anatomical variations can result in dysphagia. During the oral phase of swallowing, the food is broken down and mixed with saliva to form a bolus by the rotary and lateral movement of the tongue and mandible. The bolus is then transferred to the oropharynx through tongue movement.[84] The pharyngeal swallow is then initiated, and the following six movements occur: velopharyngeal closure, laryngeal closure, epiglottic inversion, upper esophageal sphincter opening, base of tongue retraction, and pharyngeal constriction. All of these movements occur rapidly, within 31–138 ms in a normal pharyngeal swallow.[85] After leaving the pharynx, the bolus enters the esophagus before the stomach for digestion.

Another vital component is the coordination between respiration and swallowing as the respiratory system is linked to the oropharynx via the larynx. In healthy individuals, exhalation starts prior to initiation of the pharyngeal swallow, and then there is a pause in respiration or apnea during the swallow in order to protect the airway from aspiration.[86] The exhalation is then completed after the swallow. A disruption in this pattern can impact swallow function, and evidence has demonstrated that individuals with head and neck cancer who did not initiate the swallow during the expiratory phase had a greater severity of swallowing impairment.[86,87]

Evaluation of swallow function

Multidimensional assessment as discussed earlier in this chapter is best practice and particularly critical evaluating the swallowing system. Evaluation must identify the physiological impairments, functional impairments, as well as patient goals to inform the rehabilitation plan. In addition to functional measures, PROs, patient interview, oral motor exam, and a motor speech exam, swallowing evaluation may include a clinical swallowing evaluation and/or an instrumental examination. The most commonly used instrumental examinations are a Modified Barium Swallow Study (MBSS) or Fiberoptic Endoscopic Evaluation of Swallowing (FEES). High-resolution manometry (HRM) measures pressure in the pharynx during swallowing with only emerging uptake thus far in the clinical setting. Thus, HRM will not be discussed in detail.

Clinical swallowing evaluation

During a clinical swallowing evaluation (CSE), a patient is given various consistencies of liquids/or solids depending upon the clinical scenario in addition to assessment of cranial nerve function and oral structures as described earlier.[88,89] The examination spans the oral preparatory phase including labial and lingual control as well as bolus clearance from the oral cavity. The clinician may also observe signs and symptoms of aspiration or inefficiency of the pharyngeal swallow. A clinical swallow evaluation is not as reliable as an instrumental exam as there is no direct visualization of the pharynx, but the exam can be suggestive of pharyngeal dysphagia.

There are several standardized tools that provide a clinician with benchmarks and guidelines to support clinical decision-making. Some of these instruments are the 3-ounce water screen, Yale Swallow Protocol, Toronto Bedside Swallowing Screening Test (TOR-BSST), and the Mann Assessment of Swallow Ability-Cancer (MASA-C).[90–93] The CSE can be suggestive of oropharyngeal dysphagia, determine readiness for an instrumental exam, and indicate which type of instrumental examination may be the most advantageous, in some cases, for the individual and clinical scenario.

Modified barium swallow

The modified barium swallow (MBS) is completed under videofluoroscopy and is a multidisciplinary examination that is typically completed with a speech–language pathologist and radiologist. During the exam, the patient is given bolus trials with a contrast such as barium and the swallow is visualized from the lips through the upper esophagus. The clinician rates physiological impairments as well as the safety (aspiration) and efficiency (residue) of the swallow. Additionally, the clinician may test for compensatory strategies of postures to improve the safety or efficiency of the swallow. Administering a standardized bolus protocol and implementing a validated rating instrument results in a reproducible exam.[94] Trained speech–language pathologists can have high inter- and intrarater reliability when using standardized measures.[95] There is no consensus on which measurements should be used in clinical practice and in research; Table 11.4 lists selected validated and standardized measures that can be utilized to interpret and rate the MBS, most commonly clinically adopted in cancer.

Fiberoptic endoscopic evaluation of swallowing

A fiberoptic endoscopic evaluation of swallowing (FEES) utilizes a flexible endoscope that is passed transnasally, and bolus trials are administered while directly visualizing the oropharynx. The oral phase of swallowing is not visualized during an FEES, and there is often a white out during the peak of the swallow due to epiglottic deflection. An advantage of FEES is the direct visualization of the swallowing structures (i.e., pyriform sinuses, valleculae), airway sufficiency and glottic

Table 11.4 Modified barium swallow study (MBSS) measures.

Measure	Description
Modified Barium Swallow Impairment Profile (MBSImp)[96]	17 physiological components of the oral, pharyngeal, and esophageal phase of swallowing
Dynamic Imaging Grade of Swallowing Toxicity (DIGEST)[97,98]	5-point grade of overall swallowing impairment of pharyngeal swallowing that is an interaction of swallowing efficiency and safety
Penetration Aspiration Scale (PAS)[99] [a]	8-point interval scale to rate the depth of penetration and aspiration

[a] PAS can be used with both MBS and FEES.

closure, tumor, surgical defects, postradiation effects, and cranial nerve function.[100,101] Additionally, there is no radiation exposure during the exam, which makes this instrumental exam ideal for patient biofeedback and strategy training with visualization.[102] Research has demonstrated that FEES and MBS are comparable in detecting airway penetration, aspiration, and pharyngeal residue.[103,104] Similar to MBS, there is not a consistent measure that is used in research or clinically to rate and interpret FEES. Table 11.5 describes commonly used measures.

Sources of impairment in head and neck cancer dysphagia

The underlying cause and pathophysiology of dysphagia varies across different primary sites of head and neck cancer as well as the treatment modality. Understanding how the cancer is treated and the anatomy and physiology of the structures that the tumor invades, and the structures that treatment impacts are vital to treating and understanding the potential impact on the swallowing system. Dysphagia may be present prior to treatment due to large tumor in swallowing critical structures, may develop during radiation or occur well into survivorship after radiation, or may be a result of surgical intervention. Additionally, there are patient factors that increase

Table 11.5 Fiberoptic endoscopic evaluation of swallowing (FEES) measures.

Measure	Description
Yale Residue Rating Scale[105]	5-point ordinal rating scale based on location of pharyngeal residue
Dynamic Imaging Grade of Swallowing Toxicity for Flexible Endoscopic Evaluation of Swallowing(DIGEST-FEES)[106]	5-point grade of overall swallowing impairment of pharyngeal swallowing that is an interaction of swallowing efficiency and safety
Boston Residue and Clearance Scale[107]	11-point ordinal rating scale that rates residue of three aspects of swallowing

the risk of dysphagia including sarcopenia, poor nutritional status, advanced age, pretreatment dysphagia, and smoking and/or alcohol abuse.[82,108—111]

Head and neck surgeries that involve swallowing critical structures place individuals at risk for postoperative dysphagia. There is wide variability in postsurgical outcomes that are highly dependent upon location and size of surgical resection and closure patterns (e.g., reconstruction vs. primary closure). For oral cavity cancers, advanced-stage tumor, larger surgical resections, and adjuvant therapy are risk factors for dysphagia postoperatively.[112] Patients typically experience dysphagia in the acute setting after surgery that improves as they recover from surgery.[113] Transoral robotic surgery has become a common treatment modality for tonsil and base of tongue cancers and can result in postoperative dysphagia.[114] Evaluation of swallow function in the acute care setting is critical in starting dysphagia rehabilitation especially if the patient will undergo postoperative radiation. Additionally, individuals who undergo a partial laryngectomy are at significant risk for postoperative dysphagia and often require intensive swallowing therapy to optimize outcomes.[115—117] Given the varying range of complexity head and neck surgeries that is dependent upon size and location of tumors, there is a wide range postoperative swallow function, and the clinician must have a good understanding of the surgical resection performed and potential physiological deficits when approaching a postsurgical dysphagia consult.

Radiation associated dysphagia is a serious complication from head and neck cancer and those with advanced stage and multimodality therapy are at greater risk. In the acute phase, dysphagia may result from acute edema of swallowing structures, whereas in the chronic phase, dysphagia is a result of fibrosis, change in sensation, and denervation. With swallowing intervention and resolution of the acute toxicities of treatment, swallowing impairments often improve.[76] However, late radiation-associated dysphagia (late-RAD) is more difficult to treat, presenting years after cure with a progressive course of functional deterioration expected. Early identification and intensive swallowing therapy is critical to optimize outcomes and prolong functional years.[118]

Some studies estimate that over 50% of individuals treated with chemoradiation develop dysphagia and aspiration pneumonia is the most common cause of non—cancer-related deaths.[119]Those with baseline dysphagia and a prolonged period of taking nothing by mouth (greater than 2 weeks) have elevated risk of long-term impairment.[120,121] A baseline instrumental evaluation identifies those with pretreatment dysphagia who may benefit from closer monitoring or more intensive prehabilitation strategies during radiation. Additionally, prophylactic swallowing therapy is considered best practice and is related to improved functional outcomes.[76,122]

Feeding tubes are common during radiation and the initial months of recovery and are typically temporary. Between 30% and 70% of patients receiving multimodality therapy with a primary site in the larynx, supraglottis, hypopharynx, or oropharynx have a feeding tube placed during treatment.[123] Odynophagia resulting from mucositis is the main driver for feeding tube placement and is not necessarily indicative of pharyngeal dysphagia.[124] Long-term feeding tube rates are also variable in the literature with one study reported that 11% of patients were feeding tube dependent for greater than 5 years posttreatment after radiation to the nasopharynx and another study showed an increase risk of feeding tube rate in those individuals with lower cranial neuropathy.[15,125] However, feeding tube rates cannot be directly correlated with long-term severe dysphagia as many individuals may continue to eat and drink by mouth despite complication.

Treatment of swallowing disorders

The treatment of swallowing disorders after head and neck cancer treatment is complex and often requires multidisciplinary collaboration with otolaryngologists, speech–language pathologist, nutritionists, prosthodontists, physiatrists, and gastroenterologists.[111,126] The treatment of the swallowing disorder is highly dependent upon the mechanism of injury and physiologic impairment profile and may include both medical and behavioral therapies. An underlying theme in the treatment of dysphagia in the head and neck cancer population is a "use it or lose it" philosophy as disuse atrophy and pharynx immobilization can occur in radiated patients as well as postsurgical patients who have a prolonged period of NPO status.[127–129] Early intervention promoting mobilization of the swallowing system is imperative to optimize functional outcomes.

Proactive swallowing therapy is the best practice for patients undergoing head and neck radiation.[130] Proactive swallowing therapy may decrease the risk of feeding tube use, shorten length of feeding tube use, improve subacute recovery of swallowing-related quality of life, and result in less severe dysphagia.[76,122] There is not a consensus in the literature with regard to the specific exercises or therapy techniques that should be utilized, but rather that preventative therapy appears to result in better functional outcomes and quality of life.[131]

Behavioral dysphagia management often integrates compensatory swallowing strategies promoting more effective bolus clearance, swallowing exercises such as the Masako or effortful swallow, bolus-driven therapies such as McNeil Dysphagia Therapy Program (MDTP) or EAT-RT, or device-facilitated exercises such as expiratory muscle strength training (EMST) and tongue strength devices.[74,132–134] For more severe, refractory, or progressing dysphagia, intensive therapy may integrate a number of these therapies in addition to medical management such as esophageal dilatation. The authors have published a framework for organizing more intensive swallowing therapies in an oncology setting.[135]

Conclusions

Individuals with head and neck cancer commonly develop communication and swallowing disorders that can have a significant impact on health and quality of life before, during, and after treatment. Best practice is a multidisciplinary approach in the assessment and treatment of the disorder with the patient's goals driving clinical decisions.

References

1. Sehlen S, et al. Depressive ymptoms during and after radiotherapy for head and neck cancer. *Head Neck*. 2003;25(12):1004−1018.
2. Osazuwa-Peters N, et al. Suicide risk among cancer survivors: head and neck versus other cancers. *Cancer*. 2018;124(20):4072−4079.
3. Bernacki RE, Block SD, American F. College of Physicians High Value Care Task, Communication about serious illness care goals: a review and synthesis of best practices. *JAMA Intern Med*. 2014;174(12):1994−2003.
4. Chen AY, et al. The development and validation of a dysphagia-specific quality-of-life questionnaire for patients with head and neck cancer: the M. D. Anderson dysphagia inventory. *Arch Otolaryngol Head Neck Surg*. 2001;127(7):870−876.
5. Rogers SN, et al. The physical function and social-emotional function subscales of the University of Washington Quality of Life Questionnaire. *Arch Otolaryngol Head Neck Surg*. 2010;136(4):352−357.
6. Belafsky PC, et al. Validity and reliability of the eating assessment tool (EAT-10). *Ann Otol Rhinol Laryngol*. 2008;117(12):919−924.
7. Dwivedi RC, et al. Validation of the Sydney Swallow Questionnaire (SSQ) in a cohort of head and neck cancer patients. *Oral Oncol*. 2010;46(4):e10−e14.
8. da Costa de Ceballos AG, et al. Diagnostic validity of Voice Handicap Index-10 (VHI-10) compared with perceptive-auditory and acoustic speech pathology evaluations of the voice. *J Voice*. 2010;24(6):715−718.
9. Slavych BK, Zraick RI, Ruleman A. A systematic review of voice-related patient-reported outcome measures for use with adults. *J Voice*. 2021;38(2).
10. Baylor C, Eadie T, Yorkston K. The communicative participation item bank: evaluating, and reevaluating, its use across communication disorders in adults. *Semin Speech Lang*. 2021;42(3):225−239.
11. Crary MA, Mann GD, Groher ME. Initial psychometric assessment of a functional oral intake scale for dysphagia in stroke patients. *Arch Phys Med Rehabil*. 2005;86(8):1516−1520.
12. List MA, Ritter-Sterr C, Lansky SB. A performance status scale for head and neck cancer patients. *Cancer*. 1990;66(3):564−569.
13. Mason RM, Simon C. An orofacial examination checklist. *Lang Speech Hear Serv Sch*. 1977;8(3):155−163.
14. Hutcheson KA, et al. Delayed lower cranial neuropathy after oropharyngeal intensity-modulated radiotherapy: a cohort analysis and literature review. *Head Neck*. 2017;39(8):1516−1523.
15. Aggarwal P, et al. Swallowing-related outcomes associated with late lower cranial neuropathy in long-term oropharyngeal cancer survivors: cross-sectional survey analysis. *Head Neck*. 2019;41(11):3880−3894.
16. Charters E, et al. A pilot study of intensive intervention using a novel trismus device. *Int J Speech Lang Pathol*. 2022:1−8.
17. Cardoso RC, et al. Self-Reported Trismus: prevalence, severity and impact on quality of life in oropharyngeal cancer survivorship: a cross-sectional survey report from a comprehensive cancer center. *Support Care Cancer*. 2021;29(4):1825−1835.
18. Watters AL, et al. Prevalence of trismus in patients with head and neck cancer: a systematic review with meta-analysis. *Head Neck*. 2019;41(9):3408−3421.

19. McMillan H, et al. Manual therapy for patients with radiation-associated trismus after head and neck cancer. *JAMA Otolaryngol Head Neck Surg.* 2022;148(5):418−425.

20. Hannibal R. Thinking outside of the speech box: cranial nerves made simple. *Aster J Neurosci.* 2017;1:1−11.

21. Woo P. *Stroboscopy and High-Speech Imaging of the Vocal Function.* 2nd ed. Plural Publishing; 2021:437.

22. Palmer AD, et al. The safety and efficacy of expiratory muscle strength training for rehabilitation after supracricoid partial laryngectomy: a pilot investigation. *Ann Otol Rhinol Laryngol.* 2019;128(3):169−176.

23. Jacobi I, et al. Voice and speech outcomes of chemoradiation for advanced head and neck cancer: a systematic review. *Eur Arch Oto-Rhino-Laryngol.* 2010;267(10): 1495−1505.

24. Tuomi L, Andrell P, Finizia C. Effects of voice rehabilitation after radiation therapy for laryngeal cancer: a randomized controlled study. *Int J Radiat Oncol Biol Phys.* 2014; 89(5):964−972.

25. Kang MG, et al. Effects of percutaneous injection laryngoplasty on voice and swallowing problems in cancer-related unilateral vocal cord paralysis. *Laryngoscope Investig Otolaryngol.* 2021;6(4):800−806.

26. Entezami P, et al. A systematic review and meta-analysis on the outcomes of type I thyroplasty in the irradiated neck. *Am J Otolaryngol.* 2023;44(2):103769.

27. Wu MP, et al. Risk factors for laryngectomy for dysfunctional larynx after organ preservation protocols: a case-control analysis. *Otolaryngol Head Neck Surg.* 2021;164(3): 608−615.

28. Cheung NH, Napolitano LM. Tracheostomy: epidemiology, indications, timing, technique, and outcomes. *Respir Care.* 2014;59(6):895−915. discussion 916−9.

29. Kaut K, Turcott JC, Lavery M. Passy-Muir speaking valve. *Dimens Crit Care Nurs.* 1996;15(6):298−306.

30. Holmes TR, et al. Multidisciplinary tracheotomy teams: an analysis of patient outcomes and resource allocation. *Ear Nose Throat J.* 2019;98(4):232−237.

31. O'Connor LR, Morris NR, Paratz J. Physiological and clinical outcomes associated with use of one-way speaking valves on tracheostomised patients: a systematic review. *Heart Lung.* 2019;48(4):356−364.

32. Han X, et al. Biomechanical mechanism of reduced aspiration by the Passy-Muir valve in tracheostomized patients following acquired brain injury: evidences from subglottic pressure. *Front Neurosci.* 2022;16:1004013.

33. Lian S, et al. Clinical utility and future direction of speaking valve: a review. *Front Surg.* 2022;9:913147.

34. Marvin S, Thibeault SL. Predictors of aspiration and silent aspiration in patients with new tracheostomy. *Am J Speech Lang Pathol.* 2021;30(6):2554−2560.

35. McRae RD, et al. Resistance, humidity and temperature of the tracheal airway. *Clin Otolaryngol Allied Sci.* 1995;20(4):355−356.

36. Varghese BT. Tracheostomy care during COVID 19 pandemic in a head and neck oncology unit. *Oral Oncol.* 2020;107:104810.

37. Vitacca M, et al. Breathing pattern and respiratory mechanics in chronically tracheostomized patients with chronic obstructive pulmonary disease breathing spontaneously through a hygroscopic condenser humidifier. *Respiration.* 1997;64(4): 263−267.

38. Merol JC, et al. Randomized controlled trial on postoperative pulmonary humidification after total laryngectomy: external humidifier versus heat and moisture exchanger. *Laryngoscope*. 2012;122(2):275−281.

39. Arora A, et al. Driving standards in tracheostomy care: a preliminary communication of the St Mary's ENT-led multi disciplinary team approach. *Clin Otolaryngol*. 2008;33(6): 596−599.

40. Olinde L, Evangelista L, Bewley AF. Functional laryngectomy for the dysfunctional larynx: indications and outcomes in setting of prior chemoradiotherapy. *Curr Opin Otolaryngol Head Neck Surg*. 2021;29(6):473−478.

41. Hutcheson KA, et al. Outcomes of elective total laryngectomy for laryngopharyngeal dysfunction in disease-free head and neck cancer survivors. *Otolaryngol Head Neck Surg*. 2012;146(4):585−590.

42. Shenson JA, Craig JN, Rohde SL. Effect of preoperative counseling on hospital length of stay and readmissions after total laryngectomy. *Otolaryngol Head Neck Surg*. 2017; 156(2):289−298.

43. Souza FGR, et al. Quality of life after total laryngectomy: impact of different vocal rehabilitation methods in a middle income country. *Health Qual Life Outcomes*. 2020;18(1):92.

44. Singer MI, Blom ED. An endoscopic technique for restoration of voice after laryngectomy. *Ann Otol Rhinol Laryngol*. 1980;89(6 Pt 1):529−533.

45. van Sluis KE, et al. Objective and subjective voice outcomes after total laryngectomy: a systematic review. *Eur Arch Oto-Rhino-Laryngol*. 2018;275(1):11−26.

46. Lewin JS, et al. Device life of the tracheoesophageal voice prosthesis revisited. *JAMA Otolaryngol Head Neck Surg*. 2017;143(1):65−71.

47. Lundstrom E, et al. The pharyngoesophageal segment in laryngectomees−videoradiographic, acoustic, and voice quality perceptual data. *Logoped Phoniatr Vocol*. 2008; 33(3):115−125.

48. Schwarz R, et al. Substitute voice production: quantification of PE segment vibrations using a biomechanical model. *IEEE Trans Biomed Eng*. 2011;58(10):2767−2776.

49. Moon S, et al. Changing trends of speech outcomes after total laryngectomy in the 21st century: a single-center study. *Laryngoscope*. 2014;124(11):2508−2512.

50. Gitomer SA, et al. Influence of timing, radiation, and reconstruction on complications and speech outcomes with tracheoesophageal puncture. *Head Neck*. 2016;38(12): 1765−1771.

51. Doyle PC, Damrose EJ. Has esophageal speech returned as an increasingly viable post-laryngectomy voice and speech rehabilitation option? *J Speech Lang Hear Res*. 2022; 65(12):4714−4723.

52. Isshiki N, Snidecor JC. Air intake and usage in esophageal speech. *Acta Otolaryngol*. 1965;59:559−574.

53. Berlin CI, Zobell DH. Clinical measurement during the acquisition of esophageal speech: II. An unexpected dividend. *J Speech Hear Disord*. 1963;28:389−392.

54. Gates GA, Hearne 3rd EM. Predicting esophageal speech. *Ann Otol Rhinol Laryngol*. 1982;91(4 Pt 1):454−457.

55. Schaefer SD, Johns DF. Attaining functional esophageal speech. *Arch Otolaryngol*. 1982;108(10):647−649.

56. Xi S, et al. The effectiveness of voice rehabilitation on vocalization in post-laryngectomy patients: a systematic review. *JBI Libr Syst Rev*. 2009;7(23):1004−1035.

57. Nagle KF, et al. Effect of fundamental frequency on judgments of electrolaryngeal speech. *Am J Speech Lang Pathol.* 2012;21(2):154−166.
58. Maclean J, Cotton S, Perry A. Dysphagia following a total laryngectomy: the effect on quality of life, functioning, and psychological well-being. *Dysphagia.* 2009;24(3):314−321.
59. Maclean J, Cotton S, Perry A. Post-laryngectomy: it's hard to swallow: an Australian study of prevalence and self-reports of swallowing function after a total laryngectomy. *Dysphagia.* 2009;24(2):172−179.
60. Maclean J, et al. Impact of a laryngectomy and surgical closure technique on swallow biomechanics and dysphagia severity. *Otolaryngol Head Neck Surg.* 2011;144(1):21−28.
61. Sweeny L, et al. Incidence and outcomes of stricture formation postlaryngectomy. *Otolaryngol Head Neck Surg.* 2012;146(3):395−402.
62. Scheenstra RJ, Muller SH, Hilgers FJ. Endotracheal temperature and humidity in laryngectomized patients in a warm and dry environment and the effect of a heat and moisture exchanger. *Head Neck.* 2011;33(9):1285−1293.
63. Hilgers FJ, et al. The influence of a heat and moisture exchanger (HME) on the respiratory symptoms after total laryngectomy. *Clin Otolaryngol Allied Sci.* 1991;16(2):152−156.
64. Hilgers FJ, et al. A multicenter, prospective, clinical trial evaluating a novel adhesive baseplate (Provox StabiliBase) for peristomal attachment of postlaryngectomy pulmonary and voice rehabilitation devices. *Laryngoscope.* 2012;122(11):2447−2453.
65. Leemans M, et al. Analysis of tracheostoma morphology. *Acta Otolaryngol.* 2017;137(9):997−1001.
66. Goepfert RP, et al. Symptom burden as a driver of decisional regret in long-term oropharyngeal carcinoma survivors. *Head Neck.* 2017;39(11):2151−2158.
67. Xu B, et al. Aspiration pneumonia after concurrent chemoradiotherapy for head and neck cancer. *Cancer.* 2015;121(8):1303−1311.
68. Hutcheson KA, et al. Long-term functional and survival outcomes after induction chemotherapy and risk-based definitive therapy for locally advanced squamous cell carcinoma of the head and neck. *Head Neck.* 2014;36(4):474−480.
69. Nicol AJ, et al. Predictive factors for chemoradiation-induced oral mucositis and dysphagia in head and neck cancer: a scoping review. *Cancers.* 2023;15(23).
70. Nutting C, et al. Dysphagia-optimised intensity-modulated radiotherapy versus standard intensity-modulated radiotherapy in patients with head and neck cancer (DARS): a phase 3, multicentre, randomised, controlled trial. *Lancet Oncol.* 2023;24(8):868−880.
71. Petkar I, et al. DARS: a phase III randomised multicentre study of dysphagia- optimised intensity- modulated radiotherapy (Do-IMRT) versus standard intensity- modulated radiotherapy (S-IMRT) in head and neck cancer. *BMC Cancer.* 2016;16(1):770.
72. McDowell L, Hutcheson KA, Ringash J. Dysphagia-optimised intensity-modulated radiotherapy versus standard radiotherapy in patients with pharyngeal cancer. *Lancet Oncol.* 2023;24(10):e396.
73. Massonet H, et al. Home-based intensive treatment of chronic radiation-associated dysphagia in head and neck cancer survivors (HIT-CRAD trial). *Trials.* 2022;23(1):893.
74. Hutcheson KA, et al. Expiratory muscle strength training for radiation-associated aspiration after head and neck cancer: a case series. *Laryngoscope.* 2018;128(5):1044−1051.

75. Crary MA, et al. Functional and physiological outcomes from an exercise-based dysphagia therapy: a pilot investigation of the McNeill Dysphagia Therapy Program. *Arch Phys Med Rehabil.* 2012;93(7):1173−1178.

76. Barbon CEA, et al. Adhering to eat and exercise status during radiotherapy for oropharyngeal cancer for prevention and mitigation of radiotherapy-associated dysphagia. *JAMA Otolaryngol Head Neck Surg.* 2022;148(10):956−964.

77. Rodriguez AM, et al. A scoping review of rehabilitation interventions for survivors of head and neck cancer. *Disabil Rehabil.* 2019;41(17):2093−2107.

78. McBride SM, et al. Intensity-modulated versus conventional radiation therapy for oropharyngeal carcinoma: long-term dysphagia and tumor control outcomes. *Head Neck.* 2014;36(4):492−498.

79. Ursino S, et al. Patient-reported outcomes after swallowing (SWOARs)-sparing IMRT in head and neck cancers: primary results from a prospective study endorsed by the head and neck study group (HNSG) of the Italian association of radiotherapy and clinical oncology (AIRO). *Dysphagia.* 2023;38(1):159−170.

80. Silver JA, et al. Quality of life after neoadjuvant chemotherapy and transoral robotic surgery for oropharynx cancer. *JAMA Otolaryngol Head Neck Surg.* 2023;150(1): 65−74.

81. Sher DJ, et al. Efficacy and quality-of-life following involved nodal radiotherapy for head and neck squamous cell carcinoma: the INRT-AIR phase II clinical trial. *Clin Cancer Res.* 2023;29(17):3284−3291.

82. Alexidis P, et al. Investigating predictive factors of dysphagia and treatment prolongation in patients with oral cavity or oropharyngeal cancer receiving radiation therapy concurrently with chemotherapy. *Curr Oncol.* 2023;30(5):5168−5178.

83. Liu HC, et al. Quantitative prediction of aspiration risk in head and neck cancer patients treated with radiation therapy. *Oral Oncol.* 2023;136:106247.

84. Jeri A, Logeman KAH, Starmer HM, Ciucci MR, Gibbons PJ, Tellis GM. *Logemann's Evaluation and Treatment of Swallowing Disorders.* 3rd ed. 2022:440. Pre-ed.

85. Molfenter SM, Steele CM. Temporal variability in the deglutition literature. *Dysphagia.* 2012;27(2):162−177.

86. Martin-Harris B, et al. Respiratory-swallow training in patients with head and neck cancer. *Arch Phys Med Rehabil.* 2015;96(5):885−893.

87. Hopkins-Rossabi T, et al. Respiratory-swallow coordination and swallowing impairment in head and neck cancer. *Head Neck.* 2021;43(5):1398−1408.

88. Logemann JA. The role of the speech language pathologist in the management of dysphagia. *Otolaryngol Clin North Am.* 1988;21(4):783−788.

89. Logemann JA, et al. Impact of the diagnostic procedure on outcome measures of swallowing rehabilitation in head and neck cancer patients. *Dysphagia.* 1992;7(4):179−186.

90. Suiter DM, Leder SB. Clinical utility of the 3-ounce water swallow test. *Dysphagia.* 2008;23(3):244−250.

91. Martino R, et al. The Toronto Bedside Swallowing Screening Test (TOR-BSST): development and validation of a dysphagia screening tool for patients with stroke. *Stroke.* 2009;40(2):555−561.

92. Suiter DM, Sloggy J, Leder SB. Validation of the Yale Swallow Protocol: a prospective double-blinded videofluoroscopic study. *Dysphagia.* 2014;29(2):199−203.

93. Carnaby GD, Crary MA. Development and validation of a cancer-specific swallowing assessment tool: MASA-C. *Support Care Cancer.* 2014;22(3):595−602.

94. Martin-Harris B, et al. Best practices in modified barium swallow studies. *Am J Speech Lang Pathol.* 2020;29(2S):1078−1093.

95. Clain AE, et al. Structural validity, internal consistency, and rater reliability of the modified barium swallow impairment profile: breaking ground on a 52,726-patient, clinical data set. *J Speech Lang Hear Res.* 2022;65(5):1659−1670.

96. Martin-Harris B, et al. MBS measurement tool for swallow impairment–MBSImp: establishing a standard. *Dysphagia.* 2008;23(4):392−405.

97. Hutcheson KA, et al. Dynamic imaging grade of swallowing toxicity (DIGEST): scale development and validation. *Cancer.* 2017;123(1):62−70.

98. Hutcheson KA, et al. Refining measurement of swallowing safety in the dynamic imaging grade of swallowing toxicity (DIGEST) criteria: validation of DIGEST version 2. *Cancer.* 2022;128(7):1458−1466.

99. Rosenbek JC, et al. A penetration-aspiration scale. *Dysphagia.* 1996;11(2):93−98.

100. Queija DDS, et al. Cervicofacial and pharyngolaryngeal lymphedema and deglutition after head and neck cancer treatment. *Dysphagia.* 2020;35(3):479−491.

101. Langmore SE, et al. Tutorial on clinical practice for use of the fiberoptic endoscopic evaluation of swallowing procedure with adult populations: Part 1. *Am J Speech Lang Pathol.* 2022;31(1):163−187.

102. Langmore SE. Evaluation of oropharyngeal dysphagia: which diagnostic tool is superior? *Curr Opin Otolaryngol Head Neck Surg.* 2003;11(6):485−489.

103. Labeit B, et al. Comparison of simultaneous swallowing endoscopy and videofluoroscopy in neurogenic dysphagia. *J Am Med Dir Assoc.* 2022;23(8):1360−1366.

104. Wu CH, et al. Evaluation of swallowing safety with fiberoptic endoscope: comparison with videofluoroscopic technique. *Laryngoscope.* 1997;107(3):396−401.

105. Neubauer PD, Rademaker AW, Leder SB. The Yale pharyngeal residue severity rating scale: an anatomically defined and image-based tool. *Dysphagia.* 2015;30(5):521−528.

106. Starmer HM, et al. Adaptation and validation of the dynamic imaging grade of swallowing toxicity for flexible endoscopic evaluation of swallowing: DIGEST-FEES. *J Speech Lang Hear Res.* 2021;64(6):1802−1810.

107. Kaneoka AS, et al. The Boston Residue and Clearance Scale: preliminary reliability and validity testing. *Folia Phoniatr Logop.* 2013;65(6):312−317.

108. Erul E, et al. Role of sarcopenia on survival and treatment-related toxicity in head and neck cancer: a narrative review of current evidence and future perspectives. *Eur Arch Oto-Rhino-Laryngol.* 2023;280(8):3541−3556.

109. Denaro N, Merlano MC, Russi EG. Dysphagia in head and neck cancer patients: pretreatment evaluation, predictive factors, and assessment during radio-chemotherapy, recommendations. *Clin Exp Otorhinolaryngol.* 2013;6(3):117−126.

110. Wopken K, Bijl HP, Langendijk JA. Prognostic factors for tube feeding dependence after curative (chemo-) radiation in head and neck cancer: a systematic review of literature. *Radiother Oncol.* 2018;126(1):56−67.

111. Kuhn MA, et al. Expert consensus statement: management of dysphagia in head and neck cancer patients. *Otolaryngol Head Neck Surg.* 2023;168(4):571−592.

112. Gupta DK, et al. Evaluation of swallowing in patients with T3/T4 oral squamous cell carcinoma. *Med J Armed Forces India.* 2023;79(2):181−188.

113. Ou M, et al. Perioperative change trajectories and predictors of swallowing function and swallowing-related quality of life in patients with oral cancer: a longitudinal observational study. *BMJ Open.* 2023;13(12):e075401.

114. Hutcheson KA, et al. Dysphagia after primary transoral robotic surgery with neck dissection vs nonsurgical therapy in patients with low- to intermediate-risk oropharyngeal cancer. *JAMA Otolaryngol Head Neck Surg.* 2019;145(11):1053−1063.

115. Freitas AS, et al. Residue localization and risk for aspiration in partial laryngectomy: the relevance of assertive therapeutic strategies and resources. *Einstein (Sao Paulo).* 2022;20:eAO6262.

116. Pizzorni N, et al. Swallowing safety and efficiency after open partial horizontal laryngectomy: a videofluoroscopic study. *Cancers.* 2019;11(4).

117. Lewin JS, et al. Functional analysis of swallowing outcomes after supracricoid partial laryngectomy. *Head Neck.* 2008;30(5):559−566.

118. Seth I, et al. Pre-rehabilitation interventions for patients with head and neck cancers: a systematic review and meta-analysis. *Head Neck.* 2024;46(1):86−117.

119. Szczesniak MM, et al. Persistent dysphagia after head and neck radiotherapy: a common and under-reported complication with significant effect on non-cancer-related mortality. *Clin Oncol.* 2014;26(11):697−703.

120. Cates DJ, Evangelista LM, Belafsky PC. Effect of pretreatment dysphagia on postchemoradiation swallowing function in head and neck cancer. *Otolaryngol Head Neck Surg.* 2022;166(3):506−510.

121. Rosenthal DI, Lewin JS, Eisbruch A. Prevention and treatment of dysphagia and aspiration after chemoradiation for head and neck cancer. *J Clin Oncol.* 2006;24(17):2636−2643.

122. Hutcheson KA, et al. Eat and exercise during radiotherapy or chemoradiotherapy for pharyngeal cancers: use it or lose it. *JAMA Otolaryngol Head Neck Surg.* 2013;139(11):1127−1134.

123. Ajmani GS, et al. Association of a proactive swallowing rehabilitation program with feeding tube placement in patients treated for pharyngeal cancer. *JAMA Otolaryngol Head Neck Surg.* 2018;144(6):483−488.

124. Iovoli AJ, et al. Severe oral mucositis after intensity-modulated radiation therapy for head and neck cancer. *JAMA Netw Open.* 2023;6(10):e2337265.

125. Gill G, et al. Longitudinal functional outcomes and late effects of radiation following treatment of nasopharyngeal carcinoma: secondary analysis of a prospective cohort study. *J Otolaryngol Head Neck Surg.* 2022;51(1):41.

126. Martin-Gonzalez C, et al. Oropharyngeal dysphagia in head and neck cancer: how to reduce aspiration pneumonia. *J Laryngol Otol.* 2023;137(7):820−825.

127. Burkhead LM, Sapienza CM, Rosenbek JC. Strength-training exercise in dysphagia rehabilitation: principles, procedures, and directions for future research. *Dysphagia.* 2007;22(3):251−265.

128. Hinther A, et al. Volumetric changes in pharyngeal structures following head and neck cancer chemoradiation therapy. *Laryngoscope.* 2020;130(3):597−602.

129. Patterson JM, Lawton M. Dysphagia advances in head and neck cancer. *Curr Otorhinolaryngol Rep.* 2023:1−8.

130. Starmer H, et al. Pretreatment swallowing assessment in head and neck cancer patients. *Laryngoscope.* 2011;121(6):1208−1211.

131. Beuren AG, et al. Preventive measures for the progression of dysphagia in patients with cancer of head and neck subjected to radiotherapy: a systematic review with meta-analysis. *Codas.* 2023;35(2):e20210246.

132. Carnaby-Mann GD, Crary MA. McNeill dysphagia therapy program: a case-control study. *Arch Phys Med Rehabil.* 2010;91(5):743−749.

133. Loewen I, et al. Prehabilitation in head and neck cancer patients: a literature review. *J Otolaryngol Head Neck Surg*. 2021;50(1):2.
134. Hutcheson KA, et al. Eat All through Radiation Therapy (EAT-RT): structured therapy model to facilitate continued oral intake through head and neck radiotherapy-User acceptance and content validation. *Head Neck*. 2020;42(9):2390−2396.
135. Malandraki GA, Hutcheson KA. Intensive therapies for dysphagia: implementation of the intensive dysphagia rehabilitation and the MD Anderson Swallowing Boot Camp Approaches. *Perspect ASHA Spec Interest Groups*. 2018;3(13):133−145.

Rehabilitation of communication disorders related to head and neck cancer

12

Mary E. Owens, MEd, CCC-SLP and Daniel Gonzalez, MSV

Miami Cancer Institute, Miami, FL, United States

The way we communicate with others and with ourselves ultimately determines the quality of our lives …

Tony Robbins.

Individuals diagnosed with head and neck cancer (HNC) present with unique challenges pre-and postintervention. The 5-year survival rate for individuals recovering from or living with head and neck cancer is variable depending on the site of malignancy. Based on data retrieved from the American Cancer Society website from 2012 to 2018, patients diagnosed with cancer of the head and neck involving the oral cavity, oropharynx, supraglottis, glottis, subglottis and hypopharynx had survival rates ranging from 91% for lip cancer down to 37% for hypopharyngeal cancer. This data does not consider survivorship related to head and neck cancers positive for p16 (HPV), which have a survival rate of greater than 5 years.[1] Head and neck cancer can impact critical areas involved in verbal communication. Cancers that occur within the oral cavity, pharynx, and larynx have a damaging effect on the ability of a person to produce clear speech and voicing. Thus, many individuals diagnosed with head and neck cancer may develop short-term and sometimes lifelong difficulties with their communication.

Although dysphagia is the main concern when considering the role of the speech−language pathologist (SLP) as a patient undergoes treatment for head and neck cancer, this chapter will identify the other role of the SLP: the evaluation and management of communication disorders with the ultimate goal of improving quality of life (QOL). Whether through surgical intervention or effects of chemoradiation therapy, cancer in the head and neck region leads to changes in communication, specifically in the areas of articulation, voice, and resonance. The degree of these deficits spans from mild to severe, ranging from speech that is intelligible but noticeably defective to total voice loss, or aphonia. No matter the severity, communication impairments derived from head and neck cancers negatively impact the quality of life of an individual. In a study conducted by Aggarwal et al. (2021), the responses of 906 survivors who were treated for oropharyngeal cancer responded to the MD Anderson Symptom Inventory−Head and Neck Cancer Module were

Copyright © 2025 Elsevier Inc. All rights reserved, including those for text and data mining, AI training, and similar technologies.

analyzed. Of the participants, 881 patients responded to the questions about voice and speech symptoms. Based on results, 12.8% reported moderate to severe voice symptoms and 32.7% reported mild voice and speech symptoms.[2] This data is significant because when people feel as although there is a communication disorder, the tendency is to speak less and there is an increased risk for social isolation. Several studies have been conducted in the area of QOL. Available data from a recent study published in the Journal of Clinical Oncology in 2018 concluded that HNC survivors were nearly twice as likely to die by suicide than other cancer survivors and will benefit from lifelong psychosocial interventions.[3] A systematic review of many studies identifies impairments in communication and swallowing as well as physical changes to the head and neck region as primary factors impacting the quality of life[4]; thus the SLP is a vital member of the multidisciplinary HNC team.

Overview

When a person is diagnosed with a tumor in the head and neck region, treatment will typically involve one or a combination of the following three options: surgery, radiation therapy, and systemic therapy such as chemotherapy and immunotherapy. Cases are typically presented at a tumor board with the head and neck cancer team in attendance to determine the course of treatment. While tumor eradication is primary goal, the treatment plan will largely depend on the size and extent of the tumor as well as the overall health of the patient. Risk factors, such as comorbidities and age, influence the treatment approaches. Many individuals with head and neck cancer will receive surgical resections that will alter the anatomy and physiology of the structures within the oral cavity, pharynx, and larynx. In other cases, individuals will undergo chemoradiation that may result in internal inflammation and/or tissue damage that will lead to chronic impairments in speech and voice production.

Ideally, when the patient's case is presented at a tumor board, the SLP will be present to gain knowledge of the treatment plan. It is useful for the SLP to have established clinical pathways for management of patients with head and neck cancer. These may include workflows for surgical resection, chemoradiation, and total laryngectomy (TL). All clinical pathways should include a baseline communication assessment, established followup treatment visits, as well as future follow-up/reassessment if applicable.

Baseline visit

The SLP is introduced to the patient with head and neck cancer early on in their diagnosis, before surgery and/or other treatment has commenced. As stated, the predominant role of the SLP with this population is dysphagia. This first visit serves as a baseline evaluation of swallowing skills along with speech production and voice parameters of the patient. During this initial visit, the SLP will establish a relationship with the patient and family and review the role of speech language pathology in cancer treatment. Here, the SLP will also gauge patient's understanding of their upcoming treatment and receptiveness to SLP intervention.

The components of the baseline evaluation necessary for communication include the following:

Case history: Include medical and surgical history, medications, and prior level of function. A thorough case history is pertinent in establishing goals and prognosis of maximizing communication skills.

Comprehensive assessment: Evaluation of the areas involved in speech and voice production. A thorough speech/voice assessment will include an oral mechanism examination along with measurements of speech, voice, and resonance parameters. A formal cognitive/linguistic evaluation does not necessarily need to be completed, but an informal assessment of expressive and receptive language, problem-solving, and memory skills will provide beneficial information when considering communication options postcancer treatment. The patient should also have a hearing screening and be referred to an audiologist if results are not favorable.

The data collected during the initial assessment is essential for the clinician because it serves a reference point to baseline function prior to medical intervention and therapeutic rehabilitation. Overall, the analysis of speech production and vocal function and ability is a combination of subjective and objective measurements and may predict outcomes for successful communication postcancer treatment.

Oral mechanism examination: Strength, range of movement, agility, and function of oral components are necessary for speech production and resonance. The clinician assesses the oral cavity, observing dentition, oral mucosa, and oral hygiene and may use instrumentation when available for more accurate measurements in the following areas:

Mouth opening/jaw mobility: Normal mouth opening is ∼50 mm or three of the individual's own fingers. Maximum interincisal opening (MIO) is measured as the maximal distance between the incisors of the maxilla and the mandible. MIO of 35 mm or less is considered trismus.

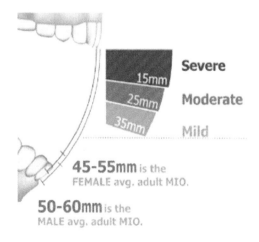

Photos from craniorehab.com

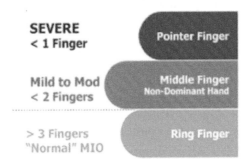

Three-Finger Basic Diagnostic

SEVERE
< 1 Finger — Pointer Finger

Mild to Mod
< 2 Fingers — Middle Finger Non-Dominant Hand

> 3 Fingers "Normal" MIO — Ring Finger

The 3-Finger method generally accounts for body size, the primary determination of MIO. Normal **MIO** is about the height of a person's pointer, middle, and ring finger on their **NON-DOMINANT** hand.

Trismus (decreased mouth opening) may be present during the initial evaluation related to the tumor itself or trismus may develop because of the cancer treatment. In the literature, trismus is reported anywhere between 10% and 50% in relation to head and neck cancer.[5] Trismus and/or decreased jaw mobility may impact speech production by impairing resonance and articulation. Trismus may also impact a person's ability to perform oral hygiene, place dentures, and place an obturator or palate augmentation device, thereby having a negative impact on communication. Knowing baseline MIO as well as planned cancer intervention will be beneficial for clinician to treatment plan and to educate the patient.

Lip/tongue strength and ROM: Inadequate lip and tongue strength/pressure may affect phoneme production. The clinician will observe labial and lingual ROM to assess for any weakness or limitation that may interfere with the production of intelligible speech. Tongue and lip strength and endurance can be measured with an instrument such as an Iowa Oral Performance Instrument (IOPI) for baseline values. Additionally, to judge labial and lingual movement, speed, and coordination, the SLP may have the individual perform alternating motion rates or diadochokinetic rates.

Palate elevation: Soft palate elevation is essential for adequate resonance. Velopharyngeal insufficiency (VPI) is the incomplete closure of the sphincter between the oral pharynx and nasal pharynx and may occur due to tumor in the palate. VPI may also be seen following surgical resection of structures in the area such as tonsils or adenoids. Additionally, VPI may also occur from immediate of late effects of radiation therapy due to soft tissue radionecrosis.[6]

The clinician will then obtain baseline values in the following areas:

Speech production: A patient's articulation skills will likely be impacted both by the resection and reconstruction of oral tumors as well as effects of chemoradiation therapy. A clinician can obtain valuable baseline information via perceptual and instrumental assessment of articulation and speech intelligibility. This assessment should include data related to speech parameters of rate, timing, and precision at the word, phrase, sentence, and conversational speech level. Standardized articulation tests that provide more accurate measures include Frenchay Dysarthria Assessment and Computerized Assessment of Intelligibility in Dysarthric Speakers.

Resonance: When a person undergoes palate resection and/or radiation to the nasopharynx it typically results in VPI causing a resonance disorder. VPI has also been noted following treatment for cancers in the oral pharynx, including the base of tongue and posterior pharyngeal wall.[7] Too little or too much nasality can have a negative impact on speech production. During the assessment, the clinician can perceptually assess resonance and note hypernasality, hyponasality, nasal emission, and/or cul-de-sac resonance. It is best practice to have a baseline measurement via instrumentation for comparative data postcancer treatment. Standard measures include nasometry, videonasendoscopy, and nasopharyngoscopy.

Voice: Dysphonia may be a clinical indicator of a tumor or other vocal pathology but is not always the result of a vocal fold lesion. Dysphonia may develop from chemo/radiation therapy due to inflammation, scarring, or nerve damage. There are many contributing factors to dysphonia, such as those pertaining to vocal hygiene. The clinician will perform a perceptual and acoustic analysis of vocal function, documenting the quality, pitch, and loudness of the voice, which are correlated with other acoustic and aerodynamic values. Vocal parameters such as fundamental frequency, frequency range, maximum phonation time, voicing percentage, vocal intensity, and acoustic perturbation can be gathered using a voice analysis software, such as the Visi-Pitch (Fig. 12.1). It is also helpful to make general observations

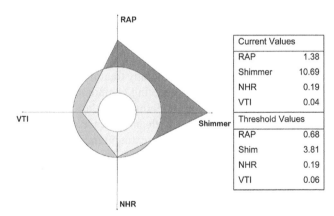

Current Values	
RAP	1.38
Shimmer	10.69
NHR	0.19
VTI	0.04
Threshold Values	
RAP	0.68
Shim	3.81
NHR	0.19
VTI	0.06

FIGURE 12.1

Voice analysis using Visi-Pitch.

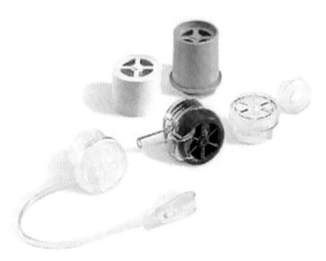

FIGURE 12.2

PMSV image courtesy of Passey-Muir Inc.

regarding respiration as a patient may be tracheotomy dependent postcancer treatment and might benefit from the use of a one-way valve such as a Passey-Muir Speaking Valve (PMSV) (Fig. 12.2) for functional communication.

If a patient is scheduled to undergo a TL, there is no need to take initial voice measurements. Instead, the session will focus on education on "the new voice." The clinical pathway for (TL) will be fully discussed later in this chapter.

Counseling and education: This first meeting also serves as a valuable counseling and education session for the patient, where the patient will be further educated on the anatomical and physiologic changes that occur with surgery and/or the possible impact cancer treatment may have on his or her ability to communicate. It is helpful to have a model of the head and neck region when providing education to patients. When reviewing anatomy and physiology with surgical patients, it is important that the patient be aware of both temporary and possible permanent effects the surgical plan will have on communication. Also, reviewing the postoperative speech therapy treatment plan may be included in this education session. For patients receiving chemoradiation therapy, education should include side effects of these treatment modalities including xerostomia and mucositis and their impact on speech and voice. Patient education should also include the long-term effects of cancer treatment including radiation fibrosis and osteoradionecrosis. Radiation fibrosis varies from patient to patient and is still an area with many unknowns. The patient may experience or report pain, trismus, neck stiffness, and tissue fibrosis, all of which can impact communication.[8] Damage to the jawbone (ORN) may also occur because of radiation therapy. Additional education may include prophylactic oral motor and voice exercises if warranted as well as compensatory strategies for speech production and voice conservation. Although the physician or dentist may have already educated the patient in oral and dental hygiene, additional education in this area should be provided as to its impact on communication.

Treatment/clinical pathways

Following the initial consultation, the clinician will remain in close contact with the patient and the cancer team. Patient follow-up will be dependent on treatment options/clinical pathways.

    Clinical pathway chemoradiation: For patients whose primary treatment is chemo- and/or radiation therapy, there may be cause to follow the patient on a weekly or biweekly basis to review home program and assist in strategy use to maximize communication. Strategies include compensatory techniques for speech production and voice conservation for dysphonia.

    Once chemoradiation therapy is completed, the patient typically requires 3–4 weeks to recover from immediate toxicities. When medically cleared for treatment, the patient initiates aggressive communication therapy.

    Clinical pathway surgery: Surgery and adjuvant therapy is typically the treatment of choice for patients[9] with oral cancers and may include resection of lips, tongue, floor of mouth, buccal mucosa, hard palate, maxilla, and mandible. The size and location of the tumor typically dictates the surgical approach and volume of mass removed. For example, an early-stage tongue cancer may be treated with a wide local excision while a more advanced tumor may require a hemiglossectomy with free flap reconstruction.

    Hard palate tumors are less common than other oral cancers. Again, depending on the volume removed, the excised area may be closed after surgery. If not, a prosthetic device such as an obturator may be required to close the affected area.

    While less common, a patient with laryngeal cancer may undergo a partial laryngectomy or vertical/hemilaryngectomy. Either option may have a negative impact on voice and/or may require temporary or permanent tracheostomy.

    The SLP should have a clear understanding of the surgical plan and refer to the operative report to identify structures removed, reconstruction efforts and future plans, whether it be chemo- and/or radiation therapy or any further surgery. The SLP may see the patient postoperatively while still hospitalized once cleared by the surgeon. At this stage, the SLP may introduce the patient to resistive oral motor exercises and begin training in compensatory strategies to improve communication skills.

    Upon discharge home, the patient will be referred for aggressive rehabilitation in an ambulatory setting, which may start as soon as 1 week postdischarge. If the plan is for adjuvant therapy, the clinical pathway for chemoradiation may instead be followed as the patient may not be clinically ready to participate in aggressive therapy until they complete chemoradiation.

Postsurgical/chemoradiation therapy treatment

Whether single or multimodality treatment, the patient will undergo a complete reassessment of oral motor, resonance, speech production, and voice parameters. The clinician will also identify any areas of inflammation, ulceration, muscle tension, and any negative behaviors that may be impacting speech and voice such as frequent throat clearing. It is also important to note any other changes such as presence of a tracheostomy tube or any prosthetic devices. In addition, it is recommended to have patient complete quality of life (QOL) scales to obtain a baseline measure of the patient's QOL. Two popular choices include Speech Handicap Index (SHI)[10] and the Voice Handicap Index (VHI).[11] Therapy goals to maximize communication skills will be established with the patient and will be dependent on various factors including, but not limited to surgical resection, adjuvant therapy type and dosage, treatment fields, comorbidities, and overall patient motivation and family support. Treatment plans are geared to the individualized needs of the patient and require multiple modalities.

Treatment options

Once the reassessment is completed and goals are established to address deficit areas, the clinician then reviews the treatment plan including patient role, clinician role, and referrals/collaboration with other healthcare providers. With all treatment plans, it is important for the patient to understand the purpose and benefits of performing each prescribed exercise as this awareness typically leads to compliance. Common treatment plans and modalities include the following:

Resistive oral motor exercises: Although there is conflicting evidence in the literature on the benefit, exercises designed to increase strength, ROM and agility of lips, tongue, cheek, jaw, and palate are often prescribed to the patient during treatment. Using principles of exercise physiology, these exercises should be performed against resistance to improve strength, ROM, agility, and endurance. Rapid alternating movements of the articulators are required to improve articulation. A recent study by Van den Steen, Baudelet et al. showed improved tongue strength after 8 weeks of training using the IOPI.[12] In addition to its use in providing assessment values of tongue strength, the IOPI is also used for treatment. When using the IOPI for exercise, the SLP sets a target to a specific value and the patient receives biofeedback each time the target is achieved. As tongue strength improves, the target value can be adjusted making this a progressive resistance exercise program. The use of an IOPI or similar devices is motivating for the patient as it provides immediate feedback on performance and progress toward the goal.

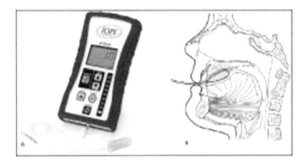

IOPI

Manual therapy

Another option for oral motor weakness is evidence-based myofascial release (MFR). Fascia is the connective tissues that cover most body parts including organs and muscles and is made up of mostly collagen. The fascia may harden over time due to trauma, in patients treated for HNC likely due to surgery and/or radiation therapy, thus restricting movement and flexibility. MFR is a type of manual therapy technique designed to stretch and loosen the connective tissue to improve mobility, breakup adhesions, and decrease pain. Trained clinicians may perform releases and techniques including transverse muscle play and fascial elongation to improve the function of muscles for speech and voice production.[13]

While most patients experience edema in the head and neck region following head and neck cancer treatment, chronic swelling may be related to lymphedema. According to the literature review, lymphedema may occur in ~75% of patients being treated with surgery and/or radiation.[14] If lymphedema is present, patients may benefit from manual lymph drainage (MLD) as part of a complete decongestive therapy (CDT). Trained clinicians may perform MLD in the head and neck regions as well as intraoral to reduce swelling and improve function. Clinicians who use this modality must be aware of contraindications to MLD including CHF, major cardiac problems, uncontrolled HTN, cellulitis, tissue breakdown, and active disease. Discuss any concerns with the referring physician prior to initiating MLD.

If oral motor weakness is due to defects from oral surgery, the goal is to maximize residual ROM of impacted structures. This can be achieved through the aforementioned therapeutic modalities. If the residual defects continue to negatively impact speech intelligibility, the SLP may contact the surgeon for any available medical management options available to patient.

Treatment for trismus

If the patient presents with trismus, treatment options include manual therapy, passive and active jaw stretching, masseter and medial pterygoid release, and neck stretches/ ROM. The patient may also benefit from the use of TheraBite/OraStretch or an Ark-J. Always seek physician clearance if there is a surgical flap prior to using a device or if there are any concerns for osteoradionecrosis (ORN). There is limited available research in the benefit of the use of a device versus a home exercise program in the treatment of trismus. However, available literature supports the benefit of adhering to a jaw mobility program. A retrospective study found gains in mouth opening using manual therapy, with the greatest gain after the first session.[15] Additionally, recent studies have found that low-level laser therapy and low-intensity ultrasound combined with an exercise program have had positive results with jaw mobility.[16]

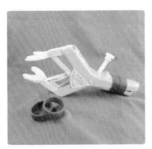

Orastretch with resistance bands for dynamic stretching, Image courtesy of Cranio Mandibular Rehab, Inc.

Speech production exercises: To improve articulation, the treatment plan includes maximizing function of articulators via oral motor exercises as well as traditional articulation therapy including direct therapy focusing on the speech parameters of place, manner, and voicing within the specific phoneme groups. The foundation of articulation therapy is the motor production of each speech sound in isolation with generalization to syllable, word, phrase, sentence, and ultimately conversation level. While several studies have shown that speech therapy is effective in improving articulation following treatment for head and neck cancer, the first acoustic analysis of speech in individuals treated for head and neck cancer showed the manner of articulation rather than place of articulation was more predictive of articulation changes posttreatment.[17] This is significant because further research in this area may change speech rehabilitation strategies following treatment for HNC.

If a patient has undergone surgery, such as a glossectomy, the treatment plan includes training in compensatory strategies including reducing rate and exaggerating articulation to maximize the residual tongue movement. It is also important to eliminate any negative compensatory behaviors early in the therapy sessions. Trial and error and extensive training to maximize use of effective strategies is advised for optimal articulation.

Prosthetic options including dentures and palatal augmentation prosthesis may also have a positive impact on articulation. A palatal augmentation device will improve tongue—palate contact during speech, improving production of lingual phonemes. The clinician works closely with the prosthodontist when designing these devices for optimal function.

Resonance: VPI may result from the surgical resection of tumors extending to the soft palate or because of toxicities from radiation therapy. VPI results in the perception of hypernasality and in some cases nasal emission. Mild cases of VPI can usually be successfully treated by the SLP with focus on palate elevation and increasing oral pressure via elevating loudness and exaggerating articulation.

For more severe cases of VPI, the patient may benefit from prosthetic options such as a palatal lift or palatal obturator. The palatal lift is designed to assist in velopharyngeal closure by elevating the soft palate. This is beneficial for patients with a structurally intact palate who may have VPI due to denervation from tumor location or radiation fibrosis. The palatal obturator is designed to close the defects in the hard and soft palate from the palate resection to prevent hypernasality and improve intraoral pressure. Unfortunately, for defects in the soft palate, the palatal obturator is not completely efficient in preventing hypernasality.

Voice: Depending on the cause and severity of dysphonia, several treatment options are available. The foundation of voice rehabilitation is behavioral modifications for voice use. Namely, voice therapy targets optimizing vocal quality, loudness, and pitch by improving the balance/coordination among respiratory, phonatory, and resonatory systems. It is useful to begin the session with tension displacement and relaxation exercises to reduce laryngeal tension. This may include head and neck stretches to promote movement and flexibility in the compromised region. Furthermore, the SLP may integrate manual therapy techniques to reduce tension and inflammation in the laryngeal area. These include myofascial release, MLD if lymphedema is present and circumlaryngeal massages and reposturing techniques. Simultaneously, these exercises also promote proprioceptive awareness and work in conjunction to improve posture, which ties directly into breath awareness and support.

During voice therapy, the SLP wants the patient to improve their inspiratory capacity by maximizing diaphragmatic breathing. In layman's terms, the SLP promotes deep breathing by instructing the patient to utilize a "lowered" breath without extensive clavicular or thoracic involvement. Additionally, the SLP trains expiratory capacity through expiratory muscle strength training (EMST) techniques. This may be trained through guided respiration activities involving verbal, visual, or tactile instructions or with devices designed to improve both inspiratory and expiratory strength. By improving both inspiratory and expiratory capacity, the patient is learning how to speak/phonate with optimal breath support.

When addressing phonation and resonance, the SLP may work on a variety of voice exercises including vocal function exercises, resonant voice techniques, and semioccluded vocal tract (SOVT) exercises. If a patient has a tracheostomy, therapy will target coordinating respiration and phonation as well as use and tolerance of PMSV. Ultimately, the goal is to promote balanced phonation without laryngeal strain or compensation as well as to improve vocal fold adduction. Because many individuals recovering from radiation therapy may present with increased inflammation in the anatomy involved in phonation, it is imperative for the individual to learn how to speak or phonate with minimal laryngeal strain or effort to achieve a more functional and healthier voice.

The patient will also benefit from education and training in voice conservation strategies and vocal hygiene awareness. This includes promoting a balance between voice use and voice rest, as sometimes managing vocal demands and vocal needs is a challenge for these patients who want to reintegrate themselves in occupational and social domains. Although the individual is encouraged to utilize their voice, they are advised to avoid straining and are dissuaded from engaging in other vocally abusive behaviors (i.e., whispering, shouting, throat clearing). Due to increased dryness in the larynx, the SLP may also encourage the patient to improve both systemic and topical hydration by increasing water intake, using a humidifier, or using portable nebulizer. Additionally, the individual will be encouraged to avoid or reduce the intake of drying agents, such as caffeine and alcohol.

If voice rehabilitation alone is not successful, the SLP may refer the patient to the ENT to discuss surgical options for dysphonia including medialization of a paralyzed vocal fold or vocal fold injection to augment area.

Clinical pathway TL: Prior to surgery, the patient is referred to speech pathology services for a presurgery counseling session. As with all precancer treatment sessions, it is important for the clinician to establish a relationship with both the patient and caregivers as well as to assess the patient's understanding of the upcoming surgery. During this initial visit, an evaluation and/or observation of communication skills is completed, assessing language, articulation, oral mechanism, hearing, reading, and writing. This is necessary to establish postoperative communication expectations and goals. Education is extremely important during this session. There are several companies that provide information and products for patients undergoing TL. Two of the more popular companies include ATOS Medical and Inhealth Technologies. Both companies provide a wealth of information for patients and caregivers, and when possible, the clinician should have information packets from these companies to provide to the patient as well as information regarding websites for reference.

It is helpful to have a model of the larynx when reviewing the anatomical and physiologic changes that will impact both communication and swallowing. Ensure clear understanding that the "voice box" will be permanently removed and that the patient will learn and use a "new voice" for communication. Additionally, the patient should be educated in neck breathing for oxygen and resuscitation and be provided information with regard to medical alert bracelet stating that the patient is a neck breather. The patient and caregiver must also be educated in the importance of postlaryngectomy pulmonary rehab via use of stoma covers and heat moisture exchange cartridge (HME). When the stoma is covered with foam or HME and when the patient exhales, the heat and moisture is trapped so there is some degree of heat and moisture upon inhalation. The clinician may show the patient an actual HME and review its benefits of 24-h use including decreasing coughing, mucous, expectoration, and need for stoma cleaning. Finally, the clinician will review stoma care, changes in taste, and smell and necessary lifestyle changes. When addressing these changes, it is important to provide handouts to the patient and caregivers, clearly stating information presented.

The patient is then introduced to the three prominent communication options following TL. The first option is the **artificial larynx** more commonly known as the **electrolarynx**. This is a portable handheld device that is typically used on the neck or cheek. There is also an intraoral adapter option available, which can be used immediately following the surgery while the operative site is healing. The electrolarynx provides vibrated air that is shaped into words from the articulators. Some advantages of an electrolarynx include its portability, and ease of learning and use. The disadvantages include robotic quality of voice, lack of loudness, and overall reduced intelligibility when communicating across a variety of settings.

A second communication option is **esophageal speech**. This method of alaryngeal speech occurs when the patient injects air into the esophagus and then expels the air to create a "burp" as air passes through the pharyngoesophageal (PE) segment. This expelled air is then used to create words, phrases, and sentences. An advantage of esophageal speech is that it offers hands-free communication and does not require any apparatus or maintenance. However, this method of "voicing" is not a popular option with patients due to difficulty learning this technique and overall reduced speech intelligibility in a variety of communication settings.

Tracheoesophageal puncture (TEP) is the third option for alaryngeal speech and currently the most preferred method. A puncture hole is formed between the trachea and upper portion of the esophagus. A voice prosthesis is then placed in this fistula tract. When the stoma is occluded, the patient can produce voice when the expelled air from the trachea passes through the one-way valve into the esophagus and through the PE segment creating sound, which is then shaped into words via the oral articulators. This fistula can be created as a primary placement during the surgery or secondary placement after the initial operation. There are pros and cons to both primary and secondary placements of the TEP. The SLP may discuss each case with the surgeon and make the best choice for each individual patient. Whether it is placed at the time of the laryngectomy or at some time after the advantages of a TEP include relative ease of learning, most natural sounding voice and option to speak hands-free with additional attachments. It is important to note that not every patient is a candidate for a TEP. The SLP will work closely with the surgeon to determine candidacy. Other disadvantages to the TEP include maintenance, cost, risk of infection, short life of voice prosthesis (VP), typically requiring change every 4−6 months.[18]

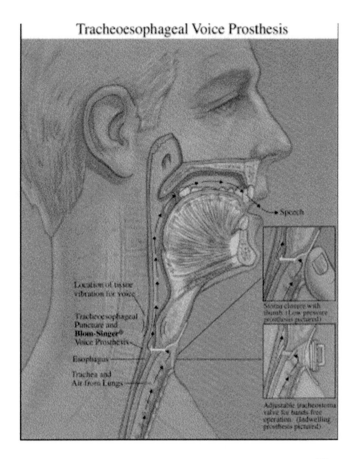

Inhealth Technology image of Tracheoesophageal Speech[18]

During this counseling session, it is also helpful for both the patient and family to meet a laryngectomized patient, if possible, watch videos of different communication methods and receive information with regard to local support groups. The SLP will remain available for the patient leading up to the surgery.

The initial postoperative encounter occurs when cleared by the surgeon while the patient is hospitalized. Communication immediately following the surgery is limited to pen and paper or whiteboard. Time spent with the patient in the hospital is utilized teaching stoma care, instruction in use of electrolarynx, placement of the HME, and reviewing home kit and ordering supplies from preferred company. If the patient had primary placement of TEP, the general recommendation is a 2-week waiting period prior to placement/use of VP.

Once the patient is discharged home, the surgeon refers the patient to ambulatory speech therapy for ongoing management/treatment of TL. This management includes reviewing information learned during the initial session. Ongoing treatment includes teaching of alaryngeal speech via one or all of the methods mentioned before.

When training in the use of the **electrolarynx**, the SLP will assist the patient in device placement and contact for optimal voice. This is typically in the anterior neck or cheek where the head of the device makes contact with the soft part of the skin or under a fold of skin. If a good seal cannot be achieved, the patient may require the use of an intraoral device. Further training includes device maintenance, use of compensatory strategies such as slow rate, exaggerated articulation, and pacing to improve intelligibility. Once these initial techniques are mastered, the patient should learn how to change pitch and volume for improved intonation.

Esophageal speech training includes teaching air injection methods via tongue movement, consonant production, or inhalation. All methods are designed to create an "air charge" by getting air into the mouth of the esophagus that will then be expelled as sound and formed into words. Once the patient can successfully produce an air charge and produce single words, the SLP works with the patient to increase utterance length, improve articulation and prosody, and avoid negative behaviors such as stoma charge, which may interfere with speech intelligibility.

The role of the therapist with a patient who has a **TEP** may include short-term therapy to optimize voice and intelligibility via coordination of breathing and speaking. Patients with TEP/VP require ongoing management, including assessing for leaks around or through the prosthesis, changing the VP, trouble shooting, and education.

All laryngectomee patients need ongoing education and training in pulmonary rehab, stoma care, and the ordering of supplies. Ambulatory speech therapy continues until the patient can produce functional speech with their preferred method of "voicing" and is independent in management of stoma care and supply management. The SLP should remain available as needed.

Augmentative/alternative communication: In some cases, functional communication may only be achieved with the use of a speech generating device, whether it is for higher demand settings or fall all communication. Devices range from low-tech such as a dry erase board, to an advanced tablet. The SLP should be aware of the available options for patients and make necessary referrals.

Posttreatment follow-up: From the initial meeting with the patient to the final ambulatory treatment session, the SLP must provide ongoing counseling and education regarding immediate and long-term changes and side effects from cancer treatment including radiation fibrosis and ORN. The SLP may include in the clinical pathways scheduled postdischarge follow-up assessments at certain intervals. These follow-ups vary and may be a phone call to check-in, a planned reassessment of communication skills, or participation in a multidisciplinary clinic at 6-month intervals.

Conclusion

HNC is complex and requires a multidisciplinary team effort to provide both immediate and long-term care. The cancer itself, along with the treatment, affects many structures that result in a negative impact on communication skills. Survival rate is favorable and continues to improve. Thus, there is a need to address quality of life concerns. The role of the SLP is essential in providing postcancer treatment therapy. It is essential that the SLP has extensive knowledge and training in this population to provide optimal treatment to improve communication skills for better quality of life. It is also essential that trained SLPs stay current with literature and treatment programs to provide best care possible. This can be achieved through continuing education, journal clubs, and participation in multidisciplinary conferences.

Case study

A 67-year-old female presented for presurgical communication and swallowing assessment with diagnosis of stage IVa right lateral tongue invasive squamous cell carcinoma well differentiated. Results from this assessment yielded normal tongue and lip strength per IOPI (anterior 64 posterior 56). Her Maximal Interincisal Opening (MIO) was 45 mm with dentures in place. Findings from examination of her oral cavity were unremarkable with exception of an ulcerated mass on the border of her tongue that did not impact strength or movement. Patient wore well-fitting dentures. All speech and voice parameters were WFL's, and speech was considered intelligible over 90% of the time across all communication settings. She underwent a wide local excision/partial glossectomy of right tongue lesion and right selective neck dissection. Pathology report was significant for invasive squamous cell carcinoma invasive to a depth of 14 mm and present 2 mm from posterior and deep margins with perineural invasion present. The right neck contents were significant for metastatic carcinoma to 2 of 28 lymph nodes. The patient was reassessed following the surgery and prior to commencing adjuvant chemoradiation therapy with weekly cisplatin. When compared with baseline session, she now presented with trismus, MIO was 45 mm fully edentulous. QOL score on SHI was 84. In general, she reported lack of desire to talk as she was not understood by family and friends. She participated in weekly follow-up sessions targeting oral motor and swallowing as well as compensatory strategies to produce intelligible speech. Upon completion of adjuvant treatment, the patient was referred for ambulatory therapy. She attended 20 treatment sessions over a 12-week period. Her treatment plan consisted of manual therapy including MLD, myofascial release, resistive oral motor exercises including maximizing lingual strength, agility, ROM, and jaw mobility. The patient also participated in direct therapy for articulation. The clinician also worked closely with the prosthodontist who fabricated dentures for the patient. The patient was also trained in a home program, which she completed daily. At discharge, the patient demonstrated an MIO of 40 mm with dentures in place, allowing her to easily place and remove dentition. She used compensatory strategies to produce intelligible speech at least 80% of the time in high demand settings such as crowded areas, with unfamiliar listeners and over the telephone. QOL score on SHI reduced to 21. The patient also received education throughout her treatment and was discharged with a home exercise program. One-year follow-up yielded no significant change in functional status. She reported she was comfortable communicating in a variety of settings and was compliant with her daily home exercise program.

Compensatory strategies for speech production

To optimize speech intelligibility following alteration, removal, or damage to the structures in the oral cavity involved in speech production, an individual can implement different compensatory strategies that include the following:

- **Slow down rate of speech.** Slowing down will provide the listener more time to perceive speech sounds and allow you coordinate motor speech sounds more effectively.
- **Overarticulate.** Exaggerate the movement of primary articulators (i.e., lips, tongue, jaw) to increase articulatory precision and range of motion.
- **Try to relax.** Speaking in a calm manner will aid in the production of "easy" speech by reducing tension in the areas involved in speech production.
- **Remember to breathe.** Support your speaking voice with diaphragmatic breathing and abdominal support.
- **Improve posture.** By maintaining an upright posture, you will improve breath support. Additionally, by facing the listener when speaking, you will increase the likelihood of being understood.
- **Choose your words wisely.** Substitute syllabically complex or challenging words for simpler words to maximize intelligibility. Similarly, use shorter sentences and shorting phrasing when appropriate.
- **Pause often.** Provide frequent pauses in speech when appropriate.
- **Avoid speaking when you are tired.** When you are fatigued, your speech will sound less precise and less energized, resulting in reduced intelligibility.
- **Modify your environment.** Speak in quiet settings when possible. Do not compete with excess noise or distraction when you are speaking. You may want to avoid speaking to multiple people at once to reduce speaking demands.
- **Avoid talking on the phone if necessary.** You may choose to send a text or an email if talking on the phone is too difficult.

In cases where speech is rendered highly unintelligible despite use of compensatory strategies, the individual may attempt to utilize alternative means of communication, including the following:

- Writing, texting
- Speech generating device (i.e., text to speech)

- Other AAC devices ranging frow low to high-tech options (i.e., communication board vs. Lingraphica)
- Gesturing, signing, or mouthing words

Ultimately, a combination of both verbal and nonverbal methods of communication will prove the most beneficial in optimizing communication skills. A total communication approach that utilizes any method of communication viable or accessible to a patient will yield the greatest outcomes.

Recommendations for vocal hygiene and wellness

Dysphonia is a common symptom present in patients who are receiving treatment for head and neck cancer or who have undergone treatment in the past. Dysphonia is primarily a result of a vocal fold pathology, and it is imperative that an individual consult with an ENT prior to initiating any voice therapy. Dysphonia, whether temporary or chronic, can negatively impact social and occupational involvement regardless of its severity; therefore, it is valuable to learn good vocal hygiene techniques or wellness practices to promote a healthier voice. Vocal hygiene constitutes the habits a person can implement to help preserve and/or improve his or her voice. Vocal hygiene can include the following:

1. **Increase systemic and topic hydration.** Stay hydrated by drinking water. Consider using a portable nebulizer for topical hydration of the throat.
2. **Limit excessive talking and singing.** The voice needs to rest, so it is important not to strain or overuse the voice.
3. **Stop vocally abusive behaviors.** Vocally abusive behaviors include coughing, throat clearing, whispering, and shouting. Use moderate voice loudness when you are communicating.
4. **Avoid alcohol use.** Alcohol consumption can reduce hydration and contribute to gastric reflux.
5. **Avoid excessive caffeine intake.** Caffeinated beverages can strip away moisture and can contribute to laryngeal dryness.
6. **Cease smoking.** Smoking is highly damaging to the vocal folds and can lead to cancer.
7. **Manage acid reflux.** Gastric reflux can irritate the vocal folds, resulting in increased hoarseness.
8. **Modify your environment.** Avoid talking in places with excess noise. Also, avoid places with poor air quality (i.e., smoky environments, chemical products, allergens).

Voice exercises can also be performed to improve expiratory airflow and forward resonance. Generally, by improving breath support and vocal placement, an individual can improve his or her vocal quality . However, a person should always seek professional help prior to initiating any vocal exercises. Some exercises that can improve voice use include the following:

1. **Head and neck stretches.** Stretching is a useful method of reducing laryngeal tension and compensation. Additionally, it aids in reducing soreness and promotes flexibility.
2. **Laryngeal and circumlaryngeal massages.** Massaging the laryngeal musculature can help reduce tension that can impact vocal quality.
3. **Breathing and relaxation exercises.** Guided respiration activities targeting inspiratory and expiratory capacity are useful in promoting improved breath support for voice production.
4. **Resonant voice exercises.** Humming and chanting can help promote a more "forward" placement of the voice, which reduces laryngeal compensation and strain.
   a. Sustain/m/consonant on various pitches, feeling vibration on the lips, cheeks, and nose
   b. Chanting/m/consonant with different vowels (i.e., "ma-ma-ma, mu-mu-mu, etc.")
   c. Reciting words, phrases and sentences that begin with/m/(i.e., "may, meat, march, Monday, etc.")
5. **Vocal function exercises.** Through sustained phonation and pitch manipulation activities, vocal function exercises help in vocal fold adduction, which can improve phonation. Vocal function sustained activities include the following:
   a. Sustain/u/vowel using minimal vocal effort on various pitches
   b. Pitch glides using/u/vowel going from low to high and high to low

References

1. Head and neck cancers: cancers of the head and neck. Cancers of the Head and Neck | American Cancer Society. https://www.cancer.org/cancer/types/head-neck-cancer.html. Accessed 4 August 2023.
2. Aggarwal P, Hutcheson KA, Garden AS, et al. Association of risk factors with patient-reported voice and speech symptoms among long-term survivors of oropharyngeal cancer. *JAMA Otolaryngol Head Neck Surg.* 2021;147(7):615. https://doi.org/10.1001/jamaoto.2021.0698.
3. Osazuwa-Peters N, Simpson MC, Zhao L, Adjei Boakye E, Olomukoro SI, Varvares MA. Suicide risk among cancer survivors: head and neck versus other cancers. *J Clin Oncol.* 2018;36(7_suppl):146−146. https://doi.org/10.1200/jco.2018.36.7_suppl.146.
4. Hammermüller C, Hinz A, Dietz A, et al. Depression, anxiety, fatigue, and quality of life in a large sample of patients suffering from head and neck cancer in comparison with the general population. *BMC Cancer.* 2021;21(1). https://doi.org/10.1186/s12885-020-07773-6.

5. Abboud WA, Hassin-Baer S, Alon EE, et al. Restricted mouth opening in head and neck cancer: etiology, prevention, and treatment. *JCO Oncol Pract.* 2020;16(10):643−653. https://doi.org/10.1200/op.20.00266.

6. Zenga J, Sharon JD, Gross J, Gantz J, Pipkorn P. Soft palate reconstruction after radionecrosis: combined anterolateral thigh adipofascial and NASOSEPTAL flaps. *Auris Nasus Larynx.* 2018;45(4):875−879. https://doi.org/10.1016/j.anl.2017.11.003.

7. Kallambettu V, Bae Y, Carrau R. Velopharyngeal function post head and neck cancer: a review. *Ear Nose Throat J.* 2022. https://doi.org/10.1177/01455613211070895. Published online 2022:014556132110708.

8. Ramia P, Bodgi L, Mahmoud D, et al. Radiation-induced fibrosis in patients with head and neck cancer: a review of pathogenesis and clinical outcomes. *Clin Med Insights Oncol.* 2022;16:117955492110368. https://doi.org/10.1177/11795549211036898.

9. Mehta S, Kuriakose MA. Principles of surgical management of oral cancer. In: *Ooral and maxillofacial surgery for the clinician.* 2021:1869−1891. https://doi.org/10.1007/978-981-15-1346-6_82. Published online.

10. Rinkel RN, Leeuw IM, van Reij EJ, Aaronson NK, Leemans CR. Speech handicap index in patients with oral and pharyngeal cancer: better understanding of patients' complaints. *Head Neck.* 2008;30(7):868−874. https://doi.org/10.1002/hed.20795.

11. Jacobson BH, Johnson A, Grywalski C, et al. Voice handicap index (VHI) development and validation. *Am J Speech Lang Pathol.* 1997;6(3):66−70. https://doi.org/10.1044/1058-0360.0603.66.

12. Van den Steen L, Baudelet M, Tomassen P, Bonte K, De Bodt M, Van Nuffelen G. Effect of tongue-strengthening exercises on tongue strength and swallowing-related parameters in chronic radiation-associated dysphagia. *Head Neck.* 2020;42(9):2298−2307. https://doi.org/10.1002/hed.26179.

13. Kelly J. Myofascial release and manual techniques in dysphagia management, a course for practicing clinicians. Miami, FL; n.d. www.ciaoseminars.com.

14. Deng J, Ridner SH, Dietrich MS, et al. *J Pain Symptom Manag.* 2012;43(2):244−252. https://doi.org/10.1016/j.jpainsymman.2011.03.019.

15. McMillan H, Barbon CE, Cardoso R, et al. Manual therapy for patients with radiation-associated trismus after head and neck cancer. *JAMA Otolaryngol Head Neck Surg.* 2022;148(5):418. https://doi.org/10.1001/jamaoto.2022.0082.

16. Chee S, Byrnes YM, Chorath KT, Rajasekaran K, Deng J. Interventions for trismus in head and Neck Cancer Patients: a systematic review of randomized controlled trials. *Integr Cancer Ther.* 2021;20:153473542110064. https://doi.org/10.1177/15347354211006474.

17. Tienkamp TB, van Son RJJH, Halpern BM. Objective speech outcomes after surgical treatment for oral cancer: an acoustic analysis of a spontaneous speech corpus containing 32.850 tokens. *J Commun Disord.* 2023;101:106292. https://doi.org/10.1016/j.jcomdis.2022.106292.

18. Pou A. Tracheosophageal voice restoration with total laryngectomy. *Otolaryngol Clin.* 2004;37(3):531−545. https://doi.org/10.1016/j.otc2004.01.009.

Nutritional considerations in head and neck cancer

13

Nicole Rittman, RD, CSO, LDN

Miami Cancer Institute, Miami, FL, United States

Introduction

Nutrition and dietary patterns are relevant in every facet of oncological care, especially in patients with head and neck cancer (HNC), who experience a continuum, reviewing the recommended dietary pattern for HNC patients, determining the appropriate prescription for nutrient needs and the application of nutrition-related interventions.

Dietary patterns

Recommended dietary patterns

Recommended dietary patterns of HNC patients should mirror those of the general population. The Dietary Guidelines for Americans (DGAs), which is released every 5 years, provide guidance to the public regarding healthy eating patterns. The most recent DGAs, released for 2020–25, encourage individuals to increase their consumption of nutrient-dense foods (items rich in vitamin, minerals, fiber, etc.), while decreasing foods that are calorie-dense with little nutritional value. To achieve this, the DGAs recommend a diet abundant in vegetables, whole fruits, grains (half of which should be whole grain), low-fat dairy, protein sources (both animal- and plant-based), and oils, as these constitute nutrient-dense foods. An attempt should be made to select primarily unsaturated and polyunsaturated fats, like those from olives, olive oils, nuts/seeds, and seed oils. In exchange, individuals should reduce foods items high in saturated fat, sodium, and added sugars.[1] Examples of these types of foods include processed meats, commercially baked desserts, frozen dinners, and sweetened beverages. Individuals should attempt to eat from all food groups every day to achieve a balanced and nutritionally complete diet pattern. More detailed information and nutrition recommendations can be found at the DGA website, www.dietaryguidelines.gov.

Head and Neck Cancer Rehabilitation. https://doi.org/10.1016/B978-0-443-11806-7.00006-0
Copyright © 2025 Elsevier Inc. All rights are reserved, including those for text and data mining, AI training, and similar technologies.

Nutrition and head and neck cancer risk

The World Cancer Research Fund (WCRF) and the American Institute of Cancer Research (AICR) have collectively analyzed multitudes of studies worldwide, as part of their Continuous Update Project (CUP), to assess the impact of nutrition, lifestyle, and physical activity on the prevention of specific cancers. The most recent CUP report conducted on HNC, which was last published in 2018, demonstrated strong evidence that alcoholic beverage consumption increased the risk of HNC.[2] A metaanalysis within the report found that each 10 g of alcohol consumed daily was associated with a 19% increase in risk for oral cavity and pharyngeal cancers. A separate metaanalysis investigating laryngeal cancer and alcohol intake found a 9% increase in cancer risk with each 10 g of alcohol consumed daily.[2] This report supports the well-recognized association between alcohol intake and increased cancer risk, especially in the HNC population. The CUP report also noted probable evidence that being overweight or obese, by assessment of BMI, waist circumference, and waist—hip ration, may increase the risk of HNC, specifically in individuals who never smoked. The mechanism behind the relationship of overweight/obesity and HNC risk is still uncertain; however, it is postulated that the chronic inflammation from obesity and metabolic impact from adipose tissue may influence cancer cell development and growth.[2]

Lastly, the CUP report indicated some evidence of an inverse relationship between nonstarchy vegetables intake and HNC cancer risk, citing that increased consumption of nonstarchy vegetables may decrease risk of certain HNCs; however, the evidence was limited.[2] Since the latest CUP report was issued, studies continue to explore the role of healthy eating patterns on HNC risk. A recent study, published in June 2023, investigated adherence to Mediterranean diet principles, vitamin C intake and the risk of head and neck cancer in 202 individuals. The study found that patients determined to have healthier diet scores (indicating alignment with the mediterranean diet principles) had a decreased probability of HNC compared with patients with an unhealthy diet score.[3] The study determined that for each 1-point increase in healthy diet adherence, an associated 12% reduction in HNC was noted.[3]

Estimating nutrition needs

Unintentional weight loss is a common issue within the HNC population, especially during treatment. Several reviews have found that 44%—57% of patients experienced severe weight loss (>5% of body weight) during radiation treatment, with the severity increasing during concomitant therapies.[4–6] Ensuring individuals with HNC achieve their nutritional needs is a critical outcome during treatment. The first step is to guide the patient toward an eating pattern that is adequate in energy, macronutrient and micronutrient intake.

Energy

There are several ways medical professionals can estimate energy needs. Conducting an indirect calorimetry (IC) assessment is considered the most accurate way to ascertain a person's individual energy requirement, especially in the oncology population, where the nutritional needs have been found to be diverse.[7,8] Unfortunately, this is not feasible or practical in the majority of healthcare settings. Several predictive energy equations exist for the estimation of energy needs (including the Harris-Benedict Equation, the Mifflin-St Jeor Equation, etc.); however, when investigated for their accuracy in predicting the energy needs in the adult oncology population, in comparison with IC, many were found to over or underestimate needs.[8-10]

As an alternative, several professional groups have adopted the use of weight-based calculations in estimating the energy needs in this population, as detailed in Table 13.1. This approach is often more practical in the healthcare setting and permits a point of reference for early assessment. It may overestimate needs in the overweight/obese population and underestimate needs in the underweight population; therefore, some clinical judgment will need to be applied in these instances. Care providers should monitor and reevaluate their patient's nutritional status over the course of treatment and adjust energy estimations as the clinical picture warrants. If a patient presents with weight loss, despite meeting the estimated energy goals, it is possible their calorie needs exceed the original estimated value and increased energy intake should be encouraged.

Currently, no consensus has been determined to specifically estimate the energy needs for individuals with head and neck cancer. One recent cohort study investigated the effectiveness of adhering to the estimated calorie intake goals stipulated in the European Society of Parenteral and Enteral Nutrition guidelines (25–30 kcal/kg) and its impact on lessening weight loss and/or muscle loss in the HNC population. The study found that patients who consumed greater than 30 kcal/kg/day experienced less muscle mass loss come day 100, compared with patients who consumed less than 30 kcal/kg/day (1% ± 0.87% muscle loss, and 7.6% ± 4.9% muscle loss, respectively).[13]

Table 13.1 Various methods to estimating energy needs in oncology population.

Estimating energy needs for oncology population[11,12]		
Oncology Nutrition DPG-AND	Inactive, nonstressed	25–30 kcal/kg/day
	To promote weight gain	30–35 kcal/kg/day
	Hypermetabolic, clinically stressed	35 kcal/kg/day
ESPEN Practical Guideline for Clinical Nutrition in Cancer		25–30 kcal/kg/day

Academy of Nutrition and Dietetics Oncology Nutrition Dietetics Practice Group (ON DPG-AND); European Society of Parenteral and Enteral Nutrition (ESPEN).

Although this study investigated a small sample size (41 patients), it ponders the question that HNC patients may require energy needs more than typically recommended for other adult oncology patients.

Macronutrients

Macronutrients are a class of nutrients comprised of dietary carbohydrates, proteins, and fats. Once digested and absorbed, these nutrients serve as energy sources in the human body. Daily energy needs should be met via a combination of these three macronutrients. The Acceptable Macronutrient Distribution Ranges for Adults (AMDR) provides recommendations on the appropriate distribution of these nutrients. It is recommended that 45%−65% of an individual's total daily calories come from carbohydrates sources, 20%−35% from dietary fat, and the remaining 10%−35% of daily calories from dietary protein.[14] For instance, for an individual with an estimated daily calorie goal of 1800 calories, the recommended distribution of macronutrients would be 203−293 g of carbohydrates, 40−70 g of fat, and 45−158 g of protein (Table 13.2).

Certain clinical instances may warrant manipulation in the typical distribution of macronutrients. For example, in ESPEN's guideline for clinical nutrition in cancer patients, it is recommended to encourage increased dietary fat intake, in exchange for decreased carbohydrate consumption, in weight losing, insulin-resistant individuals.[12] The intention is to decrease the overall glycemic intake in these patients, while taking advantage of the high energy provision within dietary fats. In this scenario, the more appropriate macronutrient distribution may be 203 g of carbohydrates, 70 g dietary fat, and 90 g protein, representing 45%, 35%, 20% of total calories for carbohydrate, fat, and protein, respectively. Patients can increase their dietary fat intake by adding avocado, olive oil, nuts and nut butters, and moderate amounts of full-fat dairy into their daily routine.

Table 13.2 Recommended distribution of macronutrients in an individual's diet.

Acceptable Macronutrient Distribution Range (AMDR)		
Carbohydrate (CHO) 45%−65% of total daily calories	Fat 20%−35% of total daily calories	Protein 10%−35% of total daily calories
Example: For an individual with daily energy goal of 1800 calories		
1800 calories × 0.45−0.65 810−1170 calories Divide by 4 calories per gram 203−293 g CHO	1800 calories × 0.2−0.35 360−630 calories Divide by 9 calories per gram 40−70 g fat	1800 calories × 0.1−0.35 180−630 calories Divide by 4 calories per gram 45−158 g protein

Protein intake

Protein is uniquely relevant in cancer patients as it is known that protein requirements are increased in this population. There are several reasons protein needs are elevated, including increased catabolism of muscle mass,[15] less efficient amino acid utilization,[12] as well as increased demands from critical illness, surgical interventions, etc. The Oncology Nutrition Dietetic Practice Group from the Academy of Nutrition and Dietetics recommends the adult oncology patients receive 1−1.5 g of protein per kilogram of body weight to meet their daily protein requirements.[11] This wide range allows for the application of clinical judgment by the medical professional, dependent on the patient's individual picture. These recommendations are also in line with ESPEN, who recommends a range of 1−1.5 g/kg.[12] In some instances, like individuals with cancer cachexia, protein needs may need to be increased toward 2 g/kg body weight or higher.[11,12] Similar to energy estimations, consideration should be taken for the overweight/obese population, as using a weight-based approach may overestimate the protein requirements in these individuals.

Protein requirements can be met through a variety of food sources, both animal-based and plant-based. Animal-based proteins, such as poultry, beef, game, dairy, and fish, have some of the highest concentrations of protein per serving. Many of these sources of protein also contain the complete profile of essential amino acids for bodily functions.[15] Eating an adequate quantity of animal-based proteins during the day can be an efficient way to meet the daily protein requirements; however, it should not be assumed as the only way. Many patients may not include animal-based proteins in their diets for a variety of reasons, whether it be related to taste aversions from treatment, personal beliefs, or socioeconomic limitations. Plant-based proteins—consisting of legumes, beans, whole grains, and soy—should still be considered a suitable opportunity for protein needs. Although some plant-based proteins make up an incomplete amino acid profile on their own, pairing different plant-based proteins together throughout the day can be an effective way to achieve all the required essential amino acids.[15]

Fluid intake

Fluid requirements align with the recommendations for the general population. There are multiple ways to calculate fluid needs, which has been summarized in Table 13.3. Individual circumstances may warrant increased fluid needs, such as promoting kidney and bladder protection for patients receiving chemotherapy with increased incidence of bladder or kidney toxicity. This includes chemotherapy such as cisplatin, which is a common treatment in the HNC population.

Micronutrient needs

Micronutrients consist of vitamins and minerals. In contrast to macronutrients, micronutrients do not function as energy sources. Instead, these nutrients are involved in supporting various metabolic processes within the body. In general,

Table 13.3 Various methods for estimating fluid needs for an individual.

Equations for calculating fluid needs[15]	
Age-based method	Age 18–55 years: 35 mL for each kilogram body weight Age 56–75 years: 30 mL for each kilogram body weight Age 75+ years: 25 mL for each kilogram body weight
Holliday–Segar method	Age 50 or less: 1500 + 20 mL for each kilogram body weight over 20 kg Age 50+: 1500 + 15 mL for each kilogram body weight over 20 kg
Energy method	1 mL fluid for each kilocalorie of energy needs

the micronutrient recommendations for HNC patients are the same as the general population and can be found by referencing the dietary reference intakes. Adjustment in recommendations should be made on an individual basis and contingent on a patient's unique clinic picture. For instance, some HNC patients receiving systemic therapy of cisplatin may require increased magnesium intake or repletion due to the increased urinary depletion of magnesium during treatment.[11]

Nutrition rehabilitation

Malnutrition

Head and neck cancer poses some of the highest rates of malnutrition in the oncology demographic. A recent comprehensive review found that 25%–65% of HNC patients met criteria for malnutrition upon initial presentation, while some studies showed upward of 80% of patients developed malnutrition over the course of treatment.[16,17] It is well documented that malnutrition has negative impacts on oncology patients, including increased rates of hospitalizations (with increased length of stay), decreased quality of life, and decreased tolerance to cancer treatments.[18] For this reason, identifying patients at high risk of developing malnutrition, or who already present with malnutrition, should be a standard practice in cancer centers.

There are several malnutrition screening tools that have been validated for the oncology population. Each screening tool has its own criteria for identifying malnutrition and has been validated in specific patient-care settings, including the inpatient setting, the outpatient setting, or both. Current validated screening tools for the adult oncology population are listed in Table 13.4. These tools are meant to be efficient and efficacious, permitting easy integration into patient care. Most screening tools are recommended to be conducted on the initial visit and upon each follow-up, allowing the provider to evaluate for malnutrition across the treatment continuum.

Although each screening tool varies slightly in its own criteria, all tools recognize the importance in evaluating an individual's overall nutritional energy intake

Table 13.4 Validated screening tools in the adult oncology population.[18,19]

Screening tool	Setting	Criteria assessed
Malnutrition Screening Tool (MST)[20]	Outpatient and inpatient setting	Weight loss, decreased appetite
Malnutrition Universal screening tool (MUST)[21]	Inpatient setting	BMI, weight loss, acuity status + poor nutritional intake
Nutrition Risk Screening 2002 (NSR-2002)[22]	Inpatient setting	BMI, weight loss, decreased dietary intake, acuity status
Mini-Nutritional Assessment (MNA)[22]	Outpatient setting	Decreased dietary intake, weight loss, mobility, acuity status/stress, neuropsychological status, BMI

and presence of unintentional weight loss. These two criteria, inadequate energy intake and weight loss, create the cornerstone of malnutrition in many patient cases and should be intervened promptly once identified.

Nutrition-impact symptoms

Nutrition-impact symptoms (NIS) describe a collection of treatment-related sides effects that can impair a patient's nutritional status, either by deterring oral intake or interfering in nutrient absorption. Many patients completing treatment for HNC will experience one or more NIS over the course of their treatment regimen and during survivorship.[23] Although there are many potential side effects from chemotherapy, radiation, and surgery, one systematic review evaluated 15 studies (encompassing 849 HNC survivors) and found the most common NIS experienced after completion of treatments were dysphagia (73%), xerostomia (36%), trismus (36%), salivary issues (36%), mucositis (13%), and oral pain (13%).[23] Although not mentioned in the study, other common NIS that may occur include taste alterations, decreased appetite, nausea and/or vomiting, constipation, and diarrhea. Table 13.5 highlights some common recommendations for the various NIS.

A recent study explored the impact of NIS on patients' oral intake and weight pattern over the course of treatment (evaluating at baseline, 7 weeks into treatment, and then 6 and 12 months posttreatment). The results revealed that the more NIS a patient experienced, the greater the weight loss trend, describing a compounding association.[24] Taking a proactive approach in the management of NIS creates a pivotal opportunity for attenuating the rates of significant weight loss and malnutrition in this population. As with most patient care, the recommendations for NIS management should be customized to the patient's individual presentation. Registered dietitians are uniquely capable of integrating dietary changes and nutrition counseling into the patient's care, while working in tandem with medical and pharmacological

Table 13.5 Common nutrition impact symptoms and their associated nutritional interventions.

Nutrition impact symptom	Nutrition management recommendations[27]
Anorexia	• Encourage small and frequent meals of nutrient-dense, high-protein foods. • Schedule times for meals, instead of waiting to "feel hungry." • If experiencing early satiety, recommend patients separate fluids from mealtimes. This will optimize intake of nourishment at meals. • As appropriate, encourage light activity to promote digestion and appetite.
Constipation	• Encourage patients to meet hydration goals. • Encourage slow increase in dietary fiber, including sources of insoluble fiber (beans, fruits with skin, whole grains, wheat bran). • Encourage light activity, as tolerated, to promote digestion.
Diarrhea	• Encourage smaller, frequent meals as opposed to two to three large meals. • Encourage a trial low-fat, low-fiber foods. Avoid spicy or overly seasoned dishes as this may worsen symptoms. • Encourage lactose-free alternatives if lactose intolerance suspected. • Reduce or eliminate caffeine, alcohol as this can exacerbate symptoms. • Reduce sources of insoluble fiber (wheat bran, beans, fruits with skin). Increase sources of soluble fiber (bananas, applesauce, potatoes, etc.). • Encourage adequate hydration to compensate for potential fluid losses.
Dysgeusia/ageusia	Accommodating taste changes is highly individualized. Some general recommendations include the following: For bitter/acidic/metallic taste, encourage the patient to do the following: • Swap out metal silverware for plastic or bamboo. • Incorporate sweet foods with meals (melons, juices, marinades). • If mucositis is not present, trial the addition of acidic elements to dishes (lemon, orange, balsamic vinegars). • Trial different protein sources, such as eggs, beans, tofu, dairy, chicken, fish. For reduced taste, encourage the patient to do the following: • Identify flavor profiles that taste best (i.e., salty, sweet) and incorporate those into dishes. • Cook with more herbs, spices, seasonings. • Marinate meats for increased flavor.
Mucositis	• Encourage softer, more moist food items. • Moisten foods with broths, gravies, nonacidic sauces, milks, cream, etc. • Avoid acidic (tomato, lemon/lemon/orange) or spicy foods. • Choose soothing foods such as melons, peaches, yogurt, milk, etc.

Table 13.5 Common nutrition impact symptoms and their associated nutritional interventions.—cont'd

Nutrition impact symptom	Nutrition management recommendations[27]
Nausea/vomiting	• Assess sensitivity to temperatures. Cool or room-temperature food items may be best tolerated. • Encourage small and frequent meals. • Avoid high-fat, highly seasoned food items. Elect for blander cooked foods, low-fiber carbohydrates (breads, crackers, dry cereals). • Assess sensitivity to strong odors. If sensitive, choose foods that are room temperature or chilled (less-associated odor).
Xerostomia	• Encourage adequate hydration during the day, taking sips of liquids frequently. • Swish carbonated water or club soda to loosen thick saliva. • Moisten meal items with gravies, sauces, broths. • Suck on sugar-free hard candies, frozen grapes, frozen melons.

interventions. Several studies have demonstrated the impact registered dietitians have in HNC patients, noting that nutrition counseling has been associated with positive outcomes in weight patterns, energy intake, treatment tolerance, and maintained or improved quality of life.[25] The National Comprehensive Cancer Network (NCCN) Guidelines for Head and Neck Cancer support the involvement of registered dietitians, recommending they be part of the multidisciplinary team throughout the course of treatment.[26] The NCCN guidelines recommend HNC patients receive nutrition counseling at the beginning of treatment and follow-up assessments should continue until the patient is determined to be nutritionally stable.[26]

Alternate nutrition support

Integrating nutrition counseling into patient care can help patients improve their nutritional status by teaching the patient to incorporate well-tolerated nutrient-dense and high protein foods into their daily pattern; however, there may be patients who struggle to achieve adequate energy intake or weight stability despite dietary counseling. In these situations, medical providers should consider the introduction of alternative nutrition support. Oral nutrition supplements (ONS) are commercially available products, typically beverages for oral consumption, which are fortified with various nutrients, including calories, protein, vitamins, and minerals. ONS are meant to be used in conjunction with dietary intake. Other varieties of ONS may include nutritional powders that can be prepared into a beverage. ESPEN recommends the use of ONS when dietary intake is not sufficient on its own.[12]

Several systematic reviews investigated the impact of different nutrition interventions, including the use of ONS, in HNC patients completing anticancer treatments. One study supported the use of nutritional counseling together with daily ONS intake, stating that the addition of two servings of ONS daily resulted in increased protein energy intake and more weight stability in patients undergoing treatment, compared with patients who received nutritional counseling alone. Another systematic review found that ONS use may improve tolerance to treatment, based on the incidence of suspension and/or interruption of anticancer therapies in the patients prescribed ONS.[28] When quality of life was assessed, some studies suggested that ONS increased quality of life scores compared with control groups without ONS use; however, the support was limited when the impact of ONS was compared with nutrition counseling alone.[28]

If a patient is unable to adequate meet nutritional needs with nutritional counseling and oral nutrition supplements, the initiation of enteral nutrition (EN) support via an enteral feeding tube should be considered. ESPEN recommends enteral nutrition support be initiated when a patient is consuming less than 50% of estimated energy needs for greater than 1 week, or less than 75% of nutritional needs for 2 weeks.[12] The NCCN Guidelines for Head and Neck Cancers follow similar recommendations, proposing alternate enteral support when a patient is anticipated to meet less than 60% of estimated needs for greater than 10 days.[26] The use of prophylactic feeding tube placement prior to the start of treatment is not recommended, unless the patient is considered at high risk for nutritional decline over the course of therapy.[26] Enteral nutrition can be provided via a nasogastric tube, for short-term nutritional provision, or via a gastrostomy tube (G-tube or PEG) if nutrition support is anticipated for greater than 1 month. There are multiple commercially available EN formulas available on the market. Many of these commercially available products are formulated to independently support the nutritional needs of an individual, providing a composition of both macronutrients and micronutrients. Recently the introduction of blenderized tube feedings (BTFs), formula made from whole food ingredients blended to a liquid consistency, has become more popular, with several companies now preparing commercially prepared products. A recent study investigated the incorporation of commercially BTF, in place of standard commercial formula, in tube-fed HNC patients on treatment. The study reported that patients experienced improvement in pain, vomiting, constipation, gas/bloating, nausea, and diarrhea after several weeks on BTF.[29] The small sample size (14 patients) should be noted; however, the study evokes some potential to the use of BTF in a population that is plagued with NIS throughout treatment. Ultimately, the role and impact of BTF will be an interesting topic to continue to assess, as more studies determine its implication in the adult oncology setting.

Considering the high volume of NIS, and the associated risk of unintentional weight loss and malnutrition, securing a route of nutrition can be advantageous to a patient's overall care. To assist medical providers better ascertain which patients would most benefit from the placement of an enteral feeding tube, the NCCN Guidelines for Head and Neck Cancer patients outlined several criteria to consider, as detailed in Table 13.6.[26]

The final avenue for alternate nutrition support is parenteral nutrition, which provides nutrients intravenously. Parenteral nutrition is recommended only when the utilization of the gastrointestinal tract is not feasible. It is considered best practice to prioritize the use of the gastrointestinal tract whenever it remains viable; therefore, the use of ONS and EN is preferred over PN whenever possible.

Table 13.6 Criteria for considering a feeding tube placement.

Criteria for consideration of feeding tube placement
• Inadequate oral intake of less than 60% of estimated energy needs for >10 days
• Weight loss of 5% or more within 1 month
• Severe mucositis, odynophagia, dysphagia
• Aspiration
• Age >60 years old
Criteria for consideration of a prophylactic feeding tube placement (prior to start of treatment)
• Severe weight loss prior to the start of treatment (5% over 1 month, 10% over 6 months)
• Persistent nutrition-impact symptoms that impair patients' ability to consume adequate calories
• Severe aspiration OR mild aspiration in older patients, those with compromised cardiopulmonary function
• Patients with significant comorbidities

Nutrition and survivorship

As mentioned earlier in the chapter, the composition and quality of the diet can have an impact on health and disease prevention. As HNC patients transition into survivorship, incorporating eating patterns that can be protective against cancer development or recurrence should be encouraged. Several professional groups have founded their mission in compiling the most recent research on nutrition, lifestyle, and physical exercise and its role in cancer prevention and survivorship. One such group, the American Institute for Cancer Research (AICR), assembled the New American Plate as an easy graphic to guide healthy eating choices for cancer prevention and survivorship. The New American Plate emphasizes the intake of plant-based food items, recommending two-thirds of the plate be derived from fruits, vegetables, whole grains, nuts/seeds, and legumes. The remaining one-third of the plate can be reserved for animal products, such as poultry, meat, seafood, and dairy.[30] The World Cancer Research Fund International (WCRF) has also published several guidelines, collectively called Cancer Prevention Recommendations, which are aimed at reducing cancer risk. Similar to the New American Plate, the WCRF recommends a diet primarily of whole grains, vegetables, fruit, and pulses (beans, lentils).[31] Animal-based foods are permitted in both groups' recommendations; however, emphasis is placed on the reduction of red meat and the avoidance of processed meats. Both professional groups recommend decreased consumption of high-fat, high-sugar foods, such as baked goods, candies, etc.[30,31]

Other lifestyle factors should be also considered as part of survivorship. Given the association with increased alcohol intake and HNC risk, medical providers should encourage HNC survivors who consume alcohol to decrease their alcohol intake or refrain from its use. Including a physical activity routine is also recommended as part of cancer prevention.

In summary, nutrition has applications in every aspect of HNC patient care. Medical providers should advocate for the importance of maintaining nutritional intake throughout treatment and adopt an interdisciplinary approach in the management of common treatment-related side effects. Prompt intervention should be taken in patients at risk for malnutrition, to preserve their functional and nutritional status. Individualized recommendations should be made, tailored to each patient's unique medical and nutritional presentation. In survivorship, patients should focus on increasing plant-based foods, particularly vegetables, whole grains, and pulses, alongside adequate intake of proteins, healthy fats, and complex carbohydrates. Nutrition should be viewed as a positive opportunity for healthful change. There are many paths to healthy eating practices, and patients should be encouraged to select the dietary pattern that is most feasible for their lifestyle and their overall health goals.

References

1. *US Department of Agriculture and US Department of Health and Human Science. Dietary Guidelines for Americans 2020 -2025.* USDA; 2020. https://www.dietaryguidelines.gov/sites/default/files/2021-03/Dietary_Guidelines_for_Americans-2020-2025.pdf.
2. World Cancer Research Fund/American Institute for Cancer Research. Diet, Nutrition, Physical Activity and Cancers of the Mouth, Pharynx and Larynx. https://www.aicr.org/wp-content/uploads/2020/01/mouth-pharynx-larynx-cancer.pdf.
3. Saka-Herrán C, Pereira-Riveros T, Jané-Salas E, López-López J. Association between the mediterranean diet and vitamin C and the risk of head and neck cancer. *Nutrients.* 2023; 15(13):2846. https://doi.org/10.3390/nu15132846.
4. Mäkitie A, Alabi RO, Orell H, et al. Managing cachexia in head and neck cancer: a systematic scoping review. *Adv Ther.* 2022;39(4):1502−1523. https://doi.org/10.1007/s12325-022-02074-9.
5. Langius JAE, Bakker SMK, Rietveld D, et al. Critical weight loss is a major prognostic indicator for disease-specific survival in patients with head and neck cancer receiving radiotherapy. *Br J Cancer.* 2013;109(5):1093−1099. https://doi.org/10.1038/bjc.2013.458.
6. Nazari V, Pashaki AS, Hasanzadeh E. The reliable predictors of severe weight loss during the radiotherapy of head and neck cancer. *Cancer Treat Res Commun.* 2021;26:100281. https://doi.org/10.1016/j.ctarc.2020.100281.
7. De Souza MTP, Singer P, Ozório GA, et al. Resting energy expenditure and body composition in patients with head and neck cancer: an observational study leading to a new predictive equation. *Nutrition.* 2018;51−52:60−65. https://doi.org/10.1016/j.nut.2017.12.006.
8. García-Peris P, Lozano MA, Velasco C, et al. Prospective study of resting energy expenditure changes in head and neck cancer patients treated with chemoradiotherapy measured by indirect calorimetry. *Nutrition.* 2005;21(11−12):1107−1112. https://doi.org/10.1016/j.nut.2005.03.006.

9. Mazzo R, Ribeiro F, Vasques ACJ. Accuracy of predictive equations versus indirect calorimetry for the evaluation of energy expenditure in cancer patients with solid tumors — an integrative systematic review study. *Clin Nutr ESPEN*. 2020;35:12−19. https://doi.org/10.1016/j.clnesp.2019.11.001.

10. Barcellos PS, Borges N, Torres D. Resting energy expenditure in cancer patients: agreement between predictive equations and indirect calorimetry. *Clin Nutr ESPEN*. 2021;42:286−291. https://doi.org/10.1016/j.clnesp.2021.01.019.

11. Oncology Nutrition Dietetic Practice Group, Voss AC, Williams V. *Oncology nutrition for clinical practice*. 2nd ed. Academy of Nutrition & Dietetics; 2021.

12. Muscaritoli M, Arends J, Bachmann P, et al. ESPEN practical guideline: Clinical Nutrition in cancer. *Clin Nutr*. 2021;40(5):2898−2913. https://doi.org/10.1016/j.clnu.2021.02.005.

13. McCurdy B, Nejatinamini S, Debenham B, et al. Meeting minimum ESPEN energy recommendations is not enough to maintain muscle mass in head and neck cancer patients. *Nutrients*. 2019;11(11):2743. https://doi.org/10.3390/nu11112743.

14. Macronutrients PO, Interpretation SO, Board N. Dietary reference intakes for energy, carbohydrate, fiber, fat, fatty acids, cholesterol, protein, and amino acids. *J Am Diet Assoc*. 2005. https://doi.org/10.17226/10490.

15. Mueller CM, Lord LM, Marian M, McClave S, Miller SJ. *The ASPEN Adult Nutrition Support Core Curriculum*. 3rd ed. 2017.

16. Bossi P, Delrio P, Mascheroni A, Zanetti M. The Spectrum of Malnutrition/Cachexia/Sarcopenia in Oncology According to different cancer types and settings: a narrative review. *Nutrients*. 2021;13(6):1980. https://doi.org/10.3390/nu13061980.

17. Martinović D, Tokic D, Mladinić EP, et al. Nutritional management of patients with head and neck cancer—a comprehensive review. *Nutrients*. 2023;15(8):1864. https://doi.org/10.3390/nu15081864.

18. Thompson KL, Elliott L, Fuchs-Tarlovsky V, Levin RM, Voss AC, Piemonte TA. Oncology evidence-based nutrition practice guideline for adults. *J Acad Nutr Diet*. 2017;117(2):297−310.e47. https://doi.org/10.1016/j.jand.2016.05.010.

19. Reber E, Schönenberger KA, Vasiloglou MF, Stanga Z. Nutritional risk screening in cancer patients: the first step toward better clinical outcome. *Front Nutr*. 2021;8. https://doi.org/10.3389/fnut.2021.603936.

20. Abbott Nutrition. Malnutrition Screening Tool (MST). Published May 2013. https://static.abbottnutrition.com/cms-prod/abbottnutrition-2016.com/img/Malnutrition%20Screening%20Tool_FINAL_tcm1226-57900.pdf.

21. BAPEN. Malnutrition Universal Screening Tool. Published 2003. https://www.bapen.org.uk/pdfs/must/must_full.pdf.

22. Kondrup J. ESPEN guidelines for nutrition screening 2002. *Clin Nutr*. 2003;22(4):415−421. https://doi.org/10.1016/s0261-5614(03)00098-0.

23. Crowder SL, Douglas KG, Pepino MY, Sarma KVS, Arthur AE. Nutrition impact symptoms and associated outcomes in post-chemoradiotherapy head and neck cancer survivors: a systematic review. *J Cancer Surviv*. 2018;12(4):479−494. https://doi.org/10.1007/s11764-018-0687-7.

24. Granström B, Holmlund T, Laurell G, et al. Addressing symptoms that affect patients' eating according to the head and neck patient symptom checklist©. *Support Care Cancer*. 2022;30:6163−6173. https://doi.org/10.1007/s00520-022-07038-x.

25. Leis C, Arthur AE, Chen X, Greene MW, Frugé AD. Systematic review of nutrition interventions to improve short term outcomes in head and neck cancer patients. *Cancers*. 2023;15(3):822. https://doi.org/10.3390/cancers15030822.

26. National Comprehensive Cancer Network. *NCCN Clinical Practice Guidelines in Oncology Head and Neck Cancer*; 2023. https://www.nccn.org/professionals/physician_gls/pdf/head-and-neck.pdf. Accessed December 28, 2023.

27. Levin, MEd, RDN, CSO, LDN, FAND R, Oncology Nutrition Dietetic Practice Group. *Managing Nutrition Impact Symptoms of Cancer Treatment*. 2nd ed. 2021.

28. Mello AT, Borges DS, De Lima LP, Pessini J, Kammer PV, Trindade EBSM. Effect of oral nutritional supplements with or without nutritional counselling on mortality, treatment tolerance and quality of life in head-and-neck cancer patients receiving (chemo)radiotherapy: a systematic review and meta-analysis. *Br J Nutr.* 2020;125(5):530−547. https://doi.org/10.1017/s0007114520002329.

29. Spurlock A, Johnson T, Pritchett A, et al. Blenderized food tube feeding in patients with head and neck cancer. *Nutr Clin Pract.* 2021;37(3):615−624. https://doi.org/10.1002/ncp.10760.

30. American Institute for Cancer Research. New American Plate. American Institute for Cancer Research. https://www.aicr.org/cancer-prevention/healthy-eating/new-american-plate/.

31. WCRF International. *About Our Cancer Prevention Recommendations | WCRF International*. WCRF International; 2022. Published April 15 https://www.wcrf.org/diet-activity-and-cancer/cancer-prevention-recommendations/about-our-cancer-prevention-recommendations/.

Peripheral nervous system dysfunction in head and neck cancer

14

Chanel Davidoff, DO [1] **and Christian M. Custodio, MD** [2]

[1]*Physical Medicine and Rehabilitation, Donald and Barbara School of Medicine at Hofstra/ Northwell Health, Hempstead, NY, United States;* [2]*Clinical Rehabilitation Medicine, Memorial Sloan Kettering Cancer Center, New York, NY, United States*

Introduction

Individuals with head and neck cancer often face a variety of neuromuscular impairments driven by either disease or its treatments. Despite peripheral nervous system dysfunction being prevalent in this population, it is frequently underreported due to diagnostic challenges. Unfortunately, peripheral nerve injuries can compound symptom burden and significantly reduce patients' quality of life, making early recognition critical for preventing future disability. In this chapter, we will focus on etiologies, mechanisms, and diagnostic approaches used to identify various neuromuscular diseases seen in individuals with a history of head and neck cancer. Additionally, we will review current evidence supporting the use of treatments and rehabilitation in managing these conditions.

Overview of peripheral nerve injuries

Peripheral nerve dysfunction encompasses injuries or insults outside the brain or spinal cord, including spinal nerve roots, brachial or lumbosacral plexus, peripheral axons and surrounding myelin sheaths, primary sensory neurons (dorsal root ganglion), neuromuscular junction, and muscles. While primary motor neurons (anterior horn cells) anatomically reside within the spinal cord, they are commonly considered part of the peripheral nervous system. Disorders of the peripheral nervous system are diverse and can stem from various etiologies, including trauma, metabolic factors, congenital conditions, inflammation, and infections. Consequently, the clinical presentations and management approaches are highly variable. For instance, nerve injuries can result in motor, sensory, and even vasomotor changes characterized by muscle weakness, pain, numbness, decreased proprioception, gait ataxia, or autonomic dysfunction.

Copyright © 2025 Elsevier Inc. All rights reserved, including those for text and data mining, AI training, and similar technologies.

The initial step in evaluating someone with suspected peripheral nerve injury is to identify symptom patterns, which involves obtaining a comprehensive medical history and performing a thorough neurologic examination. This information is critical in narrowing down potential diagnoses and guiding subsequent workups, including laboratory tests, dedicated neuroimaging, or electrodiagnostic studies. Patterns of nerve injury are typically distinguished by several factors, including the number of nerves involved (mononeuropathy or polyneuropathy), characteristics of injury (axonal and/or demyelinating), nerve fiber types (sensory, motor, large or small fibers), as well as the anatomic location (root, plexus, nerve axon, or neuromuscular junction), among others.

Peripheral nerve injuries are frequent in cancer, can arise from different mechanisms, and result in a variety of clinical manifestations. It is, therefore, difficult to ascertain the actual prevalence of nerve injuries in the general cancer population. Direct tumor compression, malignant infiltrating, leptomeningeal dissemination, acute and late side effects of systemic treatments, and surgical interventions are common complications that result in direct injury to nerves. Peripheral nerve damage can also result from indirect effects of long-term illness, underlying medical conditions, and immune reactions to cancer or cancer treatments.

Patients with head and neck cancer experience distinct nerve complications resulting from a variety of mechanisms that are specific to involved anatomical structures, surgical interventions performed, systemic treatments administered, and predisposing medical risk factors. Tumors in the head and neck region may directly compress or cause a mass effect on cranial nerves or nearby neurovascular structures. Local tumor recurrence is also possible through perineural invasion, causing disruption or damage to nearby nerves.[1] Neuronal damage to the brachial plexus and cranial nerves has also been documented following head and neck irradiation.[2] Chemotherapy and immunotherapy, among other systemic treatments, can have significant neuromuscular effects on peripheral nerves and muscles, resulting in length-dependent neuropathies or myopathies. Nerve injuries can also occur during tumor debulking, neck dissection, or reconstructive surgeries. Familiarity with affected anatomic regions, surgical procedures performed, and systemic treatments utilized can aid in identifying a management approach.

Functional impact

Neuromuscular complications in individuals with head and neck cancer can present as various symptoms, such as pain, weakness, sensory deficits, and difficulty swallowing. The severity of nerve dysfunction can vary, ranging from mild numbness to significant loss of strength, depending on the specific nerves affected, whether sensory, motor, or both. The presence of these symptoms can limit a patient's capacity to carry out daily activities, ultimately resulting in a decline in their quality of life, potentially leading to disability. In a study investigating disability and unemployment in head and neck cancer, it was found that over half of the patients experienced disability brought on by disease or its treatments. Specifically, patients who had received chemotherapy, undergone neck dissection, or reported higher pain scores had a higher risk of disability.[3] It is, therefore, essential to promptly identify and treat these complications to prevent any possible disability. Rehabilitation plays a vital role in preserving function and enhancing the overall quality of life for individuals with head and neck cancer.

The functional impact of neuromuscular injuries in head and neck cancer includes several significant clinical implications. For one, the presence of neuromuscular impairments may necessitate adjustments to the oncologic treatment plan to address specific functional limitations faced by the patient. For example, oncologists may adjust the dose or type of treatment in an effort to minimize the impact on the patient's quality of life. Precise identification of the cause of neuromuscular dysfunction holds significant importance in cancer rehabilitation as it enables rehabilitation professionals to gain insight into a patient's functional prognosis. Collaboration between healthcare providers, including oncologists, rehab professionals, and therapists, is essential to ensure patients receive appropriate care.

Disease-related nerve dysfunction
Mononeuropathy

Mononeuropathies are classified as peripheral neuropathy that affects a single nerve. In cancer, focal mononeuropathies can arise from direct infiltration or tumor compression. Although metastasis to an individual nerve is rare, perineural spreading can occur. More commonly, mononeuropathies occur indirectly. For instance, peroneal neuropathy may result from rapid weight loss manifesting as foot drop. Medial neuropathy at the wrist (also known as carpal tunnel syndrome) may arise due to overuse, particularly in the presence of proximal limb weakness, but may also occur in the presence of upper limb lymphedema. Although radial neuropathies are less frequent, they can occur from direct compression by an adjacent humeral metastasis.

In head and neck cancer, the most common mononeuropathies caused by direct tumor compression are cranial neuropathies. Cranial neuropathies can occur due to various mechanisms related to the tumor or treatments. In the context of disease-related nerve injury, cranial neuropathy may arise due to the tumor directly invading the nerve or exerting compression on adjacent soft tissue structures. Particularly facial and trigeminal nerves are commonly affected by perineural tumor spreading, which is typically observed in squamous cell carcinoma.[4] Symptoms of cranial neuropathies are determined by the location and function of the affected nerve. For example, when the trigeminal nerve is involved, patients may experience facial numbness, weakness, or neuralgia. Involvement of the glossopharyngeal nerve can result in speech or swallowing difficulties. Due to the proximity of the facial nerve and parotid gland, parotid tumors can result in facial nerve injury. The facial nerve runs through the parotid gland before branching off to innervate the muscles of the face. As a result, symptoms of facial nerve dysfunction include paralysis of the facial muscles of the affected side of the face to various degrees, depending on the extent of the injury.

A comprehensive neurologic examination is performed to assess strength, sensation, reflexes, and cranial nerves to diagnose mononeuropathies or cranial neuropathies in head and neck cancer. Diagnostic modalities are determined based on the distribution of symptoms and exam findings. To identify tumors or lesions that may be causing compression along nerves, dedicated imaging such as CT or MRI of the brain, head, and neck with and without contrast may be considered. Diagnostic ultrasound is a noninvasive imaging modality that can be used to examine entrapment sights (i.e., median nerve at the wrist, ulnar nerve at the elbow, or peroneal nerve along the fibular head) for peripheral nerve injuries. Changes on ultrasound to a nerve that has been injured may include enlargement, thickening of the nerve sheath, and increased echogenicity of the nerve or surrounding tissue. To determine if viable disease is present, positron emission tomography (PET) scans may be recommended to assess the metabolic activity of known lesions. A biopsy of the surrounding tissue may also be necessary to confirm the diagnosis and guide treatment. If peripheral nerve injury is suspected, electrodiagnostic studies may help identify and characterize the injury. In the case of facial paralysis, facial nerve stimulation may be used to localize facial nerve injury.

Management of mononeuropathies or cranial neuropathies in head and neck cancer is symptom dependent. If symptoms are due to the direct effects of cancer, the involvement of an oncologist, head and neck surgeon, and radiation oncologist for cancer-directed treatments is required. A multifaceted approach is recommended to effectively manage symptoms, which may involve utilizing physical and occupational therapy to address weakness or sensory impairments, speech therapy to manage difficulties with speech and swallowing, analgesics to alleviate pain, and specialized interventions such as targeted nerve blocks.

Radiculopathy

Radiculopathy in the cancer setting can occur due to compression or irritation of nearby nerve roots. Cancer-related radiculopathy symptoms can resemble nonmalignant radiculopathies characterized by shooting, electric-like pain within a dermatomal pattern. In cervical radiculopathies, patients may also describe concurrent neck discomfort. On exam, areflexia, weakness, and sensory deficits in a myotomal distribution may be found and are usually asymmetrical.

Radiculopathy in head and neck cancer is less common than in spine tumors. Primary malignancies such as breast, lung, prostate, colon, thyroid, and kidney cancers are more likely to metastasize to the spine via hematologic dissemination. Head and neck cancer metastasis usually occurs through the direct extension of the tumor or via lymphatic spreading. Although less common than mononeuropathies, radiculopathy can still occur due to nerve root compression or infiltration of a head and neck tumor. Cases have been reported of head and neck cancer presenting with signs and symptoms of nerve root impingement affecting the upper limbs due to locoregional lymphatic spreading or direct erosion into cervical vertebral bodies.[5,6]

If a cancer patient experiences new onset neck or back pain, urgent medical attention is required, particularly if neurologic deficits are present. Tumors involving the spine or adjacent structures are the second most common cause of radiculopathy after degenerative spinal stenosis.[7] The gold-standard imaging modality for evaluating radicular symptoms is an MRI of the spine with and without contrast. While CT scans can help assess the bony integrity of the spine, MRI provides a more detailed visualization of soft tissue structures. Electrodiagnostic studies can help identify other peripheral nerve processes, localize nerve root involvement for clinical correlation, and guide targeted treatments.

The treatment of radiculopathy in head and neck cancer may include physical therapy, with emphasis on neck and upper extremity range of motion, postural training, scapular or spine stabilization, and core strengthening. Interventional pain procedures, such as epidural steroid injections, can be considered to temporize pain symptoms from nerve root irritation. If radiculopathy is caused by direct tumor compression, a neurosurgical evaluation may be necessary. Other cancer-directed treatments, such as radiation therapy or systemic treatments, may also be considered to shrink the tumor.

Plexopathy

Plexopathy refers to a type of peripheral nerve disorder that arises from damage to a network of nerves situated in either the brachial plexus or lumbosacral plexus. The signs and symptoms of plexopathy depend on the location of the lesion in relation to the plexus. Patients generally experience radiating pain followed by weakness and sensory deficits that are not limited to a specific dermatomal or myotomal distribution since multiple nerves are involved. In severe cases, limb paralysis can occur. In the case of the brachial plexus, lower trunk involvement may result in distal limb or intrinsic hand weakness, while upper trunk lesions may cause more proximal deficits. Posterior cord lesions may affect limb extension mechanisms and shoulder movement due to the involvement of the radial and axillary nerves.

Neoplastic brachial plexopathies have a frequency of occurrence estimated at 0.43% in cancer patients, with a higher incidence noted in individuals with lung or breast malignancies.[7] Plexopathies in head and neck cancer may result from direct tumor invasion or plexus injury due to radiation therapy or surgical resection, which will be discussed in detail later in this chapter. Head and neck cancer patients with large, bulky lymph nodes in the neck near the brachial plexus could also cause nerve injury by compression or irritation. While tumor-related plexopathy can involve any location of the brachial plexus, electrodiagnostic studies have characterized a majority of neoplastic plexopathies of the brachial plexus involving the medial cord and lower trunk.[8]

CT, MRI, and PET are imaging techniques useful in assessing tumor involvement and detecting active disease. A dedicated MRI of the brachial plexus is particularly valuable in evaluating the extent of tumor involvement, the tumor's location within the plexus, or identifying findings that indicate metastatic infiltration. In the case of tumor involvement, imaging may show a lesion with ill-defined margins, with or without mass effect on nerve structures. Abnormal enhancement of nerves or surrounding intramuscular edema (finding consistent with denervation changes) may indicate nerve injury or neoplastic infiltration of nerves. Like in radiculopathies, electrodiagnostic studies can help localize damage to the plexus and determine nerve involvement while excluding treatment-related causes (i.e., radiation therapy). It is crucial to consider the timing of EMG referral with the onset of pain and weakness. It is recommended to wait until 10−14 days after symptom onset to perform electrodiagnostic studies as electrophysiologic findings of nerve damage findings in that time frame.

The prognosis of plexopathy recovery can be variable depending on the extent of tumor involvement and treatments completed. Management of plexopathies is like that of radiculopathies, focusing on alleviating symptoms and maintaining function. In severe cases where complete paralysis of a limb has occurred, braving evaluation may be beneficial to ease the discomfort of the neck/shoulder and optimize positioning. Functional bracing and splinting can be helpful in less severe cases where focal weakness is present. Occupational and physical therapy will be crucial to maintain the upper limb range of motion, given the risk of contractures with immobility.

Peripheral neuropathies

Peripheral neuropathy, also known as polyneuropathy, is a condition characterized by more widespread nerve dysfunction. When assessing polyneuropathy, it is essential to take note of the timing, symmetry, and distribution of symptoms. Electrophysiological features of axonal versus demyelinating injuries, as well as the involvement of sensory and motor nerves, are also crucial clinical considerations. Typically, the longest nerves are predominantly affected as they are the most vulnerable to injury, consistent with distal axonopathy. Isolated sensory polyneuropathy may indicate injury to the dorsal root ganglion (i.e., ganglionopathy) or small sensory nerve fibers. Polyneuropathy can cause a variety of symptoms, commonly altered sensation or motor weakness, but depend on the specific type of neuropathy. Distal axonopathy often presents in a characteristic stocking-glove distribution, affecting the longest nerves first. When large fiber nerves are involved, symptoms may also include loss of vibration sense, proprioception, light touch sensation, and gait imbalance. Small fiber involvement may result in painful dysesthesias or loss of temperature perception.

Although chemotherapy-induced peripheral neuropathy is the most frequently occurring type of neuropathy in cancer patients, it can also develop due to other factors such as disease-related nerve infiltration, metabolic or nutritional deficiencies, or paraneoplastic processes. Disease-related peripheral neuropathy in head and neck cancer is rare, although subclinical neuropathy prior to receiving treatments has been reported in the head and neck cancer population.[9] In head and neck cancer, polyneuropathies are typically due to systemic treatments, as covered later in the chapter. Peripheral neuropathies associated with nutritional deficiencies may also be present in patients with malnutrition if severe dysphagia or trismus is affecting the ability to eat. Nutritional neuropathies may result from deficiencies of various B vitamins (B12, B6, folate, B1), vitamin E, and copper.[10,11]

Investigation of suspected peripheral neuropathy starts with a thorough medical history, which includes details of symptoms such as the onset, severity, distribution, and progression of symptoms. It is also essential to review the patient's oncological treatments, evaluate their nutritional status, and inquire about any underlying medical conditions to determine the risk of neuropathy. A neurological examination should be conducted, which includes checking muscle strength, sensation (including light touch, pinprick, and temperature), and reflexes. In addition, gait patterns should be assessed, and the skin should be carefully examined.

Diagnostic tests include blood tests to check for reversible or contributing causes of neuropathy, such as diabetes, thyroid disease, nutritional deficiencies, and inflammatory or autoimmune disease. In some instances where workup and lab work is unremarkable, it may be warranted to obtain paraneoplastic antibodies. Electrodiagnostic testing is useful in characterizing polyneuropathy, but its ability to determine the precise cause of nerve dysfunction is limited. However, nerve conduction and electromyography can determine the type of nerve injury (axonal vs. demyelinating) and determine the time course of injury (acute, subacute, or chronic). If applicable, serial electrodiagnostic studies can be helpful in evaluating nerve recovery over time. An MRI of the spine can be helpful in excluding nerve root compression or spinal cord dysfunction as potential causes of similar symptoms.

Management of peripheral neuropathy depends on the underlying cause and the severity of symptoms. Addressing any underlying and reversible causes or contributing medical conditions is essential. This may include measures such as maintaining optimal blood glucose levels and addressing nutritional deficiencies through appropriate supplementation. Use of neuropathic agents such as gabapentin, pregabalin, amitriptyline, or duloxetine can be used to manage neuropathic pain; however, it may not be effective for negative symptoms of numbness. Physical therapy helps improve balance and gait patterns to reduce the risk of falls. Bracing and orthotics can provide limb support and proprioceptive feedback in severe neuropathy resulting in lower extremity weakness or sensory ataxia. TENs (transcutaneous electric nerve stimulation) and complementary therapies such as acupuncture can be useful adjuncts in managing symptoms. Referral to a nutritionist may be warranted for patients with malnutrition.

Paraneoplastic neuropathies

Paraneoplastic neurologic syndromes (PNS) refer to a collection of syndromes that cause damage to the nervous system at various levels, such as the central nervous system (including limbic encephalitis and paraneoplastic cerebellar degeneration), the neuromuscular junction (such as Lambert–Eaton myasthenia syndrome [LEMS] and myasthenia gravis), or the peripheral nervous system (for example, autonomic neuropathy and subacute sensory neuropathy).[12] PNS are rare and not directly caused by a malignant neoplasm or its treatments. Studies have shown that approximately 15% of cancer patients may develop paraneoplastic sensorimotor neuropathy, which is more commonly observed in patients with advanced or terminal disease.[13,14] Nonetheless, determining the precise prevalence of PNS is challenging due to the extensive variety of its types.

The exact pathophysiology of paraneoplastic syndromes is not completely understood, but it is believed to be an immune-mediated process. This involves an autoimmune response against the tumor and healthy neural tissue, which may occur via autoantibodies against neuronal antigens expressed by the tumor.[15] Neurologic symptoms associated with paraneoplastic syndrome can be the presenting feature of malignancy or occur in patients with known cancer. These syndromes can manifest as a wide range of clinical symptoms, including sensory or motor deficits, ataxia, autonomic dysfunction, swallowing difficulties, vertigo, cognitive changes, or seizures.

The most common cancers associated with PNS include lung, breast, ovarian, or lymphatic malignancies. Some of the most common types of PNS are linked to specific types of cancer. Lambert–Eaton syndrome is frequently associated with small-cell lung cancer, while stiff-person syndrome is often linked to breast cancer. Subacute sensory neuropathies are commonly found in patients with gynecologic malignancies, and myasthenia gravis has been linked to thymomas.

Malignant thymomas are tumors that originate in the thymus gland located in the mediastinum. Although not classified as primary head and neck cancers, they frequently spread through local invasion and can metastasize to the upper regions of the head and neck.

As mentioned previously, thymomas are associated with myasthenia gravis, a well-described neuromuscular junction disorder caused by autoantibodies to postsynaptic acetylcholine receptors located at the neuromuscular junction, impairing neuromuscular transmission. As a result, patients experience fluctuating weakness and bulbar symptoms (i.e., diplopia, dysphagia, dysarthria). In the literature, there have been a few reports of paraneoplastic neuromuscular syndromes linked to laryngeal cancer, including cerebellar degeneration, ataxia, Lambert–Eaton myasthenic syndrome, encephalomyelitis, and polymyositis.[16]

Paraneoplastic syndromes are a rare but important differential diagnosis to consider in patients with neuromuscular dysfunction, as they can indicate the presence of a new malignancy or recurrence. Diagnosis of PNS is challenging due to the diverse clinical manifestations as well as the possibility that any part of the neuroaxis is affected. The workup may involve blood tests similar to those used for peripheral neuropathy to identify more common causes. If PNS is suspected, performing an MRI of the brain and spine, CSF cytology, paraneoplastic antibody studies, and electrodiagnostic studies with or without repetitive nerve stimulation studies is recommended.

The treatment approach for PNS primarily depends on the patient's cancer status and symptoms. For individuals diagnosed with PNS, the first step in management involves detecting hidden or recurring cancer using appropriate disease-specific imaging techniques. If a new or progressive malignancy is identified, treating the underlying tumor becomes necessary. In numerous cases, immunomodulatory treatments may be required, such as steroids, rituximab, intravenous immunoglobulins (IVIG), or plasmapheresis.[12]

In certain instances, residual neurologic deficits may persist despite receiving treatment for underlying cancer or immunomodulation. In such cases, rehabilitation plays a crucial role. The goal of rehabilitation management is to optimize functional independence and enhance the overall quality of life. This is best managed through a multidisciplinary approach with specific interventions, including physical, occupational, and speech therapy. Individuals with severe motor weakness may benefit from braces or other supportive devices. In addition to therapy interventions, psychological and social support for patient caregivers may be beneficial to help cope with neurologic symptoms and navigate functional limitations.

Treatment-related nerve dysfunction
Neuromuscular dysfunction related to systemic treatments
Chemotherapy- induced peripheral neuropathy

Chemotherapy-induced peripheral neuropathy (CIPN) is a frequently encountered and debilitating side effect of chemotherapy. The likelihood of developing neuropathy is estimated to be between 30% and 70% in individuals exposed to neurotoxic chemotherapeutic agents, such as taxanes, platinum compounds, vinca alkaloids, or bortezomib.[17,18] These medications are commonly utilized for the treatment of various types of cancers. Among the neurotoxic agents mentioned, cisplatin and docetaxel are frequently employed chemotherapeutic agents in the management of head and neck cancer.[19] While the specific mechanisms of action and molecular targets of these agents may differ, their ultimate impact involves interfering with cell division, leading to cell arrest or apoptosis. This interference occurs through various mechanisms, including altered microtubule function, disruption of cellular transport, induction of oxidative stress, disturbances in cellular membrane homeostasis, and neuroinflammation.[20]

Although the prevalence of CIPN is initially high, studies have demonstrated a decrease in prevalence over time after the completion of chemotherapy—decreasing approximately 68% in the first month to around 30% at the 6-month mark.[18] Nevertheless, some patients may experience persistent and long-lasting effects associated with CIPN. Hence, regular monitoring and surveillance for CIPN following chemotherapy are crucial to identify and address any ongoing symptoms or complications. The most important risk factor for developing CIPN is cumulative drug dose exposure. Other risk factors may include preexisting neuropathy, age, sex, smoking history, renal dysfunction, comorbidities such as diabetes, or genetic predisposition.[21,22]

In clinical practice, CIPN manifests as a symmetric sensorimotor neuropathy that follows a length-dependent pattern. Typically, symptoms initially appear in the hands and feet, resembling a glove and stocking distribution, due to the neurotoxic effects on axons. Patients commonly report sensations such as numbness, tingling, and abnormal sensory perceptions. In more severe cases, CIPN can lead to motor deficits and sensory proprioceptive disturbances, resulting in impaired balance, gait abnormalities, and difficulties with manual dexterity.[20]

Symptom onset of CIPN can manifest either acutely during chemotherapy or subacutely after the completion of treatment. In some cases, a phenomenon referred to as "coasting" has been observed with certain neurotoxic agents such as vinca alkaloids or platinum-based drugs, wherein symptoms may persist or even intensify despite discontinuation of the treatment.

The diagnostic approach to CIPN is multidimensional, including clinical evaluation, patient-reported symptoms, objective assessments, and utilization of validated scales and questionnaires. The evaluation process typically begins with a comprehensive neuromuscular examination, which encompasses the assessment of strength, sensation, proprioception, vibration sense, gait, and balance. It is also important to examine the spine, cranial nerves, and muscle tone to rule out any central causes. Regular assessment of CIPN and the selection of appropriate assessment tools are crucial. Scales such as the Functional Assessment of Cancer Therapy/Gynecologic Oncology Group-Neurotoxicity (FACT/GOG-Ntx) and Total Neuropathy Score (TNS) have been recommended for clinical use.[23] These scales aid in systematically evaluating the impact of neuropathy on patients' daily functioning, quality of life, and overall well-being.

The diagnostic workup for chemotherapy-induced peripheral neuropathy (CIPN) follows a similar approach to the general workup for neuropathy, as mentioned earlier in this chapter. This may involve conducting a neuropathy panel to evaluate for reversible or contributing causes of neuropathy. Electrodiagnostic studies can provide valuable diagnostic information by assessing the severity and distribution of nerve dysfunction and determining if the pattern of injury is inconsistent with CIPN. In CIPN, the typical electrodiagnostic pattern demonstrates length-dependent sensorimotor axonal loss. Neuroimaging is generally not indicated unless there is suspicion of a central cause for the neuropathy. The focus of the workup is primarily on identifying any potentially reversible or contributing factors and assessing the characteristic features of CIPN through clinical evaluation and objective assessments.

The treatment approach of CIPN is multimodal and aims to address the symptoms that have the greatest impact on an individual's quality of life. For example, if pain is a significant issue affecting daily functioning, pharmacotherapy may be appropriate. For functional impairments without severe pain, manual therapeutic methods can be considered. Often, a combination of pharmacological and nonpharmacological approaches is utilized. Among pharmacological options, duloxetine has shown evidence of reducing pain symptoms and is recommended based on the currently available data.[24] Other neuromodulators such as gabapentin and pregabalin have been used, but the evidence supporting their efficacy is limited. The effectiveness of other systemic therapy agents in managing CIPN is inconclusive due to the lack of consistent clinical evidence.[25] It should be noted that pharmacologic agents used for the management of CIPN can have accompanying side effects, such as dizziness and increased risk of falls. In such cases, topical therapies such as capsaicin or lidocaine cream can be considered due to their lower rate of side effects and drug interactions.[25] The nonpharmacological approach to managing CIPN focuses on functional exercises and therapies that target balance, sensory function, and motor training. Therapeutic modalities such as transcutaneous electrical nerve stimulation (TENS) or ultrasound therapy can be utilized as adjuncts to support symptom management. Currently, there is no recommended agent for the prevention of CIPN, primarily due to the limited availability of high-quality studies that provide definitive evidence on preventive strategies. It is important for healthcare providers to closely monitor and manage CIPN symptoms, tailoring the treatment approach to each individual patient's needs and considering the potential benefits and risks of different interventions.

Immunotherapy-related neuromuscular dysfunction

Immunotherapy has emerged as a significant advancement in cancer treatment and is now widely used as a standard therapeutic option for various malignancies. Unlike traditional chemotherapy, which directly targets cancer cells, immunotherapy works by enhancing the body's immune response against cancer. One of the most notable classes of immunotherapy agents is immune checkpoint inhibitors (ICIs), including monoclonal antibodies such as ipilimumab, pembrolizumab, and nivolumab. These agents have revolutionized cancer treatment by helping the immune system recognize and attack cancer cells more effectively. In the head and neck population, the integration of immunotherapy into standard treatment approaches has significantly improved patient outcomes. Agents such as nivolumab and pembrolizumab have become integral components of the treatment regimen to treat head and neck malignancies.[26]

Peripheral nervous system complications related to the immune system, known as immune-related adverse events (irAE), are uncommon but acknowledged side effects of immunotherapy agents. These immune-related neuromuscular events can present as various conditions, including cranial and peripheral neuropathies, myopathies, or disorders affecting the neuromuscular junction.[27] Uncommon but potentially severe complications of immune checkpoint inhibitors (ICIs) include acute inflammatory neuropathies such as Guillain–Barre syndrome, myasthenia gravis, and myositis.[27,28] The exact mechanism underlying immune checkpoint inhibitor (ICI)–induced peripheral nerve dysfunction remains unclear. However, it is hypothesized to involve an autoimmune response in which the activated immune system mistakenly targets and damages peripheral nerves. This mechanism differs from traditional chemotherapy-induced neuropathy, which is primarily caused by direct neurotoxic effects.

The clinical presentation of an ICI-induced peripheral nerve dysfunction is comparable with chemotherapy-induced peripheral neuropathy (CIPN) in that it can manifest as sensorimotor neuropathy. However, the distinguishing factor is that ICI-induced nerve dysfunction may also present with weakness or pain in large muscle groups (indicative of myositis), fatigue and muscle weakness (resembling myasthenia gravis), or ascending paralysis +/− respiratory dysfunction (reminiscent of Guillain−Barré syndrome).[29] The specific presentation depends on the localization of the peripheral nerve dysfunction, whether it affects the muscles, nerves, or neuromuscular junction.

Regarding the timing of symptom onset, ICI-mediated neuropathy typically emerges several weeks to months after the initiation of treatment, in contrast to CIPN, which can develop during or immediately after treatment. However, in some cases, neuromuscular toxicities such as ICI-mediated myositis or acute inflammatory demyelinating polyneuropathy (Guillain−Barré syndrome) can progress rapidly, leading to a more aggressive and rapid onset of symptoms.[29]

The workup for suspected ICI-induced neuromuscular dysfunction may involve various diagnostic tests. This includes laboratory investigations to assess inflammatory markers such as ESR, CRP, or CPK, antibody testing, cerebrospinal fluid analysis, electrodiagnostic studies, and possibly diagnostic imaging such as MRI of the brain or spine or PET scan. In the case of myositis, elevated inflammatory markers may be observed, and electromyography patterns may show myopathic muscle potentials. For acute inflammatory demyelinating polyneuropathy (AIDP), CSF analysis may reveal cytoalbuminologic dissociation, and nerve conduction studies may demonstrate demyelination, characterized by missing or prolonged F-wave latency, temporal dispersion, and possible conduction block. In myasthenia gravis, positive serum AChR antibodies may be detected, and electrodiagnostic studies may reveal a pathological decrement in the affected muscle group during repetitive nerve stimulation.[29]

The management of immunotherapy-mediated neuromuscular toxicities depends on the clinical presentation and the specific type of neuromuscular dysfunction. However, due to the rarity of these toxicities and the limited evidence available, there is a lack of consensus regarding their treatment. Toxicities can vary from mild and transient symptoms to severe forms. Commonly used treatments include glucocorticoids, intravenous immunoglobulin (IVIG), and plasma exchange. In some cases, adjustments to the dose of the immunotherapy agent or discontinuation may be necessary. For severe toxicity characterized by rapid deterioration, especially with the involvement of the cardiac or respiratory system, intensive care unit monitoring and management may be required. It is worth noting that due to the limited data available, individualized treatment approaches based on the specific clinical situation is recommended. Close monitoring and collaboration between oncologists and neurologists are essential for the optimal management of these neuromuscular toxicities.

Neuropathies related to radiation therapy

Radiation-induced brachial plexopathies and cranial neuropathies

Radiation therapy (RT) is a commonly used treatment for head and neck cancer, either as a definitive or adjuvant therapy. While it effectively targets tumor cells, it can also lead to collateral damage to nearby healthy tissues, resulting in acute or delayed onset toxicity. Despite advancements in radiotherapy techniques, such as improved dose contouring and alternative radiation modalities, patients may still experience adverse side effects from treatment. The head and neck region is particularly susceptible to developing neuropathies due to its abundance of nervous tissue. The presence of vulnerable structures in this region increases the risk of brachial and cranial neuropathies as late complications of radiation therapy in individuals undergoing treatment for head and neck cancer. These neuropathies occur as a result of the radiation field encompassing or being in close proximity to the affected nerves. It is important to recognize and manage these potential complications to minimize their impact on a patient's quality of life.

Radiation-induced brachial plexopathy (RIBP) refers to a condition where damage to the brachial plexus occurs as a delayed effect of radiation therapy (RT) in areas such as the chest wall, neck, or axilla. This injury to the brachial plexus is nontraumatic in nature and occurs as a consequence of prior radiation treatment. The occurrence rate of RIBP is estimated to range from 1.8% to 4.9%.[7,30] There appears to be a correlation between the dose of radiation received and the likelihood of developing RIBP, with higher doses associated with a higher risk. However, advancements in radiation techniques have significantly decreased the incidence of brachial plexus injury as a result of radiotherapy.

Symptoms of RIBP typically manifest gradually, appearing several months to years after the completion of radiation therapy. In a case series conducted by Gu et al., RIBP was observed in 10 patients with nasopharyngeal carcinoma, with a latency period ranging from 1 to 17 years. Similarly, a retrospective study by Cai et al. reported an average latency period of 4.26 years for the onset of RIBP. Patients with head and neck cancer may experience early transient RIBP, characterized by the onset of symptoms shortly after completing radiation therapy (RT).[31,32] This phenomenon is believed to be attributed to direct effects on Schwann cells or temporary nerve compression caused by postradiation edema, resulting in reversible nerve dysfunction. It is recommended to closely monitor these patients neurologically starting from the early post-RT period.[33] Typically, the clinical presentation of RIBP begins with subjective paresthesias as the most frequently reported symptom, followed by the development of pain and weakness. Muscle fasciculations and atrophy have also been observed in certain cases.[32] In patients who underwent radiation therapy in the head and neck region, Cai et al. found that the symptoms primarily affected the brachial plexus's upper and middle trunk distribution. This observation may be attributed to the frequent involvement of the supraclavicular fossa region with radiation therapy in individuals with nasopharyngeal cancer.

The diagnosis of RIBP may involve performing diagnostic imaging of the brachial plexus or shoulder to differentiate between tumor infiltration or compression. Key findings that suggest RIBP rather than a tumor include symmetric enhancement and thickening of nerve roots without the presence of a mass. In addition, electrodiagnostic studies can be helpful in confirming a brachial plexus lesion. These studies may reveal decreased amplitudes in both sensory and motor nerve conduction. Myokymic discharges during EMG examination are considered pathognomonic for radiation-induced damage. Furthermore, EMG findings may demonstrate a combination of neuropathic and myopathic changes in specific myotomes.[32]

Radiation-induced cranial neuropathies (RICN) can occur as a complication following high-dose radiation therapy in head and neck cancer (HNC) treatment. The incidence of these neuropathies varies, with some sources describing it as rare while others suggest it may be more common than currently recognized.[2,34] A study conducted by Kong et al. revealed that the incidence of cranial neuropathy (CNP) after definitive radiotherapy for nasopharyngeal carcinoma (NPC) remains high even during long-term follow-up, and it is influenced by the radiation dose and fractionation. In their study, 98 patients (30.9%) developed CNP, with a median latent period of 7.6 years (range, 0.3–34 years). Risk factors associated with developing RICN include cranial nerve dysfunction at the time of diagnosis, chemotherapy, total radiation dose to the nasopharynx, and upper neck fibrosis, which were identified as independent risk factors for radiation-induced cranial neuropathy (RICN).[35]

Complications of RICN can have a profound impact on the quality of life for survivors of HNC. These complications often manifest as functional impairments, including hearing loss, taste disturbances, swallowing difficulties, or vision problems.[2] Among the cranial nerves, the glossopharyngeal (IX), vagus (X), and hypoglossal (XII) nerves are commonly affected by radiation treatment, leading to various impairments. While the upper cranial nerves may also be affected, their involvement is typically less pronounced compared with the lower cranial nerves.[35] These functional issues associated with RICN can be debilitating and significantly affect the overall well-being of HNC survivors.

Progress in radiation techniques and supportive care has been directed toward reducing the risks associated with radiation-induced neuropathies. The Radiation Therapy Oncology Group (RTOG) has taken the initiative to establish guidelines that set dose limits, with the goal of minimizing the occurrence of long-term brachial plexopathies. Contouring of both the brachial and cranial nerve bundles has become a primary preventive measure to mitigate the development of both RIBP and RICN.

The management of radiation-induced neuropathies aims to address symptoms such as pain, motor weakness, and sensory impairments. It is important to establish realistic expectations with patients regarding the clinical trajectory and anticipated rehabilitation process, as symptoms may be progressive. Similar to the treatments mentioned earlier, the management approach is multimodal, incorporating both pharmacological and nonpharmacological interventions. To reduce neuroinflammation, nonsteroidal antiinflammatory drugs (NSAIDs) or short-term use of steroids may be employed. Neuromodulating agents, such as anticonvulsants (e.g., gabapentin or pregabalin), tricyclic antidepressants (e.g., amitriptyline), or selective serotonin reuptake inhibitors (SSRIs) such as duloxetine, can be used to alleviate symptoms of neuropathic pain, similar to their use in CIPN.[2] Experimental combinations of pentoxifylline, tocopherol, and clodronate have been investigated, but no beneficial effects were observed specifically for RIBP. However, these drugs have shown promising effects in other radiation-induced side effects in head and neck cancer, as demonstrated by the same research group.[36] Physical therapy, occupational therapy, and speech therapy play a crucial role in the management of functional impairments resulting from radiation-induced neuropathies. For patients with motor weakness resulting from brachial plexopathy, physical therapy focuses on various aspects such as range of motion exercises, scapular stabilization, and strengthening of the shoulder girdle. These exercises help improve joint mobility, enhance stability, and strengthen the muscles surrounding the shoulder joint. Occupational therapy may concentrate on neuromuscular training, fine motor tasks, and sensory and coordination training.

In cases where weakness of the shoulder girdle is present, bracing may be utilized to prevent subluxation of the glenohumeral joint and provide support. Braces can also be used to optimize hand positioning for functional tasks, facilitating improved hand function.

The management of cranial neuropathies involves targeted therapeutic interventions tailored to the specific neurologic deficit. For individuals experiencing visual disturbances, it is important to seek evaluation by a neuroophthalmologist. Treatment options may include the use of eye patches and occupational therapy to learn compensatory strategies and optimize visual function. In cases of speech and swallowing issues, speech therapy plays a key role. Speech therapists can work with individuals to improve swallowing mechanics and develop strategies to overcome speech and swallowing difficulties. Additionally, consulting with a dietitian can help in modifying the diet to accommodate swallowing issues and ensure proper nutrition and hydration. By addressing the specific challenges associated with cranial neuropathies through these therapeutic interventions, individuals can experience improved visual function, speech clarity, and swallowing abilities, leading to enhanced overall quality of life.

As a result, radiation-induced neuropathy in head and neck cancer is a complex condition that manifests differently based on various factors such as the treatment method, anatomical location, and the patient's overall health. Close monitoring and appropriate interventions are crucial in addressing and managing these late complications in individuals undergoing radiation therapy for head and neck cancer.

Surgical- or procedural-related neuropathies

Head and neck cancers commonly spread to cervical lymph nodes. Consequently, the removal of cervical lymph nodes is crucial and has become the standard of practice for surgical treatment of head and neck cancer. The head and neck region is characterized by intricate and densely packed anatomical structures. The lymph nodes in the neck are divided into seven levels by anatomic landmarks based on nodal drainage pathways. According to the classification system of the American Academy of Otolaryngology-Head and Neck Surgery, a radical neck dissection involves the excision of levels I–V in addition to the SCM, IJV, and CN XI. The modified radical neck dissection similarly eliminates levels I–V but preserves at least one nonlymphatic structure, which may be the SCM, IJV, or CN XI.[37] When suitable, opting for modified or selective neck dissections offers the benefit of reducing functional complications in comparison with more extensive radical neck dissections.

A thorough understanding of the critical structures in these areas is key to performing safe surgeries. Comprehensive knowledge of head and neck anatomy is also crucial for rehabilitation professionals who treat these patients as it plays a vital role in screening, assessing, and treating potential impairments that may develop as a result of surgery. Potential neuromuscular complications that may occur after neck dissection include spinal accessory nerve palsy and brachial plexopathy.

Spinal accessory nerve dysfunction

One of the most common complications following neck dissection is shoulder dysfunction as a result of spinal accessory nerve (SAN) injury. In modified radical neck dissections, the reported injury rate for spinal accessory nerve is 33%, while it is intentionally sacrificed in radical neck dissections.[38,39] The mechanism of injury is suspected to be due to direct iatrogenic injury, manipulation of surrounding structures, or devascularization of nerve.[40]

The SAN is also known as cranial nerve IX, which is a motor nerve that originates in the medulla as well as the upper segments of the cervical spine. From its origin, it exits the brain through the foramen magnum and courses through the posterior triangle of the head and neck. It travels deep to the sternocleidomastoid muscle (SCM) where it innervates the upper third muscle fibers. It continues through the posterior triangle floor where it provides motor innervation to the trapezius.[40] The sternocleidomastoid (SCM) and trapezius muscles work together to coordinate movements of the head, neck, and shoulder blades. Injury or sacrifice of the SAN often results in dysfunction of the shoulder girdle due to paralysis of the trapezius muscle.

Detecting spinal accessory nerve (SAN) injury poses a challenge, often resulting in missed diagnoses. Identification of SAN palsy involves recognizing trapezius dysfunction, manifested as scapular winging or dyskinesis, along with restricted shoulder abduction. The trapezius muscle, a large posterior muscle, originates from the base of the cervical spine and attaches to the spine of the scapula and thoracic spine. It plays a crucial role in coordinating shoulder movements, stabilizing the scapula, and maintaining proper posture. Denervation of the trapezius can lead to shoulder droop, scapular winging, compromised arm movement, and altered postural mechanics.

The clinical assessment begins with an examination of the alignment of the head and spine, as well as an evaluation of muscle bulk and scapular positioning. In cases of SAN palsy, trapezius dysfunction is often indicated by lateral scapular winging, as opposed to the medial winging which is associated with serratus anterior weakness resulting from long thoracic nerve injury. Manual muscle testing might reveal weakness with shoulder shrugging against resistance; however, the levator scapulae and rhomboids may compensate for trapezius weakness during this motion.

Although not necessary for diagnosis, referral for an EMG and nerve conduction study may be indicated to confirm SAN palsy or to rule out other etiologies for shoulder dysfunction, such as brachial plexopathy.[41] Electrodiagnostic features specific to SAN palsy may include neuropathic changes (such as positive sharp waves or fibrillation potentials, reduced recruitment pattern, or long-duration, large amplitude potentials) in the trapezius muscle. Additionally, a decreased compound muscle action potential (CMAP) with stimulation of the SAN relative to the contralateral side may also be present. It's important to note that electrodiagnostic studies should be interpreted in conjunction with clinical findings.

The management of shoulder dysfunction resulting from SAN palsy typically begins with a conservative approach. This may involve initiating physical therapy to strengthen scapular stabilizers and provide postural reeducation. Additionally, manual therapy techniques can be used for joint tissue mobilization and to improve the range of motion (ROM) of the affected shoulder. Modalities like heat compression can be employed if it is associated with myofascial pain. If there is significant arm dysfunction, a prescription for adaptive equipment may be considered. In severe cases, a nerve transfer of levator scapulae and rhomboid muscles may be indicated.[42]

Brachial plexopathy
During neck dissection for head and neck cancer, the brachial plexus is a critical structure at risk of injury due to its proximity to the surgical field. As discussed earlier in this chapter, it is a complex network of nerves originating from the cervical and first thoracic roots. These nerves converge, traveling down the neck between the anterior and middle scalene, into the axilla, and down the arm. When performing neck dissections and removing lymph nodes, manipulation and traction of nearby structures can exert pressure on the brachial plexus. Improper or prolonged positioning during surgery can further heighten the risk of nerve injury. Surgeons must be meticulous and cautious to minimize this risk. While brachial plexus injuries from neck dissection surgery are rare, rehabilitation professionals should also be cognizant of the potential for nerve injury with neck dissections. The evaluation and management of intraoperative brachial plexopathy follow a similar approach to the management of radiation-induced plexus injury discussed earlier. This encompasses a multimodal approach with a focus on symptom management and functional optimization.

Conclusion

In conclusion, peripheral nerve injuries represent a significant yet often underreported challenge for individuals with head and neck cancer. These injuries, stemming from both the disease itself and its treatments, can amplify the already substantial symptom burden and impact patients' overall quality of life. Recognizing these issues early on is paramount in preventing potential long-term disability. This chapter has delved into the diverse causes, underlying mechanisms, and diagnostic strategies for identifying various neuromuscular disorders prevalent in those with a history of head and neck cancer. Moreover, we have explored various treatment and rehabilitation strategies in effectively managing these conditions. By fostering a comprehensive understanding of these complexities, healthcare providers can better prepare themselves to address the unique needs of this patient population, ultimately enhancing their overall well-being and long-term outcomes.

References

1. Tai SK, Li WY, Yang MH, Chu PY, Wang YF. Perineural invasion in T1 oral squamous cell carcinoma indicates the need for aggressive elective neck dissection. *Am J Surg Pathol*. 2013;37(8):1164−1172. https://doi.org/10.1097/PAS.0b013e318285f684.
2. Azzam P, Mroueh M, Francis M, Daher AA, Zeidan YH. Radiation-induced neuropathies in head and neck cancer: prevention and treatment modalities. *Ecancermedicalscience*. 2020;14. https://doi.org/10.3332/ECANCER.2020.1133.
3. Taylor JC, Terrell JE, Ronis DL, et al. Disability in patients with head and neck cancer. *Arch Otolaryngol Head Neck Surg*. 2004;130(6):764−769. https://doi.org/10.1001/archotol.130.6.764.
4. Dankbaar JW, Pameijer FA, Hendrikse J, Schmalfuss IM. Easily detected signs of perineural tumour spread in head and neck cancer. *Insights Imaging*. 2018;9(6):1089−1095. https://doi.org/10.1007/s13244-018-0672-8.
5. Mendes RL, Nutting CM, Harrington KJ. Residual or recurrent head and neck cancer presenting with nerve root compression affecting the upper limbs. *Br J Radiol*. 2004;77(920):688−690. https://doi.org/10.1259/bjr/16836733.
6. Revannasiddaiah S, Thakur P, Rastogi M, Madabhavi I, Bellad A, Chindi S. Posterior pharyngeal wall carcinoma presenting as sudden onset bilateral upper limb radiculopathy. *BMJ Case Rep*. 2012;2012. https://doi.org/10.1136/bcr.11.2011.5269.
7. Jaeckle KA. Neurologic manifestations of neoplastic and radiation-induced plexopathies. *Semin Neurol*. 2010;30(3):254−262. https://doi.org/10.1055/s-0030-1255219.
8. Ko K, Sung DH, Kang MJ, et al. Clinical, electrophysiological findings in adult patients with non-traumatic plexopathies. *Ann Rehabil Med*. 2011;35(6):807. https://doi.org/10.5535/arm.2011.35.6.807.
9. Roldan CJ, Johnson C, Lee SO, Ms AP, Dougherty PM, Huh B. Subclinical peripheral neuropathy in patients with head and neck cancer: a quantitative sensory testing (QST) study. *Pain Physician*. 2018;21(4):E419−E427. https://doi.org/10.36076/ppj.2018.4.e419.

10. Staff NP, Windebank AJ. Peripheral neuropathy due to vitamin deficiency, toxins, and medications. *Contin Lifelong Learn Neurol*. 2014;20(5 Peripheral Nervous System Disorders):1293. https://doi.org/10.1212/01.CON.0000455880.06675.5A.

11. Hammond N, Wang Y, Dimachkie MM, Barohn RJ. Nutritional neuropathies. *Neurol Clin*. 2013;31(2):477. https://doi.org/10.1016/J.NCL.2013.02.002.

12. Pelosof LC, Gerber DE. Paraneoplastic syndromes: an approach to diagnosis and treatment. *Mayo Clin Proc*. 2010;85(9):838. https://doi.org/10.4065/MCP.2010.0099.

13. Croft PB, Wilkinson M. The incidence of carcinomatous neuromyopathy in patients with various types of carcinoma. *Brain*. 1965;88(3):427−434. https://doi.org/10.1093/BRAIN/88.3.427.

14. Dalmau J. Carcinoma associated paraneoplastic peripheral neuropathy. *J Neurol Neurosurg Psychiatry*. 1999;67(1):4. https://doi.org/10.1136/jnnp.67.1.4.

15. Honnorat J, Antoine JC. Paraneoplastic neurological syndromes. *Orphanet J Rare Dis*. 2007;2(1):1−8. https://doi.org/10.1186/1750-1172-2-22/TABLES/2.

16. Rinaldo A, Coca-Pelaz A, Silver CE, Ferlito A. Paraneoplastic syndromes associated with laryngeal cancer. *Adv Ther*. 2020;37(1):140. https://doi.org/10.1007/S12325-019-01160-9.

17. Kolb NA, Smith AG, Singleton JR, et al. The association of chemotherapy-induced peripheral neuropathy symptoms and the risk of falling. *JAMA Neurol*. 2016;73(7):860−866. https://doi.org/10.1001/jamaneurol.2016.0383.

18. Seretny M, Currie GL, Sena ES, et al. Incidence, prevalence, and predictors of chemotherapy-induced peripheral neuropathy: a systematic review and meta-analysis. *Pain*. 2014;155(12):2461−2470. https://doi.org/10.1016/j.pain.2014.09.020.

19. Sindhu SK, Bauman JE. Current concepts in chemotherapy for head and neck cancer. *Oral Maxillofac Surg Clin North Am*. 2019;31(1):145−154. https://doi.org/10.1016/j.coms.2018.09.003.

20. Starobova H, Vetter I. Pathophysiology of chemotherapy-induced peripheral neuropathy. *Front Mol Neurosci*. 2017;10. https://doi.org/10.3389/fnmol.2017.00174.

21. Gu J, Lu H, Chen C, et al. Diabetes mellitus as a risk factor for chemotherapy-induced peripheral neuropathy: a meta-analysis. *Support Care Cancer*. 2021;29(12):7461−7469. https://doi.org/10.1007/s00520-021-06321-7.

22. Sałat K. Chemotherapy-induced peripheral neuropathy: part 1—current state of knowledge and perspectives for pharmacotherapy. *Pharmacol Rep*. 2020;72(3):486−507. https://doi.org/10.1007/s43440-020-00109-y.

23. Haryani H, Fetzer SJ, Wu CL, Hsu YY. Chemotherapy-induced peripheral neuropathy assessment tools: a systematic review. *Oncol Nurs Forum*. 2017;44(3):E111−E123. https://doi.org/10.1188/17.ONF.E111-E123.

24. Smith EML, Pang H, Cirrincione C, et al. Effect of duloxetine on pain, function, and quality of life among patients with chemotherapy-induced painful peripheral neuropathy: a randomized clinical trial. *JAMA*. 2013;309(13):1359−1367. https://doi.org/10.1001/JAMA.2013.2813.

25. Maihöfner C, Diel I, Tesch H, Quandel T, Baron R. Chemotherapy-induced peripheral neuropathy (CIPN): current therapies and topical treatment option with high-concentration capsaicin. *Support Care Cancer*. 2021;29(8):4223−4238. https://doi.org/10.1007/s00520-021-06042-x.

26. Fasano M, Corte CM Della, Di LR, et al. Immunotherapy for head and neck cancer: present and future. *Crit Rev Oncol Hematol*. 2022;174:103679. https://doi.org/10.1016/j.critrevonc.2022.103679.

27. Rossi S, Gelsomino F, Rinaldi R, et al. Peripheral nervous system adverse events associated with immune checkpoint inhibitors. *J Neurol.* 2023;270(6):2975−2986. https://doi.org/10.1007/S00415-023-11625-1/TABLES/4.

28. Gu Y, Menzies AM, Long GV, Fernando SL, Herkes G. Immune mediated neuropathy following checkpoint immunotherapy. *J Clin Neurosci.* 2017;45:14−17. https://doi.org/10.1016/J.JOCN.2017.07.014.

29. Jordan B, Benesova K, Hassel JC, Wick W, Jordan K. How we identify and treat neuromuscular toxicity induced by immune checkpoint inhibitors. *ESMO Open.* 2021;6(6). https://doi.org/10.1016/j.esmoop.2021.100317.

30. Kıbıcı K, Erok B, Atca AÖ. Radiation-induced brachial plexopathy in breast cancer and the role of surgical treatment. *Indian J Neurosurg.* 2020;9(02):099−105. https://doi.org/10.1055/s-0040-1712272.

31. Gu B, Yang Z, Huang S, et al. Radiation-induced brachial plexus injury after radiotherapy for nasopharyngeal carcinoma. *Jpn J Clin Oncol.* 2014;44(8):736−742. https://doi.org/10.1093/jjco/hyu062.

32. Cai Z, Li Y, Hu Z, et al. Radiation-induced brachial plexopathy in patients with nasopharyngeal carcinoma: a retrospective study. *Oncotarget.* 2016;7(14):18887−18895. https://doi.org/10.18632/oncotarget.7748.

33. Metcalfe E, Etiz D. Early transient radiation-induced brachial plexopathy in locally advanced head and neck cancer. *Współczesna Onkol.* 2016;20(1):67−72. https://doi.org/10.5114/wo.2015.55876.

34. Luk YS, Shum JSF, Sze HCK, Chan LLK, Ng WT, Lee AWM. Predictive factors and radiological features of radiation-induced cranial nerve palsy in patients with nasopharyngeal carcinoma following radical radiotherapy. *Oral Oncol.* 2013;49(1):49−54. https://doi.org/10.1016/j.oraloncology.2012.07.011.

35. Kong L, Lu JJ, Liss AL, et al. Radiation-induced cranial nerve palsy: a cross-sectional study of nasopharyngeal cancer patients after definitive radiotherapy. *Int J Radiat Oncol Biol Phys.* 2011;79(5):1421−1427. https://doi.org/10.1016/j.ijrobp.2010.01.002.

36. Delanian S, Porcher R, Balla-Mekias S, Lefaix JL. Randomized, placebo-controlled trial of combined pentoxifylline and tocopherol for regression of superficial radiation-induced fibrosis. *J Clin Oncol.* 2003;21(13):2545−2550. https://doi.org/10.1200/JCO.2003.06.064.

37. Thomas Robbins K, Clayman G, Levine PA, et al. Neck dissection classification update: revisions proposed by the American Head and Neck society and the American Academy of Otolaryngology-Head and Neck Surgery. *Arch Otolaryngol Head Neck Surg.* 2002;128(7):751−758. https://doi.org/10.1001/archotol.128.7.751.

38. Larsen MH, Lorenzen MM, Bakholdt V, Sørensen JA. The prevalence of nerve injuries following neck dissections − a systematic review and meta-analysis. *Dan Med J.* 2020;67(8):1−15.

39. Wistermayer P, Anderson KG. *Radical Neck Dissection.* StatPearls. Published online April 30, 2023.

40. Kelley MJ, Kane TE, Leggin BG. Spinal accessory nerve palsy: associated signs and symptoms. *J Orthop Sports Phys Ther.* 2008;38(2):78−86. https://doi.org/10.2519/jospt.2008.2454.

41. AlShareef S, Newton BW. *Accessory Nerve (CN XI) Injury.* StatPearls Publishing; 2019.

42. Romero J, Gerber C. Levator scapulae and rhomboid transfer for paralysis of trapezius. The eden-lange procedure. *J Bone Joint Surg Br.* 2003;85(8):1141−1145. https://doi.org/10.1302/0301-620X.85B8.14179.

Palliative care: Improving quality of life in head and neck cancer patients

15

Suleyki Medina, MD and Michelle Issac, MD

Palliative Medicine Attending Physician, Miami Cancer Institute, Baptist Health South Florida, Miami, FL, United States

Introduction

The World Health Organization (WHO) defines palliative care as "an approach that improves the quality of life of patients and their families facing the problem associated with life-threatening illness, through the prevention and relief of suffering by means of early identification and impeccable assessment and treatment of pain and other problems, physical, psychosocial and spiritual."[1] It also defines it as "the active and total care of a person whose condition is not responsive to curative therapy." According to a joint report by the National Cancer Policy Board and the Institute of Medicine, palliative care encompasses comprehensive, interdisciplinary management that addresses patients' physical, psychological, social, spiritual, and existential needs. It is applicable to patients with serious medical illnesses requiring patient-centered care, symptom control, family involvement, and compassionate care.

Palliative care is appropriate both at the end-of-life, and earlier during disease processes amenable to curative treatments. Palliative care seeks to support patients in living actively until death, and assisting families and caregivers in coping with serious illness and death. Palliative care also aims to affirm life and regard dying as a normal process.

Palliative care can be provided by primary care physicians and oncologists (primary palliative care), or by specialized palliative medicine teams. Specialty palliative care is delivered by a team of palliative medicine trained physicians, nurses, social workers, chaplains, and professionals from other specialties. They collaborate with other medical disciplines including medical oncology, radiation oncology, surgical oncology, and physical medicine and rehabilitation to ensure optimal symptom control and relief of suffering. Palliative medicine teams deliver comprehensive care that aligns with patients' values and goals, operating across different levels of care, including inpatient, outpatient, and home care settings.

Palliative medicine clinicians specialize in effectively managing both cancer-related pain and nonpain symptoms such as chemotherapy-induced peripheral neuropathy, nausea, vomiting, diarrhea, appetite disturbances, constipation, fatigue,

Head and Neck Cancer Rehabilitation. https://doi.org/10.1016/B978-0-443-11806-7.00002-3
237
Copyright © 2025 Elsevier Inc. All rights reserved, including those for text and data mining, AI training, and similar technologies.

insomnia, and mood disorders. The team collaborates with social workers and chaplains certified to provide counseling, education, respite, and bereavement care.

Palliative care specialists facilitate open and honest communication between patients, families, and the healthcare team. They can help patients understand their prognosis, treatment options, and assist them in making informed decisions about their care. As end-of-life approaches, palliative care teams help patients and their families make decisions about enrolling in hospice, while providing support, and facilitating a transition from disease-directed therapy to one of comfort and quality of life (QOL). Finally, they carefully document patients' end-of-life preferences in the electronic medical record.

Palliative care delivered early in the course of a serious illness has several benefits. It can improve patients' symptoms, satisfaction with care, and overall QOL. Additionally, early palliative care interventions provide increased understanding for both patients and their families of what to expect as disease progresses and death approaches. It can offer timely pain and symptom relief, enhance support for families and caregivers, reduce crises such as emergency department visits and hospitalizations, improve QOL, and in some cases improve survival.

Although palliative care and hospice care share the same philosophy, they also have several distinguishing differences. Hospice is exclusively focused on palliative care, while palliative care can begin at the time of diagnosis of a life-limiting illness and can be provided alongside curative treatments. Hospice care requires a certified prognosis of less than 6 months, and patients must forgo insurance coverage for their qualifying diagnosis. In contrast, palliative care can be delivered concurrently with disease-modifying therapies. Palliative care is provided based on patient and family needs, regardless of prognosis, and is suitable at any age or stage of a life-limiting illness. Unfortunately, both palliative care and hospice care are underutilized in the United States, with a significant number of patients receiving hospice care for less than 30 days or even a week. According to the Center to Advance Palliative Care, as of 2017, only 48% of Medicare deaths are preceded by hospice care. Among enrollees, 54% receive hospice care for less than 30 days, and 28% receive hospice care for a week or less.

Palliative care has become an integral part of the care of cancer patients, including those with head and neck cancer (HNC). Integrating palliative care with oncology care for advanced HNC patients is now acknowledged as beneficial for improving their QOL. By incorporating palliative care earlier in the disease trajectory, the overall care of HNC patients can be enhanced.

Palliative care teams can address the specific challenges and unmet needs of HNC patients and their caregivers. The impact of both the disease and its treatment on patients' lives is profound, affecting their ability to speak, swallow, and breathe. These conditions also restrict oral food intake, diminish social functioning, and impact overall QOL. Patients with HNC often end up requiring feeding tubes and tracheostomies to maintain vital functions, leading to additional challenges such as psychological distress and social isolation. Compared with the general cancer population, these patients have a higher risk of experiencing depression and suicide. Specialty palliative care teams can make a significant and positive impact on these patients' lives by offering their expertise in symptom reduction.

Considering the overall prognosis and potential for rapid decline in a significant portion of HNC patients, it is crucial to incorporate palliative care from the time of diagnosis, especially for those with advanced disease. Approximately 50% of pts with squamous cell carcinoma (SCC) of the head and neck present with advanced stage disease (III or IV), and nearly 20% of HNC patients could be eligible for palliative or hospice care at the time of diagnosis.[2] Even for patients with better prognoses, it is important to recognize and address symptoms and distress to improve QOL and treatment outcomes.

Palliative care was introduced to cancer patients as early as the 1980s, yet today, many advanced cancer patients lack access to this necessary care. The WHO estimates that approximately 40 million people worldwide need palliative care services, yet a mere 14% of those in need currently receive it. Research has shown that integrating early palliative care in the cancer trajectory leads to better QOL outcomes for cancer patients with advanced disease. Palliative care addresses the comprehensive needs of patients whose condition cannot be cured. It encompasses physical, psychological, spiritual, and symptom management for both the patient and his/her family. Palliative care recognizes dying as a natural process and aims to maintain the highest possible QOL and dignity until death, neither hasting it nor postponing it. The patient should be informed that the purpose of palliative care is to alleviate suffering, ensure ongoing QOL, and enable a peaceful death when the time comes.[3]

Integrating palliative care into head and neck oncology typically involves a multidisciplinary approach, involving collaboration between oncologists, surgeons, radiation oncologists, palliative care specialists, and other healthcare professionals. The goal is to ensure that patients receive comprehensive care throughout their cancer journey, including from the time of diagnosis, during active treatment, and in the advanced stages of the disease. By integrating early palliative care, patients can benefit from improved symptom control, enhanced communication, better emotional well-being, and a higher QOL, even during the most challenging phases of their illness.

Extensive research has been conducted to understand the impact of palliative care in the care of cancer patients. It has been firmly established that early integration of palliative care into standard oncologic care leads to improvements in various aspects, including QOL, depression, anxiety, and overall satisfaction with care. Multiple studies have provided evidence supporting the important role of palliative care in the medical management of cancer patients.

The ENABLE trial, a randomized control trial, employed four weekly educational sessions in palliative care, followed by monthly telephone follow-ups. The trial demonstrated a notable enhancement in QOL for patients with advanced cancer.[4] In the ENABLE II trial, patients with advanced cancer received early subspecialty palliative care consultations along with monthly follow-up interventions. This study not only revealed improvement in overall survival but also showed a positive impact on caregiver depression scores and stress burden.[4]

In a trial conducted by Bakitas et al., involving 322 pts, including 117 advanced lung cancer pts, participants were randomly assigned to receive usual oncologic care or usual care in addition to a palliative care intervention led by an advanced practice provider. The study demonstrated improvements in both QOL and mood.[5] Similarly, Zimmerman et al. conducted a randomized control trial at a single tertiary center, involving newly diagnosed advanced cancer patients with an estimated prognosis of 6–24 months. The study compared consultation and follow-up with a palliative care team to standard of care. The results indicated an enhancement in QOL near the end-of-life and increased satisfaction with care for those who received the palliative care intervention.

The American Society of Clinical Oncology (ASCO) advices that individuals undergoing treatment for advanced cancer and their caregivers receive palliative care services. In cases where patients have minimal symptoms and access to tumor directed therapies, a referral to palliative care can be considered when symptoms worsen or when disease progresses. Other factors influencing the decision to refer patients to palliative care include a life expectancy of less than 1 year and poor performance status, indicated by an Eastern Cooperative Oncology Group (ECOG) score of 3 or higher. Patients in earlier stages of their disease can receive primary palliative care by the primary oncology team. Primary palliative care involves including specific education on palliative care during oncology training, allowing the oncology team to introduce and provide initial palliative care services. Distress screening and monitoring patient-related outcomes (PROs) can also help integrate palliative care in oncology care, bridging the gap between the two approaches.[4]

Distress screening, required by the National Comprehensive Cancer Network (NCCN) since 1997, provides an opportunity to bridge the gap between oncologic care and palliative care. The NCCN defines distress as a complex and unpleasant experience encompassing psychological, social, spiritual, and physical aspects, which can hinder effective coping with cancer, its symptoms, and treatments. Distress screening serves as a tool to identify and address these factors and their impact on patients' well-being.[4]

PROs have gained importance in clinical practice as they provide insights into a patient's physical and mental health from their own perspective, rather than relying solely on clinician reports. In a study by Basch et al., it was found that incorporating PROs into the care of advanced cancer patients at a single tertiary care center resulted in a statistically significant improvement in overall survival. Patients who received the PRO intervention not only had longer overall survival, but were also able to continue chemotherapy for extended period of time compared with control patients. The study suggested that the use of PROs may have enabled healthcare providers to identify and manage treatment-related adverse effects more effectively and in a timely manner.[4]

Head and neck cancer epidemiology

HNC ranks as the fifth most common cancer worldwide, with an estimated 550,000 to 900,000 cases and over 400,000 deaths annually.[6] In the United States, it represents 3%–5% of malignancies, with around 66,000 new cases and 15,000 deaths each year.[6] Males are more commonly affected than females, with a ratio ranging from 2:1 to 4:1. Certain regions such as the United Kingdom are expected to experience a 50% increase in HNC incidence over the next two decades, primarily due to cases linked to the human papilloma virus.[6]

African American men have a higher incidence of laryngeal cancer, with rates approximately 50% higher compared with other populations.[6] Additionally, the mortality rates for both laryngeal and oropharyngeal cancer are significantly higher in African American men, possibly due to lower prevalence of human papillomavirus (HPV) positivity in this group.[6] Globally, poverty and socioeconomic deprivation can impact survival rates, raising concerns regarding disparities in accessing healthcare services, including palliative care provision.[6]

Cigarette smoking is a major risk factor for HNC, with heavy smokers facing a 5- to 25-fold increased risk compared with nonsmokers. Not only cigarette smoking but also other tobacco exposures such as cigar and pipe smoking are also associated with an increased incidence of HNC, even in individuals who have never smoked cigarettes.[6] The use of smokeless tobacco, including chewing tobacco and snuff, is linked to an increased risk of cancer of the oral cavity and pharynx.[6] Additionally, exposure to second-hand smoke can also contribute to the development of HNC.

Alcohol consumption is a known independent risk factor for cancer in the upper aerodigestive tract.[6] The risk of developing HNC due to alcohol intake appears to be dose dependent.[6] There is also an interactive and multiplicative effect between alcohol consumption and tobacco smoking in increasing the risk of HNC.[6] In addition, mouthwashes containing alcohol have been suggested to be associated with HNC due to the carcinogenic properties of alcohol, which is a major component of these products.[6]

Biological risk factors, including viral infections such as HPV, Epstein–Barr virus, hepatitis C virus, and human immunodeficiency virus (HIV) contribute to the risk of developing HNC.[6] Generally, individuals infected with HIV have a two- to threefold higher risk of developing SCC of the head and neck. Immunodeficiency as a result of solid organ transplantation also raises the likelihood of developing cancer in the head and neck region. HPV-related HNCs have distinct clinical and prognostic implications compared with those caused tobacco and alcohol use. They are typically associated with higher cure rates and increased overall survival. Survivorship care planning and regular posttreatment follow-up are crucial components of the care for patients who have undergone curative treatment for HPV-related HNC.

Various occupational exposures and environmental toxins have been investigated for their potential connection to HNC. Formaldehyde, which has been liked to nasopharyngeal cancer and possibly cancers of the nasal cavity and paranasal sinuses, was classified as a carcinogen in 2004.[6] Exposure to Agent Orange has also been associated with SCCs of the oropharynx, nasopharynx, larynx, and thyroid.[6] Premalignant lesions in the oropharynx occur due to prolonged exposure of the aerodigestive tract to these carcinogenic agents. Generally, HNCs can arise in the oral cavity, pharynx, larynx, nasal cavity, paranasal sinuses, thyroid, and salivary glands.

Previous radiation therapy for malignant or benign conditions has been associated with an increased risk of thyroid cancer, salivary gland tumors, SCCs, and sarcomas.[6] However, there is typically a long period of time before these cancers develop (known as latency period), and the overall risk remains low.[6]

Treatment approaches for HNCs depend on tumor site and stage, as well as the functional outcomes and morbidity associated with them. Other considerations include the patient's performance status, existing health conditions, and personal preferences. Typically, a multimodal treatment approach involving surgery, medical oncology, radiation oncology, dentistry, speech pathology, nutrition, and rehabilitation therapy is utilized. For localized, early stage disease (stages I and II), surgery, or radiation therapy alone may be sufficient. However, patients with high risk features may require a combination of treatment methods. Patients with advanced stages of disease (III, IVA, and IVB) are managed with radiation and chemotherapy. Recurrent or metastatic disease is treated with palliative systemic therapy and/or best supportive therapy. Patients with disease confined to the head and neck may benefit from surgical or radiation salvage.[6]

Despite significant progress in multimodal therapy, the effectiveness of tumor control is hindered by a high incidence of recurrence. More than half of the patients are at risk for recurrence, with 30% facing the risk of distant failure. It is worth noting that nearly all recurrences occur within 3 years of the initial treatment. The 5-year survival rate for individuals with HNCs ranges from 40% to 65%, partly due to advanced stage of the disease at diagnosis and the presence of other medical conditions. Tragically, one in every five people diagnosed with HNC will die within 12 months of being diagnosed.[6] It is advisable to incorporate concurrent palliative care into the management of advanced head and neck tumors due to their poor prognosis. Increasing awareness about the appropriate timing for specialist palliative care expertise is crucial in these cases.[6]

Symptom management

Pain

Pain is the most common and distressing symptom experienced by patients with HNCs. It affects almost 70% of HNC patients and can significantly impact their QOL.[7] Up to half of HNC patients experience pain prior to starting radiation. During treatment, approximately 80% of patients experience pain, and even 6 months after treatment, about one-third of patients continue to suffer from pain.[8]

The consequences of pain include difficulty eating, leading to weight loss, especially in severe cases where dysphagia or odynophagia is present, requiring the use of a feeding tube for nutrition. Radiation therapy (RT) often causes mucositis or inflammation in the oropharyngeal area, contributing to the pain experienced by patients.[8]

Pain may arise due to various factors, such as damage from the cancer itself, infection, or scarring related to surgery or other treatments.[2] There are currently no specific diagnostic criteria for HNC-related pain, but it can be classified based on pathophysiology, tumor location, or the underlying cause.[7]

HNC-related pain can manifest in different clinical presentations, with patients experiencing nociceptive and neuropathic pain due to radiation.[7] In some cases, radiation-induced neuropathic pain can be observed, affecting as many as 31% of HNC survivors. This type of pain occurs due to peripheral or cranial nerve injury and can lead to painful cranial neuralgia, brachial plexopathy, and cervical plexopathy. Unfortunately, neuropathic pain can be severe, persistent, and resistant to treatment.[9]

The first step in assessing pain is to conduct a comprehensive pain assessment, which includes evaluating the location, timing, quality, and factors that aggravate or alleviate the pain. Pain is typically ipsilateral to the tumor site, but may occur bilaterally in up to 30% of cases.[7] Assess the timing of when the pain occurs, whether it is constant, intermittent, or specifically related to swallowing, eating, or drinking. The quality of the pain is often described as sharp, shooting, aching, burning, stabbing, and throbbing (typically more than one of these is endorsed), and it might also radiate to other areas. The pain can also be associated with sensory and motor deficits.[7] Triggers can include mechanical, tactile, and harmless stimulation. Patients can quantify the intensity of their pain using a scale such as the numeric rating scale or visual analog scale.

It is important to perform a thorough physical examination of the head and neck area to gather more information. Observe the patient for signs of discomfort, such as grimacing, facial expressions, or changes in posture. Inspect the face and neck for any visual abnormalities or areas of swelling. Palpate the head and neck to identify any areas of tenderness or swelling. Additionally, assess the patient's range of motion, muscle strength, sensory function, and conduct a cranial nerve exam.

It is essential to evaluate how the pain is affecting the patient's functional status and overall QOL. Pain can significantly impact a patient's ability to eat, swallow, speak, and sleep, leading to potential mental and psychological repercussions. Therefore, it is crucial to screen for anxiety and depression using screening tools such as the PHQ2 or PHQ9.[10]

A multidisciplinary approach involving medical oncologists, surgeons, radiation oncologists, palliative medicine physicians, rehabilitation oncologists, (cancer rehabilitation physicians), physical therapists, speech therapists and pain psychologists if available plays a key role in the management of pain in HNC patients. Medications are typically the first line of treatment. However in cases where pain is refractory to medications, interventions may be necessary to achieve better pain control. This is especially the case due to the somatic and neuropathic nature of the pain. For mild pain, initial management may involve the use of acetaminophen or nonsteroidal antiinflammatory medications. Additionally, starting gabapentin or Lyrica prophylactically can be beneficial in reducing the need for opioids.[9] These can play a role in neuropathic pain as can tricyclic antidepressants, such as amitriptyline and nortriptyline.[7]

In cases of moderate to severe pain, opioids are commonly started with short acting opioids and adding long-acting formulations when pain becomes more persistent. Due to dysphagia or odynophagia, medications are often changed to oral solution formulations to make administration of the medications more comfortable and easier to take. Transdermal patches sublingual and buccal formulations can be used when the oral route is compromised.[11] When starting opioid analgesics, it is crucial to screen patients for the risk of substance use disorder, which can be assessed using the opioid risk tool. Interventional pain management may be necessary in the setting of refractory pain despite medications. Options may include nerve blocks as well as neurolysis procedures.[7] For some individuals, acupuncture may offer relief from pain and could be considered as an alternative or complementary approach to pain management.

Xerostomia

Xerostomia, the reduction in saliva production, is the most common long-term complication of RT and depends on the radiation dose and volume of irradiated salivary tissue. Xerostomia typically begins 4 weeks into starting radiation and may take up to 18 months to improve.[11] RT directly affects the salivary glands, causing radiation-induced sialadenitis. It is defined as the subjective sensation of oral dryness. Injury to the salivary glands secondary to radiation effects is dose dependent and the amount of salivary tissue radiated.[11] Efforts have been made to decrease radiation to the salivary glands and thereby cause less side complications.[4] The decrease in saliva production leads to dysgeusia, dysphagia, difficulties with mastication and causes infections/dental caries impacting QOL in the short term and long term.[12,13] Saliva plays many important roles including digestion, lubrication, and antibacterial properties, protecting the teeth, promoting wound healing, and contributing to the taste of foods.[11,13]

To prevent permanent salivary gland damage, selected patients can undergo parotid-sparing intensity-modulated radiation therapy, reduced radiation dose to specific salivary glands, or be considered for a submandibular salivary gland surgical transfer. Patient may also receive amifostine, which is a thiophosphate medication that protects from radiation.[13]

Healthcare providers should begin assessing HNC patients by reviewing the patient's medications and ensuring they are not taking any anticholinergics. It is important to minimize the use of anticholinergics if possible as they will contribute to further xerostomia. To note, opioid analgesics are also known to cause xerostomia.[13]

Common anticholinergic medications

Amitriptyline	Famotidine	Olanzapine
Atropine	Fluoxetine	Oxybutynin
Baclofen	Haloperidol	Paroxetine
Cetirizine	Ipratropium	Quetiapine
Citalopram	Loperamide	Risperidone
Clonazepam	Loratidine	Scopolamine
Cyclobenzaprine	Meclizine	Temazepam
Diphenhydramine	Nortriptyline	Trazodone

Patients can benefit from using an oral gel, saliva substitute every 1−2 h as needed. Therapies include salivary substitutes or salivary stimulants; however, they typically provide transient relief of symptoms. Salivary substitutes (for example, sorbitol oromucosal, xylitol products) can provide antibacterial benefits; help prevent tooth demineralization, and can improve the patient's ability to swallow.[13] Hyaluronic acid products can provide antioxidant and antibacterial benefits. Pilocarpine is a muscarinic agonist that can work on the salivary glands and increase their flow rate[13]

Other strategies to alleviate xerostomia include drinking fluids, using ice chips, sugar-free popsicles, sugarless gum, and candy to stimulate saliva. Rinsing with diet ginger ale or salt and baking soda solution can help fresh the mouth, relieve mild discomfort, and help thin out thick oral secretions[11]

Additionally, patients can benefit from avoiding smoking, caffeine, and alcohol, using a humidifier, lifting the head of the bed, and consuming soft, moistened foods. Despite potential improvement, xerostomia can have a lasting negative impact on QOL. In the case of end of life, family members should moisten a patient's mouth with a wet sponge stick or with a few drops of water from a syringe. Petroleum jelly can be applied to help keep lips moist.[14]

Anorexia

Due to cancer itself or treatment, HNC patients often experience difficulty eating and a decreased appetite. Consequently, this can lead to weight loss and malnutrition. For some HNC patients, this weight loss may be indicative of cachexia anorexia syndrome, which is characterized by systemic inflammation and a weight loss of greater than 5% within a 6-month period.[15,16]

HNC patients are especially vulnerable to cachexia anorexia syndrome due to location of the cancer affecting their ability to eat and drink. Anorexia, defined as a loss of appetite or desire to eat, is a major contributing factor to decreased calorie and nutrient intake and subsequent weight loss in these patients.[16] Moreover, cancer cachexia is described as a "complex metabolic syndrome," involving underlying illness, muscle loss, and potentially the loss of fat.[15,16]

The impact of cachexia on HNC patients goes beyond the physical symptoms—significantly affecting their QOL, treatment outcomes, and leading to higher healthcare costs. Diagnostic criteria for cachexia include a weight loss greater than 5% within 6 months or a weight loss greater than 2% in a patient with a BMI less than 20. Another related condition is sarcopenia, which refers to weight loss that falls two standard deviations below the norm and does not necessarily involve overall weight loss. Sarcopenia is the loss of weight associated with loss of muscle mass and physical function (16, NEW).[11] In HNC patients, dysphagia, caused by the cancer itself, can further exacerbate the problem of unintentional weight loss, with some patients experiencing more than a 10% decrease from their baseline weight.[11]

Symptoms of cachexia in HNC patients include dysphagia, loss of appetite, and changes in taste and smell of foods. While the exact pathophysiology of cachexia remains unclear, studies have shown that cancer patients often exhibit higher levels of proinflammatory markers such as IL6 and C-reactive protein.[16] Furthermore, radiation and chemotherapy indirectly worsen cachexia by aggravating dysphagia, dysgeusia, and xerostomia, leading to reduced oral intake.

It is important to monitor weight early in the disease trajectory to screen for early cachexia. Registered dieticians should provide individualized nutritional counseling with the goal of improving weight loss.

Feeding tube placement should be reserved for high-risk patients or those with nutritional deficiencies, while still encouraging safe oral swallowing.[11] The placement of a feeding tube needs to be in line with the goals of the patient, and discussions need to be made between healthcare providers and patients/families. In those with swallowing disorders in HNC due to mucositis, feeding tubes can be very beneficial.[16] Patients with squamous cell HNC showed improved QOL and survival when fed through a percutaneous endoscopic gastrostomy (PEG) tube. "Parenteral administration of nutrition is indicated in subjects with gastrointestinal insufficiency, where intake of food and absorption of nutrients become severely compromised" as well as in the setting of palliative care.[16] A patient is considerate a candidate for a PEG tube when there is a significant nutritional deficiency and weight loss, which may be due to obstruction of the tumor or due to dysphagia or mucositis.[8]

Weight loss and dehydration are common side effects, emphasizing the need to preserve the patient's weight during radiation therapy. Consulting a dietitian for guidance on nutrition and preventing weight loss and dehydration is recommended.

Consuming small, frequent meals with calorie-dense foods, adding calories to meals, and including a variety of foods are essential. It can be beneficial to carry small amounts of foods or snacks when leaving the house, switching to a liquid diet when swallowing becomes difficult and adding spices to enhance the flavor of foods. There are varieties of supplemental drinks (dairy and nondairy) that are widely available that can be added to patients diet for added nutrition. Exploring different foods and relying on liquids and soft foods as side effects worsen may be necessary. Severe cases of malnutrition or dehydration may require hospitalization for treatment.[11]

Glucocorticoids can be beneficial in stimulating appetite as well as improving pain and nausea symptoms. However, they are reserved for patients nearing the end of life due to the risk of troublesome side effects including immunosuppression, proximal muscle weakness, fluid retention, and delirium. Megestrol acetate is a synthetic hormone that can improve appetite but has a minimal effect on weight gain. Orexigenic medications such as dronabinol, metoclopramide, and cyproheptadine may improve appetite by alleviating nausea symptoms. However, studies do not show clear evidence for their role in anorexia—cachexia.[16]

Dysgeusia

Dysgeusia defined as the alteration in change of foods can occur due to treatment-related side effects occurring in up to 70% of HNC patients. Chemoradiation is known to destroy taste cells, change, and decrease the number of taste receptors as well as nasal epithelium receptions (leading to anosmia). The tumor itself can damage the oral mucosa where taste buds are located, leading to changes in taste. Treatments can also impede nerve transmission.

Due to the finite number of taste receptors on the tongue, foods can taste different—too spicy or too bland, food may taste metallic or too bitter, salty, or sweet. An impaired sense of smell can also affect the sense of taste. This can lead to food aversion, causing even less nutritional intake and thereby lead to weight loss.[11]

A patient's taste buds can take up to 3—12 months to completely recover and the changes in taste may improve 3—4 weeks after radiation is completed. In some cases, there are patients who never fully recover their sense of taste, especially if damage to the salivary glands occurred. Dysgeusia can contribute to a patient's nutritional status and their desire to eat. Other factors that can worsen dysgeusia include changes secondary to chemotherapy, infection, mucositis, and poor oral hygiene.[11]

There are no clear treatments for dysgeusia, but there are suggestions that may ease symptoms. Patients may find that cold or frozen foods taste better than hot foods. Spices, herbs, sauces, and lemon can be added to foods to improve taste. Patients can do baking soda salt rinses prior to eating meals to help neutralize unpleasant taste of foods. The use of glass dishes and plastic utensils can alleviate a metallic taste. Food aversions can be prevented by not eating 1—2 hours prior to or 2—3 hours after chemotherapy. If eating red meat is unfavorable, the patient can opt for other protein options such as chicken, fish, eggs, peanut butter, beans, or dairy products. Zinc sulfate products can alleviate dysgeusia in some patients.[8]

Fatigue

Fatigue is a prevalent side effect of radiation, and its effects tend to accumulate over time. The body's healing process, which restores damaged healthy cells and tissues, is on overdrive during and after radiation. This can contribute to the onset of radiation-related fatigue.[11] Furthermore, elderly patients and those with a history of hypertension may experience a drop in blood pressure during and after radiation sessions, which can also lead to fatigue. This change in blood pressure may be influenced by various factors, including weight loss and dehydration. Several other contributing factors can lead to fatigue as a result of radiation, such as pain, difficulty sleeping, anemia, and mood changes.

In managing radiation-induced fatigue, certain strategies can be considered. Adjusting antihypertensive medications can help address the drop in blood pressure. Implementing energy conservation techniques, ensuring adequate rest, and addressing the aforementioned factors may help alleviate fatigue and improve the patients' QOL.[8]

Keeping a daily fatigue log can be helpful for patients to identify patterns and focus on daily activities and tasks when their energy levels are at their highest, as indicated by the log. Maintaining a consistent exercise program and sleep schedule can also contribute to managing fatigue effectively. Additionally, staying hydrated, avoiding caffeine, and making nutritious eating choices are important aspects to consider in managing fatigue. Furthermore, it is essential to rule out other common causes of fatigue, such as hypothyroidism, anemia, and depression.[11]

Carotid blowout/bleeding

Bleeding can be a life-threatening complication in HNC patients. Bleeding can range in severity from minor bloody discharge versus completely bleeding out. Only half of HNC patients who hemorrhage tend to survive. Risk factors for bleeding include history of radiation or chemotherapy, tumor being close to major blood vessels, advanced staging, advanced age, and use of anticoagulants/antiplatelets.[11]

Patient's having undergone chemotherapy and/or radiation therapy are at a higher risk of bleeding. During radiation, free radicals damage the walls of blood vessels making them more prone to rupture. Patients with a history of radiation as well as radical next dissection increase the risk of a bleeding event by eightfold. Both chemotherapy and radiation lead to myelosuppression, leading to thrombocytopenia and thereby higher bleeding risk. The tumors can also erode into blood vessels as they grow in size, which can cause fistulas and bleeding.[11]

Carotid blowout syndrome occurs when there is rupture, leading to hemorrhage from the carotid artery. The damage can be catastrophic with a mortality rate as high as 40% and morbidity rate of 60%. It is characterized as "threatened" when the carotid artery itself is exposed and "impending" when a small number of controlled bleeds have occurred. Active bleeding of the carotid artery is categorized as "acute." In the situation that carotid blowout is suspected. A history of radiation therapy is the primary risk factor, as well as radical neck dissection.[11]

Dark colored towels/bed sheets should be easily accessible to minimize visualizing blood. Suction should also the available to clean blood around the patient's mouth or tracheostomy.

It is also important to discuss goals of care and where the patient would like to receive care in the event of a major bleeding complication. A study discussed that healthcare providers should identify those patients that are at especially high risk of bleeding and provide support and reassurances to the patient's and their families.[11]

Dyspnea

Dyspnea is a subjective sensation of breathlessness. Vitals signs often do not reflect the feeling of dyspnea they may be experiencing. An ESAS (Edmonton Symptom Assessment scale) can be used to quantify the patient's symptoms on a scale of 1–10 with 10 being the most severe. Dyspnea may be worsened by oral secretions, cough, or anxiety.

Initial management of dyspnea includes positioning with having the patient sit up and having a fan or open window to increase the movement of air around the patient. In HNC patients, dyspnea can occur due to airway obstruction (see the following section). Dyspnea that is refractory in the end of life can be managed with low-dose oral opioids. If severe or acute, it can be given parenterally every 1–2 h as needed until the patient feels relief. HNC patients often have a history of smoking leading to COPD and thereby dyspnea at baseline prior to their cancer diagnosis. A study showed that long-acting opioids can be helpful in controlling refractory dyspnea in this patient population without the risk of respiratory depression.[11] Dyspnea may be worsened by oral secretions, cough, or anxiety. In these scenarios, patients can be treated with anticholinergics, antitussives, or benzodiazepines to improve dyspnea. Supplemental oxygen can often provide comfort to patients with dyspnea.

Airway obstructions/palliative tracheostomies

A small decrease in the diameter of the trachea or glottis can lead to significant symptom burden. The patient may experience difficulty swallowing and stridor, which can lead to aspiration and pneumonia over time. Glucocorticoids can help manage upper airway obstruction; however, long-term use can lead to significant side effects including immunosuppression, muscle weakness, osteoporosis, and weight gain. Nebulized epinephrine works fast to improve stridor. In the case of laryngeal tumors, surgical debulking using a laser or microdebrider can serve as a palliative treatment. This could be a temporary solution in the case of a fast-growing tumor. The advantages of surgical debulking over tracheostomy are fewer complications, faster recovery time, and improved functional status.[11]

Patients with incurable HNC are at impending risk of airway compromise. A palliative tracheostomy may be placed to protect the airway and mitigate this risk.

Palliative tracheostomies can be prophylactically placed to counteract the impending risk of airway. A 2019 study at the Mayo Clinic found that 55% of patients believed they were not given enough information about the possible complications that could occur with a palliative tracheostomy. Besides affecting a patient's appearance, tracheostomies can also have an impact on speaking, swallowing, and breathing. They require maintenance with tube changes, which can be especially challenging in older patients. It is found that close to 50% of HNC patients live alone, and these challenges could hinder them from being safely discharged home.

Although palliative tracheostomies can help prolong a patient's life, they can also have a negative impact on their QOL. Because it can affect swallowing function, the patient may not be able to eat solid foods. Patients may be self-conscious due to the change in their appearance as well as unpleasant odors that can occur at the site. These odors can be managed with metronidazole. Palliative tracheostomies are often placed emergently under local anesthesia, which can be emotionally traumatic for patients.[11]

Due to these reasons, some patients regret undergoing a palliative tracheostomy. It is important to discuss the patient's stage, prognosis, and wishes to determine if it is the appropriate course of action. These discussions need to be held prior to airway compromise. Patients often convey fears of choking and suffocating. They should be reassured that there are medications to manage these symptoms. Patients should be prescribed opioids for dyspnea and benzodiazepines for anxiety. Early palliative medicine involvement is important to help manage HNC at the end of life.[11]

Retained secretions/mucus

Large amounts of oral secretions can be difficult to manage. This is especially the case at the end of life and very worrisome for caretakers. The first step is always to reposition the patient to one side with their upper body propped up. If symptoms persist despite repositioning, anticholinergics, such as glycopyrrolate or scopolamine, can be given every 4 h.[11] Rinses with baking soda and salt water can also be beneficial to patients.

Psychological distress

Psychological distress is a major source of suffering among advanced cancer patients, leading to a decline in their QOL. Approximately 10%–20% of cancer patients experience major depression, regardless of the stage of their cancer.[17] Differentiating between distress caused by the illness and other psychiatric disorders is crucial to ensure appropriate treatments and safeguard patients' physical, psychological, social, and spiritual well-being.[18] The American Psychiatric Association acknowledges cancer as a traumatic stressor, as it can adversely affect different areas of functioning due to negative thoughts and emotions.

Depression is a distressing emotional experience for patients and their families. When coupled with a serious illness such as cancer, it can be intensified by physical symptoms, family distress, and fear of mortality.[18] It diminishes patients' capacity to experience joy and maintain meaningful connections.[19] In addition, depression is linked to reduced adherence to medical treatments, longer hospital stays, and a decline in overall QOL. Furthermore, there is growing recognition that depression can impact survival rates in various types of cancers.

Symptoms of depression have been reported in up to 58% of patients with a diagnosis of cancer. Rates of major depression range as high as 38% among these patients.[19] Various risk factors contribute to depression in cancer including advanced disease stage, poor performance status, and poor pain control. Factors such as personality traits, coping skills, pain, prognosis, substance usage or dependence, body image concerns, prior psychiatric illness, and poor social support may be related to depression in patients with HNC.[20]

Severe depression among HNC patients can also impair their ability to make decisions regarding their treatment. This can lead to decreased acceptance of additional therapies and more unplanned interruptions in treatment, ultimately jeopardizing their chances of survival.[20] Research has indicated that depressed HNC patients are at a higher risk of experiencing disease recurrence and poorer survival outcomes.[20] This underscores the crucial significance of identifying and treating depression in these individuals. Clinical depression is characterized by feelings of hopelessness, helplessness, worthlessness, and guilt.

Depression is also a significant risk factor for suicide and requests for hastened death. Individuals with HNC are particularly vulnerable due to factors such as disfigurement, anxiety, and disabling physical and psychological symptoms. The suicide rate among HNC patients is notably high, second only to that of pancreatic cancer patients. Patients with HNC have a fourfold higher risk of suicide compared with other cancer patients, with highest rates observed in those with laryngeal cancer and hypopharyngeal cancers.[21] Despite the wide availability of screening tools, depression and anxiety often go undiagnosed and undertreated in people with cancer.

Individuals diagnosed with HNC have elevated rates of depression and anxiety compared with other patients.[20] The location of the cancer and its impact on visible body parts and critical functions such as speech, eating, swallowing, and breathing contribute to this phenomenon. The physical consequences of HNC cancers often lead to social withdrawal and difficulties in emotional expression, rendering HNC patients more susceptible to depression or anxiety than individuals with other types of cancers.[20]

Anxiety commonly arises during and after HNC treatment due to several factors. These include the fear of recurrence, diminished communication abilities, dysphagia, changes in appearance, and the challenge of adapting to dysfunctions caused by the condition.[20] The COVID-19 pandemic created notable psychological effects on both cancer patients and their healthcare providers. A national survey conducted by De Joode et al. involving 5302 cancer patients highlighted the substantial impact of the pandemic on oncological care, emphasizing the necessity for psychooncological support during this time. Researchers identified various factors contributing to the increased occurrence of anxiety and depression in patients during the pandemic including limited social support, medical comorbidities, gender, age, and occupational stability.[20]

Neurovegetative symptoms used to denote depression in noncancer populations, such as change in weight, sleep disturbances, and loss of appetite, are likely to be disease or treatment-related in people diagnosed with cancer, and therefore are not good indicators of depression in this population. Instead, cognitive symptoms such as worthlessness or guilt, low self-esteem, depressed mood, and difficulty concentrating or making decisions should be monitored to detect depression in this population. Patient-reported outcome measures (PROMs) such as the Patient Health Questionnaire-9 (PHQ-9) and the Major Depression Inventory, which focus less on neurovegetative symptoms, may be more suitable for assessing depression in patients with HNC. The PHQ-9 and the Self-Rating Depression Scale are recommended for evaluating depression in the HNC setting due to their comprehensive content coverage relevant to HNC. The PHQ-9 is considered one of the most suitable PROMs for assessing anxiety and depression in the HNC population. Consulting with an experienced psychiatrist or psychologist may be beneficial in complex situations, as symptoms of severe illness and depression can overlap (i.e., fatigue, anorexia, sleep disturbance, poor concentration, social withdrawal, hopelessness).[20]

Deciding whether medical treatment for depression is necessary depends on the duration, intensity, and impact and daily functioning. Treatment should be considered when depression significantly outweighs other emotions and hinders the ability to experience enjoyment in life.

Spiritual and existential distress

Individuals facing life-limiting illnesses, including cancer, encounter a range of challenges and concerns. These concerns span various aspects of well-being, such as emotions, psychology, cognition, physical health, and spirituality.[22] The distress experienced by cancer patients can occur during any stage of their illness, including the palliative and end-of-life phase. Patients often feel isolated and may experience regret and a heightened sense of existential distress, which can even lead to thoughts of suicide. However, patients who manage to overcome these existential challenges can find solace and use the end-of-life period as an opportunity for psychological growth and to build stronger connections with their loved ones.

The literature emphasizes the importance of addressing QOL and palliative care—related topics early on, particularly during the care planning stage following the diagnosis. Among these topics, depression emerges as a significant factor affecting QOL for individuals with cancer and those in the terminal phase of illness. Depression and its symptoms are closely linked to a cancer diagnosis, with a negative impact on overall well-being, especially in patients experiencing functional decline, uncontrolled pain, and other severe symptoms. Patients with life-threatening illnesses have also expressed the importance of addressing social, emotional, and existential aspects of care alongside receiving treatments for physical symptoms such as pain. A significant percentage of patients, ranging from 86% to 91%, have expressed a need for spiritual support.[23,24] Recognizing the strong connection between symptom burden and existential distress, it becomes crucially important to meet this specific need for spiritual care. Providing spiritual care to HNC patients is an important aspect of their overall well-being, as it addresses their emotional and existential needs. Coping with a cancer diagnosis can be a profoundly challenging experience, and many patients turn to spirituality and faith for support. Some key points that need to be examined prior to offering spiritual care are as follows: respecting patients' beliefs, assessing their needs, listening to their concerns, providing reassurance, facilitating spiritual practices and connecting patients with spiritual resources, and collaborating with the healthcare team.

A qualitative study by Murray et al. revealed that patients with cancer faced increased isolation from family and friends due to the stigma associated with cancer, as well as the physical limitations that altered relationship dynamics. The study identified four specific time periods when patients experienced heightened psychological distress: at the time of diagnosis, treatment cessation, disease progression, and during the terminal stages of the disease. The spiritual needs of patients varied based on their religious background, with some finding comfort in the notion of transition. The study highlights the growing need for multidisciplinary approaches to support patients in all aspects of care, given the inevitable role of palliation in the management of HNC.

The significance of spiritual care extends to caregivers who play a vital role in providing day-to-day care and psychological support to their loved ones.[25] Caregivers of HNC patients often experience high levels of distress, fatigue, and sleep disturbances. Their own illness-related distress can also limit their ability to provide care, further exacerbating their distress. Exploring the aspects of spirituality and mindfulness in both HNC patients and their caregivers could be a potential future direction to consider in efforts to enhance their overall QOL and well-being.

Family and caregiver support/caregiver burnout

The integration of early palliative care in the management of advanced cancer patients has become more prevalent, as initially shown by Temel et al..[26] This study demonstrated that patients diagnosed with metastatic non–small-cell lung cancer who received early palliative care services experienced an enhanced QOL and reduction in symptom burden. Palliative care physicians provided support through counseling and symptom management, which complemented oncologic care. This added layer of support also ameliorated caregiver burden, potentially leading to improved well-being for patients. This improvement in caregiver burden will likely also hold true for HNC patient caregivers, as they too experience a significant amount of burnout.

Family and caregiver support play a vital role in the patient's cancer experience.[27] Several studies highlight a significant prevalence of depression, anxiety, irritability, guilt, and anger among caregivers of HNC patients.[28] Poor social functioning and spiritual distress are also prevalent and concerning in this population. Furthermore, high levels of depression and anxiety can persist in caregivers for up to 2 years after the patient's death. One study found that 30% of caregivers reported depression and 43% reported anxiety during bereavement. Studies have also found a positive correlation between caregiver distress and the physical and psychological distress experienced by patients at the end of life. Studies emphasize the importance of providing support to caregivers to potentially enhance their self-efficacy and reduce their psychological distress. Strategies to alleviate burnout in HNC caregivers entail that support from family and friends be offered to them. Allowing caregivers some respite time from caregiving functions may also ameliorate this problem. Encouraging caregivers to prioritize their self-care and well-being will likely be helpful as well. Allowing them time to engage in self-care activities such as exercise and relaxation may be of utility as well.

From a palliative care standpoint, effective communication among clinicians, patients, families, and caregivers prior to the end-of-life phase can also play a significant role in reducing caregiver distress. Conducting family meetings in this setting is particularly helpful as they promote collaboration and open communication, shared-decision making, emotional support, patient-centered care, goals of care discussions, and advance care planning.

Advance care planning

Understanding the goals of patients within the context of their cancer journey is crucial for healthcare providers to align their care with what most matters to the patients. Regular discussions about patients' goals, values, and preferences facilitate informed decision-making, patient-centered care, and early planning for end-of-life care.[29] Unfortunately, these high-quality discussions are often lacking when completing an advance directive (AD), a document that patients complete while they still have decision-making capacity to guide treatment decisions in the event they become incapacitated.[29] Different types of ADs, such as healthcare power of attorney or durable power of attorney for healthcare, allow patients to designate a surrogate or proxy decision-maker.

Various documents exist to outline patients' preferences for future medical care. These include living wills, FIVE Wishes, and Physician Orders for Life-Sustaining Treatment (POLST), which provide specific instructions regarding cardiopulmonary resuscitation and other medical interventions such as antibiotics and artificial nutrition and hydration. Out-of-hospital Do Not Resuscitate (DNR) forms are also available to prevent unwanted resuscitation attempts for terminally ill patients residing at home or in hospice facilities.[19]

Advance care planning (ACP) goes beyond completing and AD and emphasizes ongoing conversations among patients, their families, caregivers, and healthcare providers. It involves exploring goals, values, beliefs, illness understanding, treatment options, prognosis, and future plans. These conversations should be documented in the electronic medical record and integrated into routine care, and revisited throughout the disease trajectory. They are particularly important during critical transition points, such as before undergoing potentially high-risk treatments or when there are indications of limited life expectancy. Primary care physicians or oncologists who have provided extensive continuity of care to cancer patients are best suited to initiate ACP discussions. ACP discussions are associated with higher satisfaction with medical care, reduced stress, anxiety, and depression, and improved patient outcomes. In cases requiring more complex goals of care and end-of-life discussions and planning, consultation with specialty palliative care is recommended.

End-of-life

End-of-life care, as defined by the National Council of Palliative Care in the United Kingdom, aims to support patients with progressive, incurable illness in maintaining their dignity, and QOL until they die. It involves addressing the palliative care needs of both patients and their families, including pain and nonpain symptom management, as well as attending to psychological, social, and spiritual concerns.[30] In the United Kingdom, the General Medical Council (GMC) considers patients to be approaching the end-of-life when they are likely to die within the next 12 months. In contrast, the United States' Medicare system defines the need for hospice care during the past 6 months of life if the disease takes its natural course.[30]

The management of HNC remains challenging despite notable advancements in cancer treatments. A significant obstacle is that approximately 50% of patients newly diagnosed with squamous cell carcinoma (SCC) of the head and neck already have advanced disease (stages III and IV). It is estimated that up to 20% of HNC patients are eligible for palliative care or hospice at the time of diagnosis.[6] As HNC progresses to unmanageable and untreatable stages, the focus of the decision-making process should shift toward providing comfort and dignity for the patient. The roles of family, physicians, and caregivers transition from a curative or life-prolonging approach, to a comfort-based one, with the goal of enhancing QOL.

Healthcare professionals, particularly oncologists, need to prioritize the needs of HNC patients as they approach the end of their lives. Collaboration with palliative care or hospice specialists is crucial to ensure optimal care. It is important to recognize the limitations of further therapeutic interventions that may not provide additional benefits, and instead, initiate timely and appropriate supportive care.[31] In the context of chemotherapy, it has been acknowledged that administering chemotherapy when death is anticipated within 30 days is futile and should be avoided. Palliative chemotherapy at the end-of-life does not improve survival and is associated with increased complications, intensive care management, and potentially early death.[32] Studies focusing on patients with oral cancer in the end-of-life stage have shown that extensive and aggressive cancer-directed care negatively impacts the quality of remaining life and interferes with preparations for death. Additionally, lower rates of hospice utilization have been observed when chemotherapy is administered within 2 weeks of death.[32] To meet patients' needs during this crucial period and achieve the best possible outcomes, communication between patients, families, caregivers, and medical teams should be at the forefront.

Effective and compassionate communication is crucial when discussing the incurable nature of HNC with patients, their families, and caregivers. It is important to provide a realistic overview of the expected progression of the illness and the events that may transpire during the dying process.[31] Choosing the appropriate setting for hospice services is also important, as HNC patients often have a very high symptom burden and require intensive nursing care that may not be adequately provided in hospital or outpatient settings. Inpatient care in a hospice unit, where intensive nursing treatments such as tracheostomy care and percutaneous gastrostomy can be provided, is often the most appropriate choice. Palliative care teams can assist in managing symptoms such as pain, dyspnea, and delirium while providing comfort to family members. Preparing families for potential major events that can lead to death such as airway obstruction or bleeding can help reduce the shock and long-term impact on family members. It is important to discuss patients' goals and to elicit patients' wishes regarding interventions such as tracheostomy in advance, to avoid making any decisions during a time of crisis.[33] In addition, decisions regarding nutrition delivery, pain management, and other treatments should also be made in advance through an advance care plan, anticipating hospice enrollment.[32]

Excellent end-of-life care entails that healthcare professionals respect the dignity of patients and their families, and honor their wishes. It is essential that the care provided aligns with patients' choices and values and that their right to refuse treatments is also respected. As patients enter the final stages as life, clinicians should assist them and their families in finding a balance between maintaining hope and discussing end-of-life preparation. The focus should be on what can be done for patients, rather than dwelling on what is not possible. It is recommended to reframe hope for a cure, to hoping for more time; and from symptom relief, to hoping for a comfortable and dignified death. Patients should be assured that if they desire hospice care, the hospice team will approach them and their families with a caring attitude, guide them through the transition to the end of life, and help them achieve their goals for closure as life comes to an end.

As patients reach the final stages of their illness, opportunities may arise for patients to engage in reflection, life review, priorities, and goal setting. Examples of important priorities reported by patients as their lives come to an end include[34]:

1. Receiving adequate symptom management
2. Achieving spiritual peace
3. Having their affairs in order
4. Strengthening relationships with loved ones
5. Finding meaning and sense of purpose in their lives
6. Bringing closure to personal affairs
7. Reviewing beliefs, values, and hopes

Transition to hospice

Despite increased availability of hospice and palliative care services, there are still significant obstacles to delivering high quality end-of-life care to cancer patients. The primary barrier is decreased communication between patients and medical oncologists. Studies show that oncologists have limited conversations with their patients about prognosis, disease progression, managing expectations, and end-of-life preparations.[4] Research indicates that less than one-third of oncologists discuss end-of-life issues with their patients.[4] Unfortunately, studies also reveal that the absence of these discussions is linked to higher utilization of chemotherapy and intensive care unit (ICU) services in the final month of life. Additionally, advancements in medical technology and interventions aimed at prolonging life often create challenges in striking the right balance between the quantity and QOL. Failure to recognize impending death is also a challenge.

Recognizing the signs of approaching death is essential to facilitate the mobilization of services required to deliver compassionate end-of-life care in hospice. There are significant events that occur in the months leading up to death, such as increased infections, frequent hospitalizations, less time between hospital trips, and multisystem complications.[35] Patients may show decreased interest in socialization and will sleep more in the weeks preceding death.[35] They may experience symptoms such as shortness of breath, confusion, and decreased tolerance to food.[35] To ease symptom burden, additional medications and frequent dosage adjustments may be required. In the days prior to death, patients may exhibit labored breathing, fevers, restlessness, and decreased food and fluid intake.[35] In the final hours of life, physical changes may include mottled skin, increased perspirations, changes in breathing patterns, and decreased awareness.[35] Signs of imminent death include terminal secretions (death rattle), mandibular breathing, cyanosed extremities, and pulselessness.[36] In end-stage HNC, patients experience a rapid deterioration that leads to somnolence and eventually a comatose state, which can persist for several days until the patient dies. When the dying process begins, nurses attend the patients 24 h a day. The common causes of death in these cases are cardiorespiratory arrest and renal failure. Recognizing these signs and symptoms is crucial for providing appropriate timely care and support during the end-of-life phase.

Hospice utilization has increased over the past decade, with Medicare spending $10.4 billion on hospice in 2014 compared with $2.3 billion in 2000.[29] However, there is a concerning and alarming trend of shorter hospice lengths of stay (LOS) in recent years. In 2009, 28.4% of patients had hospice LOS of only 3 days, and a significant number of late hospice referrals were preceded by hospitalization.[37]

A study involving privately insured patients with HNC found that only 3.5% of patients were enrolled in hospice, and 21.3% spent minimal time in hospice before death, indicating aggressive end-of-life care and increased reliance on hospital-level of care near the end-of-life. "Schwam et al. found that only 14.6% of HNC patients with distant metastases received palliative care services."[37] These findings highlight the need to improve access to and utilization of hospice and palliative care for HNC patients.

Younger patients, especially those under 65 years of age, have shown a trend toward decreased LOS in Hospice. "O'Connor et al. demonstrated that cancer patients below the age of 65 and male patients in particular, are more likely to have hospice LOS of only 3 days."[37] This trend was also observed in patients with lung cancer, where a lower percentage of patients under 65 years enrolled in hospice compared with those who were 65 or older. Similar statistics may apply to HNC patients. Lastly, according to a UK study, the median survival time in hospice for HNC patients was only 19.5 days.[37]

Patients with HNC who enroll in hospice late tend to have higher end-of-life costs, mainly due to increased inpatient admissions and associated costs. This highlights the importance of earlier hospice enrollment to provide more high-value care. Further research is needed to explore whether earlier hospice enrollment, along with concurrent palliative care, can help reduce the need for intense EOL care and improve quality-of-life outcomes for HNC patients.

Transitioning to hospice care, or shifting from aggressive treatments to a comfort-based approach, is appropriate in several situations. This includes when a patient's cancer has advanced despite multiple treatment attempts, when further treatments are no longer desired or aligned with the patient's goals, or when a significant decline in performance status prevents the continuation of disease-directed therapies. Hospice care is also appropriate for patients who prioritize QOL over quantity of life. In these cases, hospice provides a supportive and compassionate environment that focuses on addressing symptoms and enhancing overall well-being.[37]

Inclusion criteria for hospice admission often consider prognostic indicators, with performance status being the most important factor. Patients who spend more than 50% of their time sitting or lying down typically have an estimated prognosis of 3 months or less.[38] As additional physical symptoms develop, survival time tends to decrease. An ECOG score of 2 or 3, indicating significant limitations in daily activities, and a Palliative Performance Scale (PPS) score of 70% or less, indicating a decline in functional ability, also support hospice eligibility.[38] Patients with a PPS score of 70% or lower are typically unable to carry on normal activities, have limited mobility, and may spend a significant amount of time in bed or a chair.[38] They may also show significant evidence of disease, reduced nutritional intake, and limited ability for self-care.[38] Generally, patients with metastatic disease at diagnosis or disease progression from an earlier stage to metastatic disease are eligible for hospice. Furthermore, patients who experience progressive decline despite the best available disease-directed treatments or those who refuse further disease-directed therapies also suitable for hospice.[38]

The Medicare Hospice Benefit is a government program in the United States designed to provide comprehensive end-of-life care to eligible individuals. It covers 100% of the cost of care related to the hospice eligible diagnosis. Medicaid coverage will vary by states. Patients must meet specific eligibility criteria to enroll. They must be eligible for Medicare Part A and have a prognosis of 6 months or less if their illness runs its natural course. Covered services include medical care, pain and non-pain symptom management, nursing care, medical equipment and supplies, prescription drugs related to the terminal illness, and emotional and spiritual counseling. Care is typically delivered by an interdisciplinary team that includes doctors, nurses, social workers, and chaplains. The team works together to manage physical, emotional, and spiritual needs of the patients and their family. If a patient's condition improves or stabilizes, the patients can still continue to receive services beyond 6 months as long as a doctor recertifies their eligibility. Patients can revoke hospice at any time, for instance, if they want to resume disease-directed treatments. Hospice provides bereavement support to the patient's family for up to 13 months following a patient's death. A DNR order is not required to receive hospice services, although encouraged as it aligns with a comfort-based approach.

The hospice benefit includes four levels of care[38]:

1. Routine home care—homecare provided at patients' residences
2. Continuous home care—provides home nursing care up to 24 h at the bedside when medically necessary to manage acute symptoms
3. Inpatient hospice care—provided in a free-standing inpatient unit or contract bed in a hospital or nursing facility for patients whose symptoms cannot be adequately managed at home
4. Respite care—provides up to five consecutive days for a patient in an inpatient setting to relieve caregiver stress for a short period of time

While hospice plays a significant role in providing palliative care, it is concerning that 50% of patients are referred to hospice less than 3 weeks before death, and 20% within 1 week. Efforts are being made to establish palliative care services in teaching and community hospitals, aiming to integrate these skills into the practice of oncology. This shift is necessary to move away from the late referrals and the perception that there is nothing else that can be done, which can lead to a sense of abandonment for patients. The concept of palliative care as an essential component of head and neck oncology throughout the disease trajectory should replace this notion, emphasizing its availability and importance in providing comprehensive care.[33]

Conclusion

Palliative care is a philosophy of care focused on improving the QOL for patients and families dealing with life-limiting illnesses. Its main goal is to prevent and alleviate suffering. Palliative care specialists are skilled at managing physical and psychological symptoms, building relationships with patients and caregivers, discussing difficult news, exploring treatment goals, and providing education about the illness. They work in collaboration with various healthcare professionals to ensure comprehensive care. The American Society of Medical Oncology recommends early integration of palliative care in standard oncologic treatment for patients with metastatic cancer or high symptom burden. Studies support the positive impact of early palliative care, in oncology care, leading to improved QOL, and the reduction of aggressive end-of-life care. It is crucial to continue educating medical professionals to better care for end-stage HNC patients, addressing their unique needs and challenges. Access to hospice care is essential for these patients to receive dignified and compassionate end-of-life support for themselves and their families.

References

1. www.who.int/cancer/palliative/definition/en. In.
2. Nilsen ML, Johnson JT. Potential for low-value palliative care of patients with recurrent head and neck cancer. *Lancet Oncol.* 2017;18:e284—e289.
3. Schrijvers D, Charlton R. Palliative care and end-of-life issues in elderly cancer patients with head and neck cancer. *Front Oncol.* 2022;12:769003. https://doi.org/10.3389/fonc.2022.769003.
4. Tan I, Ramchandran K. The role of palliative care in the management of patients with lung cancer. *Lung Cancer Manag.* 2020;9(4):LMT39. https://doi.org/10.2217/lmt-2020-0016.
5. King JD, Eickhoff J, Traynor A, Campbell TC. Integrated onco-palliative care associated with prolonged survival compared to standard care for patients with advanced lung cancer: a retrospective review. *J Pain Symptom Manag.* 2016;51(6):1027—1032. https://doi.org/10.1016/j.jpainsymman.2016.01.003.
6. Stenson KM. *Epidemiology and Risk Factors for Head and Neck Cancer.* UpToDate; 2023. https://www.uptodate.com/contents/epidemiology-and-risk-factors-for-head-and-neck-cancer.
7. Khawaja SN, Scrivani SJ. Head and neck cancer-related pain. *Dent Clin North Am.* January 2023;67(1):129—140. https://doi.org/10.1016/j.cden.2022.07.010.
8. Brook I. Early side effects of radiation treatment for head and neck cancer. *Cancer Radiother.* July 2021;25(5):507—513. https://doi.org/10.1016/j.canrad.2021.02.001.
9. Jiang J, Li Y, Shen Q, et al. Effect of pregabalin on radiotherapy-related neuropathic pain in patients with head and neck cancer: a randomized controlled trial. *J Clin Oncol.* January 10, 2019;37(2):135—143. https://doi.org/10.1200/JCO.18.00896.
10. Myers JN, et al. *Cancer of the Head and Neck.* Wolters Kluwer; 2017.
11. Weaver A, Smith M, Wilson S, Douglas CM, Montgomery J, Finlay F. Palliation of head and neck cancer: a review of the unique difficulties. *Int J Palliat Nurs.* July 2, 2022;28(7):333—341. https://doi.org/10.12968/ijpn.2022.28.7.333.
12. Nathan CO, Asarkar AA, Entezami P, et al. Current management of xerostomia in head and neck cancer patients. *Am J Otolaryngol.* March 28, 2023;44(4):103867. https://doi.org/10.1016/j.amjoto.2023.103867.
13. Li Y, Li X, Pang R, et al. Diagnosis, prevention, and treatment of radiotherapy-induced xerostomia: a review. *J Oncol.* August 27, 2022;2022:7802334. https://doi.org/10.1155/2022/7802334.
14. Periyakoil VS, et al. *Primer of Palliative Care.* American Academy of Hospice and Palliative Medicine; 2019:87—89.

15. Mäkitie AA, Alabi RO, Orell H, et al. Managing cachexia in head and neck cancer: a systematic scoping review. *Adv Ther.* April 2022;39(4):1502–1523. https://doi.org/10.1007/s12325-022-02074-9.

16. Muthanandam S, Muthu J. Understanding cachexia in head and neck cancer. *Asia Pac J Oncol Nurs.* August 27, 2021;8(5):527–538. https://doi.org/10.4103/apjon.apjon-2145.

17. Bruera E, Dalal S. *The MD Anderson Supportive and Palliative Care Handbook.* 5th ed. Houston, USA: UT Printing and Media Services. The University of Texas Health Science Center at; 2015.

18. Periyakoil V, Denney-Koelsch E, White P, Zhuvosky D. *Primer of Palliative Care.* 7th ed. American Academy of Hospice and Palliative Medicine; 2019.

19. Goldstein NE, Morrison RS. *Evidence-based Practice of Palliative Medicine.* Elsevier; 2013.

20. Shunmugasundaram C, Rutherford C, Butow PN, Sundaresan P, Dhillon HM. What are the optimal measures to identify anxiety and depression in people diagnosed with head and neck cancer (HCN): a systematic review. *J Patient-Rep Outcomes.* 2020;4:26. https://doi.org/10.1186/s41687-020-00189-7.

21. Liu J, Lingling Y, Qiu T, et al. Comparison of anxiety and depressive symptoms of head and neck cancer patients in a closed-loop management system before and during the 2019 coronavirus pandemic: a comparative study. *Ann Palliat Med.* 2022;11(9):2871–2879. https://doi.org/10.21037/apm-22-1013.

22. Lehto RH. The challenge of existential issues in acute care: nursing considerations for the patient with a new diagnosis of lung cancer. *Clin J Oncol Nurs.* 2012;16(1):E4–E11. https://doi.org/10.1188/12.CJON.E1-E8.

23. Sun V, Kim JY, Irish TL, et al. Palliative care and spiritual well-being in lung cancer patients and family caregivers. *Psycho Oncol.* 2016;25(12):1448–1455. https://doi.org/10.1002/pon.3987.

24. Murray SA, Kendall M, Grant E, Boyd K, Barclay S, Sheikh A. Patterns of social, psychological and spiritual decline toward the end of life in lung cancer and heart failure. *J Pain Symptom Manag.* 2007;34(4):393–402. https://doi.org/10.1016/j.jpainsymman.2006.12.009.

25. Cho D, Kim S, Durrani S, Liao Z, Milbury Z. Associations between spirituality, mindfulness, and psychological symptoms among advanced lung cancer patients and their spousal caregivers. *J Pain Symptom Manag.* 2021;61(5):898–908. https://doi.org/10.1016/j.jpainsymman.2020.10.001.

26. Kochovska S, Ferreira DH, Luckett T, Phillips JL, Currow DC. Earlier multidisciplinary palliative care intervention for people with lung cancer: a systematic review and meta-analysis. *Transl Lung Cancer Res.* 2020;4:1699–1709. https://doi.org/10.21037/tlcr.2019.12.18.

27. Lekka D, Pachi A, Zafeiropoulos G, et al. Pain and anxiety versus sense of family support in lung cancer patients. *Pain Res Treat.* 2014;2014:1–7. https://doi.org/10.1155/2014/312941.

28. Siminoff LA, Wilson-Genderson M, Baker S. Depressive symptoms in lung cancer patients and their family caregivers and the influence of the family environment. *Pscyhoon-cology.* 2010;19(12):1285–1293. https://doi.org/10.1002/pon.1696.

29. Silveira MJ. *Advance Care Planning and Advance Directives.* UpToDate; October 12, 2021. https://www.uptodate.com/contents/advance-care-planning-and-advance-directives.

30. Lim RBL. End-of-life care in patients with advanced lung cancer. *Ther Adv Respir Dis.* 2016;10(5):455−467. https://doi.org/10.1177/1753465816660925.
31. Sesterhenn AM, Folz BJ, Bieker M, Teymoortash A, Werner JA. End-of-life care for terminal head and neck cancer patients. *Cancer Nurs.* 2008;31(2).
32. Sciubba JJ. End-of-life care in the head and neck cancer patient. *Oral Dis.* 2016;22: 740−744. https://doi.org/10.1111/odi.12506.
33. Cleary JF. Integrating palliative care into head and neck oncology. *Int J Radiat Oncol Biol Phys.* 2007;69(2 Supplement):S83−S85. https://doi.org/10.1016/j.ijrobp.2007. 06.018.
34. Irwin SA, Fairman N, Hirst JM, Siegel JD, Montross-Thomas L. *Essential Practices in Hospice and Palliative Medicine: UNIPAC 2: Psychiatric, Psychological, and Spiritual Care.* 5th ed. American Academy of Hospice and Palliative Medicine; 2017.
35. Kramlinger M. Making the Most of the Time We Have Left: Caring for a Loved One at Life's End. VITAS Healthcare.
36. Morita T, Ichiki T, Tsunoda J, Inoue S, Chihara S. A prospective study on the dying process in terminally ill cancer patients. *Am J Hosp Palliat Care.* 1998;15:217−222. https:// doi.org/10.1177/104990919801500407.
37. Chen MM, Rosenthal EL, Divi V. En-of-life costs and hospice utilization in patients with head and neck cancer. *Otolaryngol Head Neck Surg.* 2019;161(3):439−441. https:// doi.org/10.1177/01945998/9846072.
38. VITAS Healthcare. (n.d.). Hospice Eligibility Guidelines for End-Stage Cancer Patients. https://www.vitas.com/for-healthcare-professionals/hospice-and-palliative-care-eligibility-guidelines/hospice-eligibility-guidelines/oncology.

Survivorship in head and neck cancer

16

Patrick Martone, DO [1], **Cristina Kline-Quiroz, DO** [2], **Krytal Lee, DO** [3] and
Marielle Araujo, MD [4]

[1]*Cancer Rehabilitation Medicine, Department of Physical Medicine and Rehabilitation, Northwell Health, Zucker School of Medicine at Hofstra University, Bay Shore, NY, United States;* [2]*Cancer Rehbilitation Medicine, Department of Physical Medicine and Rehabilitation, Vanderbilt University Medical Center, Nashville, TN, United States;* [3]*Cancer Rehabilitation Medicine, Department of Physical Medicine and Rehabilitation, Northwell Health, Zucker School of Medicine at Hofstra University, Hempstead, NY, United States;* [4]*Department of Physical Medicine and Rehabilitation, Northwell Heath, Zucker School of Medicine at Hofstra University, Hempstead, NY, United States*

Introduction

Survivorship in head and neck cancer (HNC) encompasses living with, through, and beyond cancer. It begins at the time of diagnosis and focuses on the physical, emotional, and social well-being of individuals who have been diagnosed and treated for HNC. In 2023, it is estimated there will be 66,920 new cases of HNC.[1]

Survivorship is not only about being free from the disease but also about addressing the long-term effects of cancer and its treatment. HNC survivorship brings unique challenges due to the complex nature of the disease, its impact on various functions, and the potential for significant morbidity. Some of these complications include dysphonia, dysphagia, trismus, cervical and shoulder dysfunction, neuropathy, and cancer-related fatigue. As new research and treatments emerge survivorship increases, making the need for addressing long-term effects and comorbidity care even more essential.[2]

Financial burdens, impaired quality of life, and psychosocial issues are commonly encountered by survivors. Harm effects include greater symptom burden, decreased adherence to treatment recommendations, and increased mortality risk. To manage the financial burden patients adopt coping mechanisms including treatment noncompliance, medication discontinuation, deferment of medical care, avoidance, use of savings, decrease in leisure activities, and working more. A study in 2019 showed 40% of head neck cancer patients experience high financial toxicity and 60% use savings or loans to pay for treatments.[3]

Social determinants of health, including access to healthcare, socioeconomic status, and cultural factors, can also influence survivorship outcomes. Additionally, barriers to care, such as limited resources, lack of awareness, and inadequate follow-up,

Head and Neck Cancer Rehabilitation. https://doi.org/10.1016/B978-0-443-11806-7.00018-7
Copyright © 2025 Elsevier Inc. All rights are reserved, including those for text and data mining, AI training, and similar technologies.

can hinder optimal survivorship care. To address these challenges, guidelines have been developed to support healthcare providers in delivering high-quality survivorship care to individuals affected by HNC. These guidelines encompass surveillance, screening for secondary malignancies, management of long-term effects, psychosocial support, and coordination of care to enhance the overall well-being and long-term outcomes of HNC survivors.[4,5]

A case

We will utilize a case scenario throughout this chapter to demonstrate how to approach rehabilitation and survivorship in HNC survivors.

History of present illness:

A 66-year-old female with a history of squamous cell carcinoma of the left tongue presents to the clinic 4 months posttreatment. She underwent a left glossectomy with bilateral neck dissection and free-flap reconstruction. This was followed by radiation therapy to the tongue and neck.

She is still having difficulty with swallowing and is on a modified diet, with PEG tube feeding for additional nutrition. She reports having some swelling and tightness in her neck and shoulders, worst on the left side. She has persistent tiredness since her treatment, but is sleeping well. She states sometimes she still feels sad when thinking back on her treatment and due to the way she is feeling now.

Physical examination findings:

Skin: Early signs of fibrosis in her cervical region.

Cervical: Reduced range of motion in cervical extension and rotation.

Lymph: Pitting edema noted in her submental region.

Shoulders: Reduced left shoulder abduction and flexion, left scapula winging, positive left Hawkin's sign.

Jaw: Reduced jaw ROM, measuring 25 mm.

Strength: 4+/5 throughout in extremities.

Sensation: Intact in extremities, but reduced in the left anterior cervical region with dysesthesia to light touch.

Assessment/plan:

Our patient is presenting with multiple signs and symptoms, which are a sequelae of her treatment, including the following:

Dysphagia, lymphedema, scapular winging/shoulder impingement, trismus, fatigue, cervical dystonia, neuropathic pain, and depression.

Posttreatment evaluation should screen for all of these symptoms to identify them early and provide interventions.

As the chapter continues, we will return to this case to discuss our patient's interventions.

Ongoing survivorship supportive care model

HNC survivors commonly experience long-term sequelae resulting from their cancer and its treatment.[6] These are wide ranging and commonly multifaceted including neuromuscular, musculoskeletal, visceral, and psychosocial late effects.[7] This chapter will highlight the role of rehabilitation providers in addressing these complications. The National Comprehensive Cancer Network has highlighted the important role of a multidisciplinary team for optimal treatment and follow-up.[8] Additionally the American Cancer Society (ACS) has published guidelines regarding ongoing surveillance and care.[5] These publications emphasize the need for a collaborative comprehensive interdisciplinary team to best serve and support HNC survivors.

Cancer rehabilitation should be integrated throughout oncology care[9] and is essential for HNC survivors. Rehabilitation providers partner with survivors to optimize physical, psychosocial, and vocational function through cooperative, interdisciplinary, patient-centered care.[10] Just as oncology care is a team based endeavor, cancer rehabilitation involves collaboration among rehabilitation disciplines including physiatry, physical therapy, occupational therapy, neuropsychology, and speech—language pathology. Furthermore, given the complexity of HNC survivorship, these authors also advocate for partnership and communication between the rehabilitation team and oncology care team.

The ACS guidelines recommended that HNC survivors have a physical examination every 1—3 months for the first year after treatment, every 2—6 months in the second year, every 4—8 months during years 3—5, and annually after 5 years.[5] Physiatrists have an essential role to provide a thorough physical exam to assess for potential neuromusculoskeletal long term and late effects including cervical dystonia, shoulder dysfunction, spinal accessory neuropathy, cervical and brachial plexopathies, trismus, lymphedema, and dysphagia (Table 16.1).[7] Survivors should also continue regular evaluation with an otolaryngologist for a focus exam with nasopharyngolaryngoscopy.[5]

Ongoing surveillance and screening are a key component to survivorship care. Survivors should receive education regarding common signs and symptoms of recurrence. Within 6 months of completion of treatment, survivors should obtain a posttreatment baseline imaging.[5] The optimal frequency of surveillance to provide a survival advantage remains to be defined.[11] HNC survivors are not only at risk for recurrence but also at risk for a second primary malignancy. Approximately 23% develop at least one second primary cancer with the head and neck region, esophagus, and lung at higher risk.[12] As such, it is recommended they receive screening according to the ACS Early Detection Recommendations. Additionally, based on smoking history, HNC survivors may need to be screened for lung cancer with low-dose CT.[5]

Table 16.1 Head and neck cancer symptom screening and interventions.[5]

HNC Survivors Should Be Screened For:	• Intervention:
Dysphagia	•Refer to Speech Language Pathology
Spinal Accessory Nerve Palsy	•Refer to Physical Therapy
Cervical Dystonia/Muscle Spasms	•Refer to Physical Therapy, Consider Neuropathic Pain Agent or Botulinum Toxin Injection
Trismus	•Refer to Speech Language Pathology or Physical Therapy, consider Jaw stretching device
Fatigue	•Counsel/Consider Aerobic/Supervised Exercise Program, Evaluate For Reversible Causes, Consider Stimulant Medication
Depression	•Refer to Psychology and Psychiatry for Evaluation
Lymphedema	•Refer to a Certified Lymphedema Therapist for Manual Lymphatic Drainage and Compression Garments
Neuropathy/Neuropathic Pain	•Consider Nerve Stabilizing Medication

Survivors should be screened for medical comorbidities

Potential medical comorbidities also require monitoring. Gastroesophageal reflux disease (GERD) should be identified and treated.[5] GERD can inhibit healing following radiation therapy. It is also associated with higher risk of HNC recurrence as well as developing a second primary malignancy. Treatment may include lifestyle modifications including tobacco cessation, refraining from alcohol consumption, limiting eating 3 h before sleep and sleeping on a wedge pillow. Patients may require medical management with antacids or proton pump inhibitors.[5]

Thyroid dysfunction is common among HNC survivors impacting almost 60% long-term.[13] Hypothyroidism may develop within weeks of treatment or a decade later. The median time to onset of hypothyroidism is 1.8 years.[14] Thus, HNC survivors should have thyroid-stimulating hormone levels checked every 6–12 months and when hypothyroidism is identified, treated with thyroid hormone replacement.[5]

Sleep disturbances and in particular obstructive sleep apnea frequently occur in HNC survivors.[15] This may be related to long-term swelling of the tongue and larynx following radiation as well as postsurgical changes related to reconstructive flaps.[15] Furthermore, as radiation fibrosis syndrome progresses, tissues and range of motion may become more restricted, further compromising airway positioning during sleep.

When sleep apnea is suspected, a referral to a sleep specialist and polysomnography is recommended for additional evaluation and potential treatment with continuous positive airway pressure.[5,15] Additional treatments may include nasal decongestants, nasal strips, cool-mist humidifiers, and sleeping with a more elevated head position.[5]

Dental care is crucial to help prevent and treat dental caries and gingival disease. HNC survivors are at increased risk of dental caries.[16,17] For daily care brushing with a soft toothbrush, using remineralizing toothpaste, the use of dental floss, and fluoride use are recommended. HNC survivors should follow regularly with a dental professional, ideally one specialized in the care of individuals with a history of cancer.[18] Lifestyle modifications include avoiding tobacco, alcohol, sugar-containing chewing gum or soft drinks, and acidic foods.[5]

Survivors should be screened for dysphagia, dysgeusia, xerostomia, odynophagia, and speech impairments

Dysphagia refers to difficulty swallowing and is a common symptom impacting ~45% of HNC survivors at 2 years.[19] Risk factors include oropharyngeal tumors, treatment with higher dose radiation to swallowing structures, and lymphedema[20,21] Speech—language pathologists (SLP) have a critical role in the care of dysphagia, and referral is recommended for HNC survivors with dysphagia, unexplained weight loss, or postprandial cough. A video fluoroscopic swallow study is considered first-line for evaluation and helps identify silent aspiration and strictures.[5] When strictures, a common sequela, are identified, survivors should be referred to specialist for consideration of esophageal dilation. Ideally, dysphagia is identified early with prompt referral to SLP for swallow therapy.[22,23] A metaanalysis confirmed the benefit of swallowing-based exercises to improve swallowing function and mouth opening,[24] and a randomized control trial demonstrated that oral exercises decreased aspiration.[25] Additional interventions utilized include biofeedback, posture changes, and changing food/liquid consistencies.[26–28] Additionally, potential protocols for exercise-based prevention programs are being investigated and have included effortful swallow, Mendelsohn's, Shaker, and Masako maneuvers.[29]

Dysgeusia also frequently impacts HNC survivors and their quality of life.[30] This taste alteration tends to peak around 2 months following radiation therapy.[5] Over the subsequent years, partial recovery can be anticipated. Evidence for management is sparse.[7] Investigational agents have included zinc, selenium, delta-9-tetrahydrocannabinol, taste and smell training, and "miracle fruit" (*Synsepalum dulcificum*).[31] The ACS recommends survivors meet with a registered dietician for counseling and assistance in seasoning food, avoiding unpleasant foods and exploring dietary options (Table 16.2).[5]

Xerostomia, or dry mouth, is present in up to 50% of HNC survivors treated with radiation therapy.[32] This is not only symptomatically burdensome to patients but can also deleteriously contribute to dental caries, taste alterations,

Table 16.2 Management strategies for dysguesia.[91]

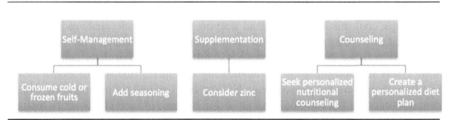

and dysphagia.[33] The ACS recommends use of alcohol-free rinses, dietary modifications, and avoiding dehydration.[5] Medications including pilocarpine and cevimeline can be considered to help enhance oral hydration and salivary flow.[5] Additional interventions investigated include acupuncture[34] and photobiomodulation.[35] Mucosal lubricants and saliva substitutes can be utilized for short-term symptomatic relief.[36]

Odynophagia occurs in nearly all by the end of treatment, but for most HNC survivors, improves over several months following treatment.[37] Mucositis, radiation, and chemotherapy may contribute to this pain.[7] Management may include topical agents including anesthetics, morphine-based mouthwashes, doxepin, sodium bicarbonate, and diphenhydramine−lidocaine−antacid mouthwash.[38−40] However, systemic medication may be required including gabapentin and for severe refractory cases opiates.[41]

Communication disorders are another common sequelae for which survivors should be referred to SLPs for voice rehabilitation and prosthesis management.[5] However, for new or progressive dysarthria or dysphonia in HNC survivors, evaluation by the oncology care team is critical to rule out recurrence or a second primary cancer.[5] Other etiologies for dysarthria include lower cranial neuropathies. Dysarthria refers to difficulty speaking due to motor components of speech, while dysphonia refers to disordered sound production at the larynx.[42] HNC survivors postlaryngectomy for laryngeal cancer have higher rates of severe impairment.[43] Early speech−language pathology evaluation and management are favored.[44] Following a laryngectomy, use of a valved voice prosthesis improved speech and quality of life.[45] For palatal defects, prosthetic obturators can improve speech.[46]

Return to case scenario:
Our patient was demonstrating deficits in swallow function.
Intervention:
She was referred to an SLP and had further evaluation with videofluoroscopic swallow evaluation.

Survivors should be screened for signs and symptoms of lymphedema

Lymphedema is the accumulation of protein-rich fluid, which can result from surgery and/or radiation therapy after HNC treatments. Lymphedema initially presents due to lymph stasis/vessel remodeling, which then can progress ultimately to fibrosis. These chronic inflammation and fibrosclerotic changes can affect function and quality of life due to their impact on range of motion restriction, contracture, and dysphagia. Studies reporting the prevalence of lymphedema in head and neck survivors vary, but more recent analysis favors a high prevalence with some demonstrating 90% of patients will be affected. Lymphedema in the HNC population can be underdiagnosed and left untreated, which has a significant impact on a survivor's quality of life because this is a condition, which is progressive, resulting in lymphedema-related fibrosis. Early intervention may mitigate some of these late-term effects, and thus, surveillance and early identification is crucial in HNC survivorship.[47]

Lymphedema in HNC survivors can affect both internal structures, such as the larynx/pharynx, and external structures, including the face and neck/shoulder region. The diagnosis of lymphedema in the HNC population can be difficult as there is no standard diagnostic criteria. Often, diagnosis is determined based upon physical examination and clinical history; however, there are tools that can be utilized to describe or measure lymphedema. Subjective symptoms, which can be elicited from patients on history, may include a sense of fullness or tightness. On physical examination, inspection for edema in the soft tissue of face, neck, and submental region should be performed. Strategies for measurement/assessment of external lymphedema in the head and neck region can include tape measurements, such as the MD Anderson approach, ultrasound evaluation, and near-infrared fluorescence. Internal lymphedema can be evaluated utilizing endoscopy and the Patterson Scale.[48]

If clinical signs and symptoms of lymphedema are identified, interventions should be performed for the management and treatment of this condition. Complete decongestive therapy should be prescribed and performed for HNC survivors presenting with lymphedema. Complete decongestive therapy involves manual lymphatic drainage, custom compression garments, exercise, and skin care. Manual lymphatic drainage is performed by a lymphedema therapist and includes soft tissue massage, stretching, and joint manipulation. Cases that are refractory to rehabilitation interventions can consider surgical management such as lymphaticovenular anastomosis (LVA). This is a microvascular surgery that produces a functional drainage pathway by identifying functional lymphatic vessels and surgically anastomosing them to venules.[49]

Return to case scenario:

Our patient was having symptoms of early edema in her submental region.

Intervention: She was diagnosed with lymphedema and educated on the cause, her risk factors, and treatment. She was referred for complete decongestive therapy with manual lymphatic drainage and was given a prescription for a compression garment.

Survivors should be screened for shoulder dysfunction

One common and significant complication that can arise from HNC and its treatment is shoulder pain and dysfunction. Shoulder dysfunction refers to a range of impairments and limitations in the shoulder joint's movement and function, leading to pain, weakness, and reduced range of motion. Shoulder dysfunction is seen in up to 70% of patients who underwent neck dissection. Most often pain and dysfunction are attributed to damage of the spinal accessory nerve (SAN) during these procedures. Other treatments such as radiation can cause damage to the SAN as well as fibrosis of the tissues surrounding the shoulder joint.[5]

The muscles of the shoulder girdle include the trapezius, levator scapulae, rhomboids, serratus anterior, pectoralis minor, and subclavius. Together these muscles control the movement and position of the scapula, allowing for proper shoulder joint function. Following neck dissection, the spinal accessory nerve is often impacted and potentially leading to SAN palsy. The SAN innervates the trapezius and sternocleidomastoid. The trapezius is responsible for scapular elevation, retraction, and superior rotation. Injury to the trapezius causes loss of muscle opposition, and patients can develop lateral scapular winging. Lateral winging refers to the prominence of the lateral border (axillary border) of the scapula away from the back.[50,51]

Muscle imbalances due to trapezius weakness, decreased shoulder stabilization, and poor shoulder joint mechanics puts patients at risk of developing impingement syndromes and rotator cuff pathologies. Overcompensation and increased stress on other muscles of the shoulder girdle (rhomboids, serratus anterior, levator scapulae, etc.) may lead to the development of myofascial pain. Muscle weakness and fibrosis can lead to decreased ROM and potential adhesive capsulitis.[5,51]

Baseline assessment of the shoulder joint should occur prior to treatment. Assessment includes range of motion with use of goniometer and strength testing. Patients with SAN palsy often have difficulty abducting the shoulder beyond 90° and weakness noted on resisted shoulder shrug. Lateral scapular winging can be more subtle than medial winging. It is best assessed on inspection from the posterior. In lateral winging, the inferior angle of the scapula is rotated laterally. Abducting the shoulder can accentuate the winging on inspection.[5,51]

Therapy interventions for shoulder dysfunction include progressive resistance training, passive and active ROM exercises, and proprioceptive neuromuscular facilitation. Exercises should include rotator cuff stretching, strengthening and scapular stabilization exercises. Current research is ongoing to identify the optimal therapy regimen. Other modalities including acupuncture and ultrasound therapy have some possible benefits. Based on clinical symptoms, rehabilitation procedures including trigger points, capsular distension, and intraarticular injections can play a role in treatment planning.[52]

Understanding the underlying causes, impact, and management strategies for shoulder dysfunction is crucial for healthcare professionals involved in the care of these patients. Providers should take a proactive approach through patient education and awareness of postoperative risks of shoulder pain. In addition, patients should be monitored for the development or worsening of symptoms. Monitoring shoulder ROM, strength, impingement signs, and scapular kinesiology will allow for earlier therapeutic intervention with the overall goal to improve quality of life.

Return to case scenario:

Our patient was demonstrating decreased shoulder range of motion. Further inspection identified impingement signs and scapular winging.

Intervention:

She was referred to physical therapy with a focus on improving shoulder range of motion and scapular stabilization exercises.

Survivors should be screened for cervical dystonia, neuropathic pain, and radiation fibrosis

HNC survivors are susceptible to long-term and chronic pain syndromes, which can emerge months to years after treatment. In one study, at a median of 6.6 years after diagnosis, 45.1% of survivors reported pain.[53] Given the prevalence of pain, which impacts quality of life, survivors should be routinely screened for such syndromes, one of which is cervical dystonia.

Cervical dystonia in HNC survivors can be a sequelae of neck dissection and radiation therapy and is characterized by painful dystonic cervical muscle spasm. The most common muscles impacted include the sternocleidomastoid, scalenes, and trapezius. Given the nature and etiology of dystonia in HNC survivors, this process can be progressive, hence signifying the need for early identification and intervention. Dystonic symptoms can include cervical rotation/flexion and shoulder elevation.[5]

In addition to dystonic symptoms, survivors may also experience neuropathic pain and fibrosis of muscles, tendons, and ligaments. As a result of treatment, damage can occur to the cervical plexus resulting in neuropathic pain in the distribution of the supraclavicular, greater auricular, transverse cervical, and/or lesser occipital nerves.[7] Radiation fibrosis syndrome is the progressive fibrotic sclerosis of tissues and the clinical symptoms associated with this process. Radiation fibrosis is typically a late complication of treatment and can occur months to years after treatment. As cervical dystonia and fibrosis progresses, fixed contracture and sustained contraction of anterior cervical muscles can occur.[54]

Rehabilitation specialists should screen for cervical dystonia, cervical neuropathic pain, and radiation fibrosis syndrome in HNC survivors. If identified, interventions including rehabilitation, medication management, and/or interventional procedures should be prescribed. Physical therapy is a mainstay of treatment. Therapeutic interventions should include techniques such as myofascial release, joint mobilization, and manual therapy. Focus on neuromuscular reeducation and postural training should be employed in addition to therapeutic exercises to improve range of motion and strength. Cervical orthotics can be prescribed, especially in cases of cervical extensor muscle weakness or "dropped-head syndrome." Medications, such as gabapentin, duloxetine, and pregabalin may be utilized to control neuropathic pain and spasm.[55] Botulinum toxin injections may also be considered in the treatment of cervical dystonia and fibrosis symptoms to reduce pain and improve cervical range of motion.[56]

Return to case scenario:

Our patient was demonstrating decreased cervical range of motion with neuropathic pain in her cervical region.

Intervention:

She was referred to physical therapy to focus on cervical range of motion, stretching, and manual therapy/myofascial release. She was also started on neuropathic pain agents to improve her sensitivity to better tolerate her therapies.

Survivors should be screened for chemotherapy-induced peripheral neuropathy

Chemotherapy-induced peripheral neuropathy (CIPN) is a complication from chemotherapy that results in damaged peripheral nerves. There are many cytotoxic drugs that can cause CIPN in HNC survivors, including platinums and taxanes.[57] The prevalence of CIPN ranges from 19% to over 85% depending on the agent, duration of treatment and cumulative dose.[58] Patients are more likely to develop CIPN if they have an underlying preexisting neuropathy prior to treatment.

Screening for neuropathies is important because CIPN affects function and quality of life including activities of daily living (ADLs) and gait. Screening and diagnosis of CIPN includes subjective and objective measurements. There are multiple scales that are used to screen for CIPN, such as the Total Neuropathy Score (TNS) and National Cancer Institute Common Terminology Criteria for Adverse Events (CTCAE) (formerly known as common toxicity criteria). The TNS includes motor symptoms, autonomic symptoms, pin sensation, vibration, strength, and tendon reflexes that are scored from 0 to 4 with 0 being normal.[59–61]

Diagnosis of CIPN is mostly clinical, and patients may have hyporeflexia, distal extremity weakness, and distal loss of vibratory sensation and proprioception. There can also be changes in their perception of temperature and pinprick sensation, in addition to autonomic symptoms. Survivors treated with platinum agents may experience coasting phenomenon with symptoms progressing up to 6 months after treatment cessation.[62] Even though CIPN is a clinical diagnosis, nerve conduction studies (NCS) can be used as an extension of our physical exam to further evaluate for concomitant conditions.[63]

Treatment of CIPN can include medications, interventions such as physical therapy, acupuncture, and modalities such as scrambler therapy. There is intermediate evidence and moderate recommendation for the use of duloxetine for CIPN. Other medication options include gabapentin, pregabalin, and amitriptyline. More recent studies show potential benefits of scrambler therapy, acupuncture, and exercise for CIPN, but further research needs to be conducted.[64] Regimens in therapy should include a combination of muscle strengthening, stretching, range of motion, balance training, and fall prevention. Therapists can also use compression gloves, heated mittens, resting wrist splints, and desensitization techniques with their patients.[65,66] Acupuncture can be trialed to decrease pain and sensory symptoms. There are minimal side effects with acupuncture, but it is recommended not to place the needle in the area of active malignancy or infection.[67] Scrambler therapy is similar to transcutaneous electrical nerve stimulation (TENS) except that it converts pain signals into nonpain signals by stimulating C-fibers with electrical impulses. Scrambler therapy and acupuncture may be utilized for patients with concern for falls secondary to side effects of oral medications.[68,69] Cognitive behavioral therapy, including self-guided interventions for pain management, is another modality, which can be utilized to manage pain symptoms associated with CIPN.[70]

Survivors should be screened for trismus

Trismus is defined as decreased jaw range of motion that can occur after radiation secondary to masseter fibrosis, damage to the soft tissues, postsurgical scarring, and/or tumor growth. There is increased risk with high radiation doses to the pterygoid and masseter muscles.[71,72] Trismus occurs most rapidly 1−9 months after treatment.[71] The prevalence of trismus after conventional radiation and intensity-modulated radiation is 25.4% and 5%, respectively. When chemotherapy and radiation are combined, the prevalence increases to 30.7%.[73]

Screening is essential since atrophy and fibrosis of muscles and soft tissues can be irreversible after treatment. Screening first involves patient education on early signs such as decreased mouth opening, difficulty chewing, pain, and/or tightness in the masseter area. Patients should be taught the finger test. If they cannot fit two to three fingers in their mouth, then they should notify their provider. A baseline maximum mouth opening should be obtained prior to treatment and monitored post-treatment. Patients are diagnosed with trismus if they have decreased maximum mouth opening around 35 mm or less. Patients can also have decreased lateral jaw excursion and jaw protrusion. Patients may have difficulty with mastication, speech, and breathing. There can be involuntary spasms, tight masseter muscles, pain, and poor dental hygiene.[74,75] Examination of the temporomandibular joint (TMJ) and cervical region should be performed. There should also be a focused neurological exam to evaluate for cranial nerve injury. If there is concern for tumor progression or other etiologies for trismus, then imaging such as CT and/or MRI can be ordered.[76]

It is also important to consider first bite syndrome (FBS) in addition to trismus for HNC patients especially if they had upper neck or parotid surgery. There is pain with the first bite in the area of their parotid gland that improves as they continue to chew. The severe pain lasts from seconds to minutes and only happens when eating and/or salivating. They will also describe the pain as cramping, spasm, stabbing, or electric shock-like.[77]

The treatment for trismus is a combination of physical therapy, jaw mobilization devices, and botulinum toxin. It is important to start treatment as early as possible because muscles and soft tissue can become atrophic and fibrotic after treatment, which can be irreversible. Physical therapy should be attempted first, and various techniques can be used, including active range of motion, manual stretching, and joint distraction. Jaw stretching devices may also be utilized to augment therapy and home stretching.[78,79] Botulinum toxin is another tool that can be used to help patients with trismus. Botulinum toxin can also ameliorate pain secondary to trismus and should be performed in conjunction with stretching to optimize potential gain in range of motion. The masseter muscle is commonly targeted. Additionally the medial pterygoid and temporalis muscles can also be targeted if appropriate.[80,81]

Return to case scenario:

Our patient was demonstrating decreased jaw range of motion, consistent with trismus.

Intervention:

She was referred to speech therapy to learn jaw range of motion exercises. She was also prescribed a jaw stretching device and educated on performing a home exercise program.

Survivors should be screened for fatigue

Cancer-related fatigue syndrome (CRFS) is defined as "an ongoing level of exhaustion disproportionate to activity output."[82] Prevalence of CRFS ranges from 50% —90% and can happen at any time including many years following treatment.[83]

Screening is essential because CRFS is often underreported and can significantly affect a patient's quality of life. Educating and counseling patients about CRFS is important because symptoms are more likely to persist and reoccur if left unmanaged.[84,85] There are many scales or questionnaires that are used for screening, but there is no universal validated protocol. At the minimum, patients should be asked their level of fatigue at routine follow-up appointments. Commonly used scales to screen for CRFS are the Bidimensional Fatigue Scale (BFS) (also known as the Chalder Fatigue Scale or the Fatigue Questionnaire) and the Functional Assessment of Cancer Therapy-Fatigue (FACT-F).[86] A focused physical examination and review of systems should be performed on patients if screening is suspicious for CRFS.[87]

CRFS is managed with physical activity, energy conservation, psychosocial interventions, and medications. There is evidence that exercise helps CRFS. Patients should be encouraged to do aerobic exercises with moderate intensity around 150 min per week. Patients can work with therapists to create exercise regimens and provide guidance on how to conserve their energy. There is also evidence for psychosocial interventions such as cognitive/behavioral therapy and psychoeducational therapy/educational therapies. In person or virtual groups, counseling and journal writing can be helpful. If CRFS is not manageable with nonpharmacologic interventions, then methylphenidate and modafinil can be considered.[87]

Return to case scenario:

Our patient was demonstrating signs of CRFS.

Intervention:

She was counseled on a home exercise program with focus on aerobic activity and low resistance strength training. She was also referred to physical therapy for a supervised exercise program.

Survivors should be screened for psychological symptoms and mood disorders

Throughout survivorship, patients are susceptible to psychosocial effects due to their disease and its treatment. Visible disfigurement from treatment and fear of recurrence can result in psychological morbidity, including depression, anxiety, and body image disturbances. Survivorship guidelines recommend screening for depression, anxiety, and body image concerns at a minimum of 3 months posttreatment and annually.[2]

75% of HNC patients experience body image disturbance. This self-perceived discontent of appearance leads to social isolation, depression, and decreased quality of life. The Body Image Scale has shown clinical validity for assessing body image changes in cancer patients; however, there is no gold standard. This highlights the importance of the psychologist in the survivorship care team.[2,88]

Suicidal ideation were reported in 16% of HNC patients within the first year. Screening tools such as the Patient Health Questionnaire (PHQ-9) and the Hospital Anxiety and Depression Scale (HADS) can be utilized to assess depressive symptoms and anxiety levels, respectively. Mental health resources are often underutilized. Given the higher risk of depression, it is integral to involve psychologists and psychiatrists. Mental health providers can be utilized prior to treatment to evaluate for preexisting risk factors of depression/anxiety. A trial showcasing use of prophylactic escitalopram demonstrated >50% risk reduction of depression in HNC patients.[2,89]

These tools help healthcare professionals identify patients who may require further evaluation or intervention such as referral to mental health specialists or support groups. Referrals to social work can help with financial burdens and other social barriers to healthcare. By implementing systematic psychological screening, healthcare providers can identify patients in need of targeted support, leading to improved psychological well-being, enhanced coping strategies, and better overall quality of life for HNC patients.

Return to case scenario:

Our patient was demonstrating symptoms of adjustment disorder and depression.

Intervention:

She was referred to psychology for cognitive behavioral therapy.

Survivors should be educated on healthy lifestyle

Health promotion and education have shown value in the general patient population and even more so in the more vulnerable patient population such as cancer survivors. As survivorship increases, patients are still susceptible to age-related conditions in addition to long-term complications of HNC. By raising awareness about risk factors, symptoms, and the importance of early detection, health promotion efforts can contribute to timely diagnosis and prompt interventions. Additionally, educating patients about the various treatment options, potential side effects, and supportive care measures empowers them to make informed decisions and actively participate in their own care. Furthermore, promoting healthy lifestyle choices, such as tobacco cessation, limiting alcohol consumption, oral hygiene, exercise, and adopting a nutritious diet, can reduce the risk of recurrence and enhance overall well-being.[2]

It's reported that 58% of HNC patients were smokers at time of diagnosis and >50% continue to smoke after diagnosis. Smoking is a risk factor for HNC recurrence and development of a secondary cancer. Overall continued smoking increases mortality; therefore, smoking cessation and abstinence is recommended. Patients should be provided with cessation resources and education on the negative impact of smoking (Table 16.3). In addition, it is recommended to screen for primary lung cancer with CT chest in HNC patients with smoking history or who continue to smoke.[2,5]

Physical activity and nutrition work hand in hand to address the long-term effects of cancer including weight loss, fatigue, and muscle mass loss. Survivorship guidelines recommend avoiding inactivity and resuming daily activities as soon as possible. Aerobic exercise is recommended for 150 min/week of moderate intensity or 75 min/week of vigorous intensity. Strength training should also be included two to three times per week. Malnutrition is common in HNC survivors making it difficult to maintain healthy weight. Malnutrition arises from loss of taste, dysphagia, and odynophagia. The ideal diet would include high vegetable, fruit and whole grain content, and minimization of sucralose and alcohol consumption. Early integration of dietician and speech pathology can assist monitoring adequate caloric intake.[5,90]

The survivorship guidelines emphasize the importance of a team approach to patient care, with recommendations for providers to be in communication with oncology, patients, and caregivers. Providers need to identify and facilitate the proper referrals to subspecialists such as dental, PM&R, psychiatry, OT/PT/SLP, and nutrition. By emphasizing the significance of regular follow-up appointments, screening tests, and adherence to prescribed treatments, health promotion and

Table 16.3 Smoking cessation strategies.[92]

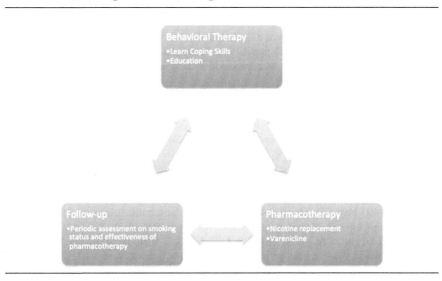

education contribute to long-term survivorship and improved quality of life for HNC patients. Together, these efforts pave the way for better patient outcomes, increased awareness in the community, and ultimately, a reduction in the burden of this challenging disease.[4,5]

References

1. Siegel RL, Miller KD, Wagle NS, Jemal A. Cancer statistics, 2023. *CA A Cancer J Clin.* 2023;73(1):17−48. https://doi.org/10.3322/caac.21763.
2. Goyal N, Day A, Epstein J, et al. HNC survivorship consensus statement from the American Head and Neck Society. *Laryngoscope Investig Otolaryngol.* 2021;7(1):70−92. https://doi.org/10.1002/lio2.702.
3. Mady LJ, Lyu L, Owoc MS, et al. Understanding financial toxicity in HNC survivors. *Oral Oncol.* August 2019;95:187−193. https://doi.org/10.1016/j.oraloncology.2019.06.023.
4. Nekhlyudov L, Lacchetti C, Davis NB, et al. HNC survivorship care guideline: American Society of Clinical Oncology Clinical practice guideline endorsement of the American Cancer Society Guideline. *J Clin Oncol.* 2017;35(14):1606−1621. https://doi.org/10.1200/JCO.2016.71.8478.
5. Cohen EE, LaMonte SJ, Erb NL, et al. American Cancer Society HNC survivorship care guideline. *CA A Cancer J Clin.* 2016;66(3):203−239. https://doi.org/10.3322/caac.21343.

6. Nori P, Kline-Quiroz C, Stubblefield MD. Cancer rehabilitation: acute and chronic issues, nerve injury, radiation sequelae, surgical and chemo-related, Part 2. *Medical Clinics.* 2020;104(2):251−262.

7. Parke SC, Langelier DM, Cheng JT, Kline-Quiroz C, Stubblefield MD. State of rehabilitation research in the HNC population: functional impact vs. impairment-focused outcomes. *Curr Oncol Rep.* 2022;24(4):517−532. https://doi.org/10.1007/s11912-022-01227-x.

8. Pfister DG, et al. Head and neck cancers, version 2.2020, NCCN clinical practice guidelines in oncology. *J Natl Compr Cancer Netw.* 2020;18(7):873−898.

9. Silver JK, Baima J, Mayer RS. Impairment-driven cancer rehabilitation: an essential component of quality care and survivorship. *CA A Cancer J Clin.* 2013;63(5):295−317. https://doi.org/10.3322/caac.21186.

10. Kline-Quiroz C, Nori P, Stubblefield MD. Cancer rehabilitation: acute and chronic issues, nerve injury, radiation sequelae, surgical and chemo-related, part 1. *Medical Clinics.* 2020;104(2):239−250.

11. Morton RP, Hay KD, Macann A. On completion of curative treatment of HNC: why follow up? *Curr Opin Otolaryngol Head Neck Surg.* 2004;12(2):142−146.

12. Morris LG, Sikora AG, Hayes RB, Patel SG, Ganly I. Anatomic sites at elevated risk of second primary cancer after an index HNC. *Cancer Causes Control.* 2011;22:671−679.

13. Miller MC, Agrawal A. Hypothyroidism in postradiation HNC patients: incidence, complications, and management. *Curr Opin Otolaryngol Head Neck Surg.* 2009;17(2):111−115.

14. Tell R, Lundell G, Nilsson B, Sjödin H, Lewin F, Lewensohn R. Long-term incidence of hypothyroidism after radiotherapy in patients with head-and-neck cancer. *Int J Radiat Oncol Biol Phys.* 2004;60(2):395−400.

15. Zhou J, Jolly S. Obstructive sleep apnea and fatigue in HNC patients. *Am J Clin Oncol.* 2015;38(4):411−414.

16. Epstein JB, Thariat J, Bensadoun R, et al. Oral complications of cancer and cancer therapy: from cancer treatment to survivorship. *CA A Cancer J Clin.* 2012;62(6):400−422.

17. Kumar S, Ram S, Navazesh M. Salivary gland and associated complications in HNC therapy. *J Calif Dent Assoc.* 2011;39(9):639−647.

18. Epstein JB, Güneri P, Barasch A. Appropriate and necessary oral care for people with cancer: guidance to obtain the right oral and dental care at the right time. *Support Care Cancer.* 2014;22:1981−1988.

19. Hutcheson KA, Nurgalieva Z, Zhao H, et al. Two-year prevalence of dysphagia and related outcomes in HNC survivors: an updated SEER-Medicare analysis. *Head Neck.* 2019;41(2):479−487.

20. Pezdirec M, Strojan P, Boltezar IH. Swallowing disorders after treatment for HNC. *Radiol Oncol.* 2019;53(2):225.

21. Jeans C, Ward EC, Brown B, et al. Association between external and internal lymphedema and chronic dysphagia following HNC treatment. *Head Neck.* 2021;43(1):255−267.

22. Murphy BA, Gilbert J. In: *Dysphagia in HNC Patients Treated with Radiation: Assessment, Sequelae, and Rehabilitation.* Vol 19. Elsevier; 2009:35−42.

23. Cousins N, MacAulay F, Lang H, MacGillivray S, Wells M. A systematic review of interventions for eating and drinking problems following treatment for HNC suggests a need to look beyond swallowing and trismus. *Dysphagia.* 2014;29(2):290.

24. Banda KJ, Chu H, Kao CC, et al. Swallowing exercises for HNC patients: a systematic review and meta-analysis of randomized control trials. *Int J Nurs Stud.* 2021;114:103827.

25. Hsiang CC, Chen AWG, Chen CH, Chen MK. Early postoperative oral exercise improves swallowing function among patients with oral cavity cancer: a randomized controlled trial. *Ear Nose Throat J.* 2019;98(6):E73−E80.

26. Benfield JK, Everton LF, Bath PM, England TJ. Does therapy with biofeedback improve swallowing in adults with dysphagia? A systematic review and meta-analysis. *Arch Phys Med Rehabil.* 2019;100(3):551−561.

27. Alghadir AH, Zafar H, Al-Eisa ES, Iqbal ZA. Effect of posture on swallowing. *Afr Health Sci.* 2017;17(1):133−137.

28. Steele CM, Alsanei WA, Ayanikalath S, et al. The influence of food texture and liquid consistency modification on swallowing physiology and function: a systematic review. *Dysphagia.* 2015;30:2−26.

29. Loewen I, Jeffery CC, Rieger J, Constantinescu G. Prehabilitation in HNC patients: a literature review. *J Otolaryngol Head Neck Surg.* 2021;50(1):1−11.

30. Baharvand M, ShoalehSaadi N, Barakian R, Jalali Moghaddam E. Taste alteration and impact on quality of life after head and neck radiotherapy. *J Oral Pathol Med.* 2013; 42(1):106−112. https://doi.org/10.1111/j.1600-0714.2012.01200.x.

31. Sevryugin O, Kasvis P, Vigano M, Vigano A. Taste and smell disturbances in cancer patients: a scoping review of available treatments. *Support Care Cancer.* 2021;29(1): 49−66. https://doi.org/10.1007/s00520-020-05609-4.

32. Chiu YH, Tseng WH, Ko JY, Wang TG. Radiation-induced swallowing dysfunction in patients with HNC: a literature review. *J Formos Med Assoc.* 2022;121(Part 1):3−13. https://doi.org/10.1016/j.jfma.2021.06.020.

33. Pinna R, Campus G, Cumbo E, Mura I, Milia E. Xerostomia induced by radiotherapy: an overview of the physiopathology, clinical evidence, and management of the oral damage. *TCRM.* 2015;171. https://doi.org/10.2147/TCRM.S70652.

34. Bonomo P, Stocchi G, Caini S, et al. Acupuncture for radiation-induced toxicity in head and neck squamous cell carcinoma: a systematic review based on PICO criteria. *Eur Arch Oto-Rhino-Laryngol.* 2022;279(4):2083−2097. https://doi.org/10.1007/s00405-021-07002-1.

35. Louzeiro GC, Teixeira D da S, Cherubini K, de Figueiredo MAZ, Salum FG. Does laser photobiomodulation prevent hyposalivation in patients undergoing head and neck radiotherapy? A systematic review and meta-analysis of controlled trials. *Crit Rev Oncol Hematol.* 2020;156:103115. https://doi.org/10.1016/j.critrevonc.2020.103115.

36. Jensen SB, Vissink A, Limesand KH, Reyland ME. Salivary gland hypofunction and xerostomia in head and neck radiation patients. *JNCI Monographs.* 2019;2019(53): lgz016. https://doi.org/10.1093/jncimonographs/lgz016.

37. Barnhart MK, Robinson RA, Simms VA, et al. Treatment toxicities and their impact on oral intake following non-surgical management for HNC: a 3-year longitudinal study. *Support Care Cancer.* 2018;26(7):2341−2351. https://doi.org/10.1007/s00520-018-4076-6.

38. Mirabile A, Airoldi M, Ripamonti C, et al. Pain management in HNC patients undergoing chemo-radiotherapy: clinical practical recommendations. *Crit Rev Oncol Hematol.* 2016;99:100−106. https://doi.org/10.1016/j.critrevonc.2015.11.010.

39. Judge LF, Farrugia MK, Singh AK. Narrative review of the management of oral mucositis during chemoradiation for HNC. *Ann Transl Med.* 2021;9(10):916. https://doi.org/10.21037/atm-20-3931.

40. Saunders DP, Epstein JB, Elad S, et al. Systematic review of antimicrobials, mucosal coating agents, anesthetics, and analgesics for the management of oral mucositis in

cancer patients. *Support Care Cancer*. 2013;21(11):3191−3207. https://doi.org/10.1007/s00520-013-1871-y.

41. Bar AV, Weinstein G, Dutta PR, et al. Gabapentin for the treatment of pain syndrome related to radiation-induced mucositis in patients with HNC treated with concurrent chemoradiotherapy. *Cancer*. 2010;116(17):4206−4213. https://doi.org/10.1002/cncr.25274.

42. Cohen S, Elackattu A, Noordzij J, Walsh M, Langmore S. Palliative treatment of dysphonia and dysarthria. *Otolaryngol Clin*. 2009;42:107−121. https://doi.org/10.1016/j.otc.2008.09.010.

43. Arenaz Búa B, Pendleton H, Westin U, Rydell R. Voice and swallowing after total laryngectomy. *Acta Otolaryngol*. 2018;138(2):170−174. https://doi.org/10.1080/00016489.2017.1384056.

44. Tuomi L, Andréll P, Finizia C. Effects of voice rehabilitation after radiation therapy for laryngeal cancer: a randomized controlled study. *Int J Radiat Oncol Biol Phys*. 2014;89(5):964−972. https://doi.org/10.1016/j.ijrobp.2014.04.030.

45. Xi S. Effectiveness of voice rehabilitation on vocalisation in postlaryngectomy patients: a systematic review. *Int J Evid Base Healthc*. 2010;8(4):256−258. https://doi.org/10.1111/j.1744-1609.2010.00177.x.

46. Marunick M, Tselios N. The efficacy of palatal augmentation prostheses for speech and swallowing in patients undergoing glossectomy: a review of the literature. *J Prosthet Dent*. 2004;91(1):67−74. https://doi.org/10.1016/j.prosdent.2003.10.012.

47. Stubblefield MD, Derek W. Under recognition and treatment of lymphedema in HNC survivors—a database study. *Support Care Cancer*. 2023;31(4):229.

48. Starmer H, et al. Assessment of measures of head and neck lymphedema following HNC treatment: a systematic review. *Lymphatic Res Biol*. 2023;21(1):42−51.

49. Tyker A, et al. Treatment for lymphedema following HNC therapy: a systematic review. *Am J Otolaryngol*. 2019;40(5):761−769.

50. Chen YH, Huang CY, Liang WA, Lin CR, Chao YH. Effects of conscious control of scapular orientation in oral cancer survivors with scapular dyskinesis: a randomized controlled trial. *Integr Cancer Ther*. 2021;20. https://doi.org/10.1177/15347354211040827.

51. Didesch JT, Tang P. Anatomy, etiology, and management of scapular winging. *J Hand Surg Am*. 2019;44(4):321−330. https://doi.org/10.1016/j.jhsa.2018.08.008.

52. Almeida KAM, Rocha AP, Carvas N, Pinto ACPN. Rehabilitation interventions for shoulder dysfunction in patients with HNC: systematic review and meta-analysis. *Phys Ther*. October 30, 2020;100(11):1997−2008. https://doi.org/10.1093/ptj/pzaa147.

53. Cramer JD, Johnson JT, Nilsen ML. Pain in HNC survivors: prevalence, predictors, and quality-of-life impact. *Otolaryngology-Head Neck Surg (Tokyo)*. 2018;159(5):853−858.

54. Stubblefield MD. Radiation fibrosis syndrome: neuromuscular and musculoskeletal complications in cancer survivors. *PM&R*. 2011;3(11):1041−1054.

55. Stubblefield MD. Clinical evaluation and management of radiation fibrosis syndrome. *Phys Med Rehabil Clin*. 2017;28(1):89−100.

56. Bach C-A, et al. Botulinum toxin in the treatment of post-radiosurgical neck contracture in HNC: a novel approach. *Eur Annals Otorhinolaryngol Head Neck Dis*. 2012;129:6−10.

57. HNCs: evidence-based treatment. In: Argiris A, Ferris RL, Rosenthal DI, eds. *Demos Medical*. New York: Springer Publishing; 2018.

58. Zajączkowska R, Kocot-Kepska M, Leppert W, Wrzosek A, Mika J, Wordliczek J. Mechanisms of chemotherapy-induced peripheral neuropathy. *Int J Mol Sci.* 2019; 20(6).

59. Cavaletti G, Frigeni B, Lanzani F, et al. The total neuropathy score as an assessment tool for grading the course of chemotherapy-induced peripheral neurotoxicity: comparison with the national cancer institute-common toxicity scale. *J Peripher Nerv Syst.* 2007; 12(3):210–215.

60. Binda D, Cavaletti G, Cornblath DR, Merkies IS, CI-PeriNomS study group. Rasch-Transformed Total Neuropathy Score clinical version (RT-TNSc(©)) in patients with chemotherapy-induced peripheral neuropathy. *J Peripher Nerv Syst.* September 2015; 20(3):328–332.

61. Miller TP, Fisher BT, Getz KD, et al. Unintended consequences of evolution of the common terminology criteria for adverse events. *Pediatr Blood Cancer.* 2019;66(7).

62. Albany C, Dockter T, Wolfe E, et al. Cisplatin-associated neuropathy characteristics compared with those associated with other neurotoxic chemotherapy agents (Alliance A151724). *Support Care Cancer.* February 2021;29(2):833–840.

63. Desforges AD, Hebert CM, Spence AL, et al. Treatment and diagnosis of chemotherapy-induced peripheral neuropathy: an update. *Biomed Pharmacother.* 2022;147:112671.

64. Loprinzi CL, Lacchetti C, Bleeker J, et al. Prevention and management of chemotherapy-induced peripheral neuropathy in survivors of adult cancers: ASCO guideline update. *J Clin Oncol.* October 1, 2020;38(28):3325–3348.

65. Wen-Li L, Wang R-H, Fan-Hao C, I-Jung F, Ching-Ju F. The effects of exercise on chemotherapy-induced peripheral neuropathy symptoms in cancer patients: a systematic review and meta-analysis. *Support Care Cancer.* 2021;29(9):5303–5311.

66. Andersen Hammond E, Pitz M, Steinfeld K, Lambert P, Shay B. An exploratory randomized trial of physical therapy for the treatment of chemotherapy-induced peripheral neuropathy. *Neurorehabil Neural Repair.* 2020;34(3):235–246.

67. Fink J, Burns J, Perez Moreno AC, et al. A quality brief of an oncological multisite massage and acupuncture therapy program to improve cancer-related outcomes. *J Altern Complement Med.* 2020;26(9):820–824.

68. Childs DS, Le-Rademacher JG, McMurray R, et al. Randomized trial of scrambler therapy for chemotherapy-induced peripheral neuropathy: crossover analysis. *J Pain Symptom Manag.* 2021;61(6):1247.

69. Ahuja D, Bharati SJ, Gupta N, Kumar V, Bhatnagar S. Scrambler therapy: a ray of hope for refractory chemotherapy-induced peripheral neuropathy. *Indian J Cancer.* 2020; 57(1):93–97.

70. Jones KF, et al. Pharmacological and nonpharmacological management of chemotherapy-induced peripheral neuropathy: a scoping review of randomized controlled trials. *J Palliat Med.* 2022;25(6):964–995.

71. Wang CJ, Huang EY, Hsu HC, Chen HC, Fang FM, Hsiung CY. The degree and time-course assessment of radiation-induced trismus occurring after radiotherapy for nasopharyngeal cancer. *Laryngoscope.* 2005;115(8):1458–1460.

72. Karlsson O, Karlsson T, Pauli N, Andréll P, Finizia C. Jaw exercise therapy for the treatment of trismus in HNC: a prospective three-year follow-up study. *Support Care Cancer.* July 2021;29(7):3793–3800.

73. Bensadoun RJ, Riesenbeck D, Lockhart PB, et al. A systematic review of trismus induced by cancer therapies in HNC patients. *Support Care Cancer.* 2010;18:1033–1038.

74. Weber C, Dommerich S, Pau HW, et al. Limited mouth opening after primary therapy of HNC. *Oral Maxillofac Surg*. 2010;14:169–173.

75. O'Leary MR, Trismus M. Modern pathophysiological correlates. *Am J Emerg Med*. 1990;8:220–227 Issue.

76. van der Geer SJ, van Rijn PV, Kamstra JI, et al. Criterion for trismus in HNC patients: a verification study. *Support Care Cancer*. 2019;27:1129–1137.

77. Steel SJ, Robertson CE. First bite syndrome: what neurologists need to know. *Curr Pain Headache Rep*. 2021;25(5).

78. Dijkstra PU, Sterken MW, Pater R, Spijkervet FKL, Roodenburg JLN. Exercise therapy for trismus in HNC. *Oral Oncol*. 2007;43(4):389–394.

79. Buchbinder D, Currivan RB, Kaplan AJ, Urken ML. Mobilization regimens for the prevention of jaw hypomobility in the radiated patient: a comparison of three techniques. *J Oral Maxillofac Surg*. 1993;51(8):863–867.

80. Hartl DM, Cohen M, Juliéron M, Marandas P, Janot F, Bourhis J. Botulinum toxin for radiation-induced facial pain and trismus. *Otolaryngology-Head Neck Surg (Tokyo)*. 2008;138(4):459–463.

81. Stubblefield MD, Levine A, Custodio CM, Fitzpatrick T. The role of botulinum toxin type a in the radiation fibrosis syndrome: a preliminary report. *Arch Phys Med Rehabil*. 2008;89(3):417–421.

82. Dolgoy ND, O'Krafka P, McNeely ML. Cancer-related fatigue in head and neck cancer survivors: energy and functional impacts. *Cancer Treat Res Commun*. 2020;25:100244.

83. Fauci AS, Hauser SL, Jameson JL, Kasper DL, Longo DL, Loscalzo J. *Harrison's Principles of Internal Medicine*. 19th ed. New York, NY: Mcgraw-Hill's AccessMedicine; McGraw-Hill Education LLC; 2015.

84. Malik S, Sadaf A. Impact of cancer-related fatigue on psychological semiology among cancer patients. *Pak J Med Res*. 2018;57(1):20–23.

85. Weis J, Horneber M. *Cancer-Related Fatigue*. Heidelberg: Springer Healthcare; 2014.

86. Alexander S, Minton O, Stone PC. Evaluation of screening instruments for cancer-related fatigue syndrome in breast cancer survivors. *J Clin Oncol*. 2009;27(8): 1197–1201.

87. Berger AM, Mooney K, Alvarez-Perez A, et al. National comprehensive cancer network. Cancer-Related Fatigue. *J Natl Compr Cancer Netw*. August 2015;13(8):1012–1039.

88. Hopwood P, Fletcher I, Lee A, Al Ghazal S. A body image scale for use with cancer patients. *Eur J Cancer*. January 2001;37(2):189–197. https://doi.org/10.1016/s0959-8049(00)00353-1.

89. Lydiatt WM, Bessette D, Schmid KK, Sayles H, Burke WJ. Prevention of depression with escitalopram in patients undergoing treatment for HNC: randomized, double-blind, placebo-controlled clinical trial. *JAMA Otolaryngol Head Neck Surg*. July 2013; 139(7):678–686. https://doi.org/10.1001/jamaoto.2013.3371.

90. Bye A, Sandmael JA, Stene GB, et al. Exercise and nutrition interventions in patients with HNC during curative treatment: a systematic review and meta-analysis. *Nutrients*. October 22, 2020;12(11):3233. https://doi.org/10.3390/nu12113233.

91. Togni L, et al. Treatment-related dysgeusia in oral and oropharyngeal cancer: a comprehensive review. *Nutrients*. 2021;13(10):3325.

92. Shields PG, et al. Smoking cessation, version 3.2022, NCCN clinical practice guidelines in oncology. *J Natl Compr Cancer Netw*. 2023;21(3):297–322.

Psychosocial considerations in head and neck cancer

17

Eileen H. Shinn, PhD [1] **and Deepti A. Chopra, MD** [2]

[1]*Department of Behavioral Science, University of Texas MD Anderson Cancer Center, Houston, TX, United States;* [2]*Department of Psychiatry, University of Texas MD Anderson Cancer Center, Houston, TX, United States*

Introduction

Head and neck cancer refers to a diverse group of cancers that together account for less than 4% of all incident cancer types in the United States.[1] In 2023, over 66,000 new cases of head and neck cancer were diagnosed. Head and neck cancer affects up to twice as many men as women.[2] The median overall age for non—HPV-associated head and neck squamous cancer ranges from 63 to 66 years[2] whereas the median age of HPV-associated head and neck cancer is 53 years.[3] The increasing incidence of HPV-associated head and neck cancer has been well documented, with the global rate expected to increase to 1.08 million new cases annually by 2030.[4,5]

Head and neck cancer types are categorized by anatomical location, the most common incidence occurring in the pharyngeal/laryngeal region. Other types include lip and oral cavity, paranasal sinus and nasal cavity, salivary gland, and thyroid cancer. Depending on the site and extent of disease spread, treatment can result in specific functional and appearance changes, which affect long-term quality of life (QOL) in survivors. This chapter focuses on the psychosocial considerations unique to certain cancers in the head and neck region, especially those affecting long-term swallowing functions and facial appearance. While survivors' structural and functional changes are highly specific to disease site, effective treatment of resulting psychological distress and coping deficits generally employs principles of psychosocial assessment and treatment that are often used in non-cancer populations. The psychosocial challenges specific to certain head and neck cancer types will be discussed first, followed by a description of validated methods of assessment and evidence-based treatment in patients with head and neck cancer.

Copyright © 2025 Elsevier Inc. All rights reserved, including those for text and data mining, AI training, and similar technologies.

Overview of psychosocial concerns in head and neck cancer patients and survivors

Quality of life

Quality of life has been studied extensively in the head and neck cancer population. People with this cancer report having very poor QOL during[6–8] and long after treatment.[9,10] In an oft-cited comparison of distress levels among 4996 patients newly diagnosed with cancer of 14 separate anatomical sites, patients with head and neck cancer were among those with the highest average levels of distress, similar to those with lung, pancreatic, liver and brain cancer.[11] When measured 1 year posttreatment, marital and sexual functioning QoL domain scores were significantly more impaired than those found with lung, colon, or breast cancer survivors who were at least 1-year posttreatment.[12] For some survivors, surgery and radiation at the tumor site may result in loss or impairment of critical functions such as breathing, swallowing, and talking. More commonplace experiences include severe dry mouth and severe, prolonged pain.[6,13] Despite advances in radiation and surgical techniques, data continue to show that compared with patients with other cancers, long-term swallowing dysfunction and dry mouth were worse for those with head and neck cancer.[14]

QOL during treatment for pharyngeal/laryngeal cancer. Because the majority of all oropharyngeal cancer patients are diagnosed at an advanced stage, high-dose radiation treatment is nearly always a primary component of treatment. For oropharynx cancer, the radiation field encompasses the salivary parotid glands and key swallowing structures including the base of tongue, pharyngeal constrictors, and strap muscles.[15] Radiation results in painful and disabling complications ranging from trismus,[16] aspiration,[17,18] mucositis,[19] xerostomia,[20] loss of taste, and fibrosis of the skin and soft tissue (see Figs. 17.1 and 17.2).[13] Limiting total radiation dose under 30 Gy (1 Gy = 1 J per kilogram) prevents permanent xerostomia

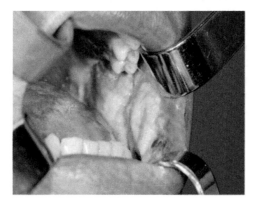

FIGURE 17.1

Mucositis.

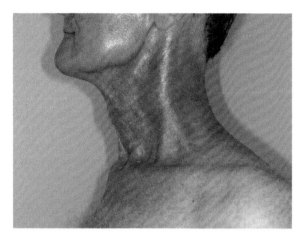

FIGURE 17.2

Radiation sunburn.

Photos courtesy of William Morrison, MD.

and dysphagia,[21,22] but most oropharynx and larynx cancer patients receive much higher total doses, between 69 and 72 Gy due to advanced stage of disease. In addition, concurrent cisplatin chemotherapy is standard, further increasing the risk for long-term dysphagia and trismus.[23]

Accordingly, the symptom burden during radiation is considerable: patients report very poor QOL, with scores equivalent to the bottom 18th percentile within the range of normal functioning.[24,25] Compared with other patients with other pharyngeal/laryngeal cancers, patients with oropharyngeal cancer report either slightly worse or similar QOL and significantly higher depressive symptomatology.[26,27] In a study assessing 40 consecutive patients with head and neck cancer outpatients, pain was experienced by 100% of the sample, and severe pain being experienced by approximately half of the sample.[13]

Swallowing function in pharyngeal/laryngeal cancer. While overall 5-year survival is relatively high across all stages, 68%,[2] up to 45% of all throat cancer survivors experience permanent sequelae, including trismus (inability to open the mouth widely)[2] and dysphagia (inability to eat normally due to scarring of swallowing muscles).[28] The severity of dysphagia ranges from not being able to swallow foods without liquid assist, to being completely dependent on percutaneous gastrostomy (PEG) tube feeding.[29–35] While typically underappreciated at the time of cancer diagnosis and treatment, dysphagia is devastating to QOL and is the key driver of decisional regret in long-term survivors.[17,36,37] In a study comparing tongue swallow and strength in oropharyngeal and oral cancer patients with age- and sex-matched controls, many of the patients had significantly impaired swallowing 2 months posttreatment. For example, the majority of the cancer patients refused to try swallowing a bolus of peanut butter, and rates of aspiration were very high among those who did attempt the swallow.[38]

In studies with long-term head and neck cancer survivors, QOL remains compromised in several domains. Three years after treatment, a mixed sample of 317 head and neck cancer patients experienced significantly worse swallowing, pain, and dry mouth 3 years after treatment, compared with norms taken from a sample of general population sample of 871 age- and sex-matched people.[39] In a study of 36 oropharyngeal patients 5 years after treatment, 100% of the sample still experienced xerostomia (severe dry mouth), 76% experienced swallowing difficulty, 48% experienced decreased energy, and 43% significant pain.[26] The two symptoms causing the most distress were also the most prevalent, xerostomia and difficulty swallowing, both of which interfere drastically with the ability to eat normally.[32] Pourel et al. followed 119 long-term oropharyngeal cancer survivors for 3 years after treatment. They reported improvements in overall physical functioning and health-related QOL, but emotional and social functioning remained profoundly impaired. After controlling for stage of disease, type of treatment, and sociodemographic factors, the sample's emotional functioning was more than 20 points lower on the European Organization for Research and Treatment of Cancer Quality of Life Questionnaire-H&N35 (EORTC-H&N) compared with general population norms, and residual symptoms such as dry mouth and inability to eat socially were more than 30 points lower.[9]

Social support mediating impact on QoL. A number of studies have shown that social support has a generally protective effect on the development of depression in cancer patients during treatment.[40] Closer examinations of the role of social support on subsequent depression in head and neck cancer patients have uncovered mixed findings. While living alone has been found to be predictive of the development of depression in HNC patients on treatment, other studies found no effect.[41–43] Other prospective studies found that the greater the number of sources of available support, the less depressed HNC patients became during treatment, and during the posttreatment period.[44] Other correlational studies have found that the impact of global and received social support is mediated by the number of physical complaints and by high levels of pain.[27,40] Qualitative interviews may be more helpful in delineating the impact of treatment on subsequent relationships and quality of social interactions: These studies show that treatment itself profoundly affects some survivors' social lives. Analysis of interview data with long-term cancer survivors revealed themes of refusing to eat in public places or with friends, due to heightened self-consciousness about eating.[45] Patients also reported a loss of confidence and greater dependence on their spouses, who tended to act as translators for those who could no longer understand the patients' speech.

While social support plays an important role in ameliorating depression, head and neck cancer patients may not receive the type of social support they need, especially if they become depressed during treatment. Clinical depression is often poorly understood by the lay public as a condition that can be overcome by sheer force of will. Without education on the nature of depressive illness, spouses and caregivers may not be emotionally inclined to lend support to their depressed counterparts. Even well-meaning partners and caregivers may lack the basic knowledge of what is helpful versus enabling behavior. Finally, living with and caring for a clinically depressed person is challenging and distressing, to such a degree that spouses or caregivers would benefit from counseling focused on their own distress and sense of burden.[46,47]

Suicidality and depression

Suicidality. Studies have consistently shown that head and neck cancer survivors in the United States are more likely to be suicidal than survivors of other types of cancer, with a recent SEER analysis showing that HNC survivors were twice as likely to commit suicide as other survivors, and 3.6 times more likely than adults unaffected by cancer.[48] The reasons for this elevated risk are multifactorial, including the persistence of elevated symptom burden and development of late effects after chemoradiation, higher male-to-female ratio of completed suicides in the general population, and premorbid risks such as substance abuse disorder.

Depression in pharyngeal/laryngeal cancer. Depression is a significant problem among head and neck cancer patients but is often underrecognized within oncological settings. The range of clinically significant depression as defined by scoring above the cutoff on a validated instrument for depressive symptoms is between 21%[45] and 42%.[44] Two studies have used measured DSM-based criteria to measure the prevalence of depressive disorders in head and neck cancer patients. Morton et al. assessed 48 buccopharyngeal cancer survivors who were within 3 years posttreatment and found a high prevalence, 40%, of those who met DSM criteria for major depression.[49] Kugaya et al. found a much lower prevalence, 17%, among 107 newly diagnosed Japanese head and neck cancer patients.[50] Whereas the earlier study assessed patients during a time when cure rates for head and neck cancer were much lower, the latter study used a controversial approach of eliminating somatic symptoms in the determination of the presence of depressive illness, an approach that has been found to underestimate the true prevalence rate.[51] Longitudinal data consistently show that depressive symptoms tend to increase as treatment progresses, peaking during the second month of treatment and decreasing gradually in the months and years thereafter.[9,44] For example, deLeeuw et al. found that 20% of head and neck cancer survivors scored in the clinical range on the Center for Epidemiological Studies (CESD), compared with general population norms of around 10%.[44] Hammerlid et al. reported that 33% of head and neck cancer survivors had high levels of depression 1 year after treatment.[52] Even after 7–11 years after treatment, Bjordal et al. reported that 31% of 2070 head and neck cancer survivors scored in the clinically meaningful range of depression on the EORTC-H&N.[53] The reason for the prolonged impairment in emotional functioning is unknown; some authors have hypothesized that patients experience burnout in coping with ongoing physical problems and permanent changes in social activities.[54] As a group, head and neck cancer patients may also have poorer premorbid psychological functioning compared with other cancer patient profiles in which alcohol dependence is not an etiological factor.

There are a number of factors that are associated with depressive symptoms in head and neck cancer patients. Among the most consistent are advanced stage of disease, worse functional outcomes, worse pain, younger age, and social support. Low self-perceived QOL and being female have also been reported to be related to depression scores in head and neck cancer patients.[55] Prospective studies consistently show that elevated levels of depressive symptoms at baseline are the most important factor in predicting subsequent depression.[44] Premorbid and ongoing alcohol and tobacco use, which itself is an important risk for pharyngeal cancers,[56] has also been associated with subsequent development of elevated levels of depression in patients undergoing treatment for head and neck cancer.[57] Unfortunately, many of these factors may also serve as barriers to receiving appropriate treatment for depression. Patients with poor physical functioning or those without social support may feel too ill or too inconvenienced to travel regularly to their medical center for depression treatment.[58,59]

Tobacco and alcohol use. Current tobacco use and high levels of alcohol consumption are highly prevalent in the head and neck cancer population. Analysis of 20 years of National Health Survey Data found that head and neck cancer survivors were more likely to be current smokers and/or heavy drinkers compared with other cancer survivors.[60] Depending on the assessment method, rates of alcohol dependence ranges from 39% for alcohol dependence (33%) to 5.2%—6% for alcohol abuse; between 24.6% and 33% met the criteria for nicotine dependence. Up to 75% of the sample reported drinking more than three drinks per day for a median of 29 years.[50,57]

Risk and detection of dysphagia: Patients getting tumoricidal doses of radiation for laryngeal/pharyngeal cancers are at high risk for dysphagia.[61,62] In head and neck cancer and especially oropharyngeal cancer, swallowing function tends to remain compromised after radiation therapy. Three years after radiation treatment, a mixed sample of 317 head and neck cancer patients experienced significantly worse swallowing, pain, and dry mouth, compared with 871 age- and gender-matched people.[39] While IMRT is a means of delivering radiation dose in a more precise manner than conventional radiotherapy, a study examining 3-year toxicity outcomes in 69 advanced head and neck cancer found no improvement for IMRT with various toxicity measures. For example, 36% of those treated with conventional radiotherapy were completely feeding-tube dependent 3 years after radiation compared with 40% for IMRT.[63] In a study of 36 oropharyngeal patients 5 years after treatment, 100% of the sample still experienced xerostomia, 76% experienced swallowing difficulty, 48% experienced decreased energy, and 43% significant pain. These were also the symptoms that caused the most distress.[26] Pourel et al. also found impaired functioning in 119 oropharyngeal cancer survivors 3 years after treatment and concluded that future rehabilitation research should target impaired emotional functioning, dry mouth, and difficulties with eating.[9]

Currently, there is no reliable method to predict who will develop long-term dysphagia or trismus in throat cancer patients.[64–66] Furthermore, noninvasive screening procedures for early detection of radiation-associated fibrosis do not yet exist. Instead, fiberoptic endoscopic evaluation of swallowing (FEES) and gold-standard modified barium swallow tests are typically ordered after the patient begins to complain of difficulties with swallowing.[36] Unfortunately, once fibrosis of the swallowing muscles has fully developed, there is little hope of restoring normal function.[67-69]

Body image in facial cancers

Facial appearance is an important means of identity and for communication with others.[70] Cancers involving the facial region are categorized as upper aerodigestive tract tumors or other cutaneous cancers that may impact different parts of the face such as eyes or ears. Changes to the face are difficult to cope with because they may impact many routine activities, and these could occur at any time during or after cancer treatment.[71,72]

Body image is a dynamic and multidimensional construct. Cash et al. define it as "perceptions, thoughts, and feelings about body and bodily experience."[73] Body image develops over time and is the interaction between self and the society.[73] Illness such as cancer is life-threatening and life-altering, which may result in changes that may be difficult to adjust to. White proposes that degree of body image investment in a specific function/appearance and discrepancy between self and ideal perception of appearance or functioning results in body image concerns.[74] For patients with facial changes, various authors explain the process of adaptation, for example, Newell's fear avoidance model explains how the thought of fear or disgust when interacting with others or other's reaction to visible change results in avoidant behavior.[73] On the other hand, how different psychological factors could moderate adaptation to various physical and functional changes with cancer or its treatment.[75] In the early postoperative phase, Dropkin et al. identified various coping behaviors to help with reintegration into activities.[76] Another group of researchers suggested various reintegration behaviors,[70] which would help the nursing staff in the postoperative phase. During survivorship, physical changes may persist for example, dry mouth, lockjaw, lymphedema, and ongoing functional concerns.

To mitigate these adverse effects on body image, some authors have considered psychosocial interventions. These interventions range from being appearance focused, fitness related, education material, or psychological interventions.[77] Data regarding impact of psychosocial interventions is mixed.[78-83] Among the various psychological interventions, specifically cognitive behavioral therapy has been more promising in patients with facial cancers.[84] In this section, we will outline clinically relevant approaches to help patients with body image adjustment during different phases of treatment trajectory.

At the time of diagnosis or before treatment: Information about anticipated physical changes should be discussed in detail, if possible, prior to initiation of specific treatment. If unable to discuss changes, then written information could be shared with patients. Aforementioned education will help set realistic expectations about upcoming treatment. Additionally, it may help relieve some of the anticipated anxiety.

Immediately after surgery: Patient experienced significant distress when they noticed changes in comparison with image of previous surgery status. Additionally, seeing themselves in the mirror can be challenging. Hence, offering support (if they are open to) when they see themselves in the mirror may help some patients. Support may take the form of helping them understand the nature of immediate physical changes, offer practical strategies such as use of a small size mirror first, and manage emotional response to these changes. Interaction between healthcare providers and patients during this time is extremely important.[85] Healthcare providers may need to be more sensitive to the physical changes and be mindful of their own desensitization due to chronic nature of focused patient care. It is important for healthcare providers to take an explorative stance to understand patient's concerns in the context of their lifestyle and avoid negative connotation words like disfigurement.[77,86]

Patient's commonly have swelling which may impact functioning of different parts. It is important for patient to start working with speech and occupational therapy early during their recovery. Some patients may need a feeding tube, so working with a dietitian becomes important too.

Late after surgery: During this phase, patients experience anticipatory anxiety about resuming their routine. Specific concerns include reaction of others, interaction with family members, and eating in public places. Stigma is a common concern.[87] To help overcome the aforementioned concerns, behavioral strategies that help with desensitization, being aware about verbal and nonverbal cues related to body language, and ways to respond to others can be considered.[88] Many times, mental health professionals will be called after patients have viewed themselves in the mirror. At that time, reframing the experience also helps the patient. If the degree of emotional distress is severe and warrants psychotropic management, then referral to appropriate resource such as psychiatry is recommended. With radiation, chemotherapy, and immunotherapy, relevant body image concerns include weight loss or weight gain, and hair loss. These are visible and unwanted side effects.

Assessment

Patient-reported outcomes. There is a wealth of validated patient self-report measures that can be reliably administered in clinical settings to measure a wide range of symptoms and unexpected side effects; these instruments can provide insight as to whether treatment gains are outweighed by side effect burden or conversely accompanied by improvement in disease-related symptoms. Commonly referred to as patient-reported outcomes (PROs), they also provide an alternative reporting method for patients to disclose sensitive information they may not feel comfortable discussing with their treatment team. While the following list is not exhaustive, the following list of potentially useful PROs has been reviewed for quality, patient burden, reading level, availability in multiple languages, and cost.

Symptom burden

The MD Anderson Symptom Inventory measures 13 common core symptoms and 6 interference items with a 10-point Likert response format ranging from 0 (not present) to 10 (as bad as you can imagine).

The **Brief Pain Inventory (BPI)** is a nine-item self-report measure specifically designed to assess pain in cancer and to provide information regarding pain severity and pain interference. Patients rate their pain severity on a Likert-type scale (0 = no pain to 10 = pain as bad as you can imagine) at the time of responding, and at its worst, least, and average over the previous week. Patients rate pain interference on a Likert-type scale (0 = no interference to 10 = interferes completely) as to how much pain interferes with activity, mood, walking, work, relations with others, sleep, and enjoyment of life. An interference score is derived as the mean of these scores. Because of the variability of pain, the BPI has been demonstrated to have better test–retest reliability over short intervals than long intervals. Validity data are from studies examining the use of the instrument with prostate cancer patients and patients with other diseases.[89]

The **Brief Fatigue Inventory (BFI)** is a nine-item self-report measure similar in format to the BPI. Three items ask patients to rate the severity of their fatigue at its "worst," "usual," and "now" during normal waking hours. Participants rate their fatigue on a Likert-type scale (0 = no fatigue to 10 = fatigue as bad as you can imagine). Six items assess the amount that fatigue has interfered with different aspects of the patient's life with general activity, mood, walking ability, normal work, relations with others, sleep, and enjoyment of life. An interference score is derived as the mean of these scores.[90] The BFI is an internally stable and reliable measure with an internal consistency of 0.96. It is correlated with measures of performance status (patients who are more ill report higher levels of fatigue) and with physiological markers of anemia (hemoglobin) and nutritional status (albumin) known to be associated with fatigue.[90]

PRO-CTCAE. The National Cancer Institute has developed a PRO measurement system to evaluate symptom toxicities in clinical trials. Validated in over 30 languages and publicly available without cost, individual modules assessing 78 symptoms from among 14 general categories are downloadable from the NCI's Pro-CTCAE form builder: https://healthcaredelivery.cancer.gov/pro-ctcae/instrument.html. Each symptom module evaluates frequency, severity, interference with daily activities, and presence or absence. The severity, frequency, and interference scores are meant to be used descriptively in graphs or summary statistics (i.e., cutoff scores have not yet been validated against other research instruments).

Quality of life

The Functional Assessment of Cancer Therapy-Head and Neck (FACT-HN) is a 38-item questionnaire consisting of the four subscales of the Functional Assessment of Cancer Therapy-General (physical, social, functional, and emotional well-being) and a subscale measuring concerns specific to head and neck cancer. Overall, the FACT-HN has good test–retest and internal reliability and demonstrated good convergent, divergent, and criterion validity with the Beck Depression Inventory, the Performance Status Scale for Head and Neck Cancer Patients, and the University of Washington Quality of Life Scale.[42,91]

Alcohol Abuse Screening (**AUDIT**) is a 10-item, 5-point Likert response screening tool developed by the World Health organization to identify hazardous drinkers (those at risk of developing alcohol-related problems), harmful drinkers (those with recent physical or mental harm from drinking), and people with alcohol dependence. The self-report version of the AUDIT includes a visual reference guide for defining one "standard drink" for different alcohol beverages (beer, wine, hard liquor). AUDIT subscale scores have shown concordant validity with other established alcohol dependence screening measures.[92]

Depression

The Patient Health Questionnaire-9 item (PHQ-9) is a 9-item self-administered version of the DSM-based Prime-MD, which asks about the nine criteria for major depression.[93] For each of the items, patients indicate whether during the previous 2 weeks, the symptoms occurred "not at all," "several days," "more than half the days," or "nearly every day." It can be used as a diagnostic instrument and can yield information about depression severity. The PHQ-9 yielded a 76% positive predictive value against a structured diagnosis of major depression in primary care populations,[94,95] an extremely high value compared with other screening instruments, which have yielded PPVs in the ranges of 27%–35%.[96,97] It is important to note that the question asking about presence and severity of suicidal ideation may be reliably deleted from the scale if timely clinical follow-up is not consistently available for patients who endorse suicide ideation.[98]

Swallowing function and swallowing-related quality of life

The Performance Status Scale for Head and Neck Cancer (PSS-H&N) is a modified visual analog scale instrument consisting of three discrete subscales: *normalcy of diet* (the patient chooses from 12 different types of diet and food categories listed in descending order from "full diet, no restrictions" to "nonoral feeding (tube fed)"), *public eating* (the patient chooses from seven categories listed in descending order starting with "No restriction, eats out at any opportunity" to "Nothing per mouth"), and *understandability of speech* (five categories ranging in descending order from "Always understandable" to "Never understandable, may use written communication"). The PSS-H&N yields a total of three ratings, one of each subscale. PSS-HN demonstrated good internal when used either as a clinician-rated instrument or as a self-administered questionnaire (kappa coefficient ranged from 0.65 to 0.84 for normalcy of diet and eating in public) and was able to detect differences in stage, treatment type, and extent of surgery in head and neck cancer patients based on the extent of their surgery.[8,99–101]

MD Anderson Dysphagia Inventory (MDADI): The MDADI measures swallowing-related QOL in patients with swallowing dysfunction. It evaluates the patient's physical (P), emotional (E), and functional (F) perceptions of swallowing dysfunction. This instrument has high internal consistency (0.85−93) and demonstrated good construct validity with the SF-36 subscales.[102]

Treatment

Pharmacotherapy for radiation-related anxiety

Radiation treatment is commonly associated with anxiety, which is mostly with immobilization while wearing a mask.[103] Hence, it is important to screen for anxiety both before and after radiation treatment especially if someone has preexisting history of claustrophobia or posttraumatic stress disorder.[104] Both general (support, music therapy, and involvement of the radiation oncology team) and specific (relaxation techniques, interrupt usage of mask, anxiolytic medication, and education about mask related concerns) measures to address anxiety should be considered.[105,106] Anxiolytic therapy includes benzodiazepines and atypical antipsychotics. Prior history of substance use or current use of opiates may limit use of benzodiazepines. Hence, olanzapine may be considered by some.[56]

Psychological treatment for depression in cancer patients. Despite the availability of effective treatments, treatment rates for depressed cancer patients are woefully low. In one study, only 3% of patients with validated diagnoses of clinically significant depression were being professionally treated at time of assessment.[107] In another study, only 14% for patients with validated diagnoses of major depression were receiving treatment.[108] Cancer patients themselves cite several reasons for rejecting referral for antidepressant treatment, including concerns with antidepressant side effects[109] and preference for psychotherapy.[43] While there are anecdotal reports that prescription for antidepressant medication is on the rise, pharmacologic interventions may not be sufficient. One controlled trial comparing different modes of treatment in depressed cancer patients found that a structured psychotherapy treatment combined with antidepressant medication was clearly superior compared to antidepressant medication alone.[44]

Regarding drug-free psychotherapy, studies have shown that professional psychotherapy may appeal to a limited demographic: white, middle-class, and college-educated patients.[110] And, cancer patients with more severe cancer-related symptoms and poorer functioning are less likely to agree to psychotherapy, citing their reluctance to commit the time and effort needed to attend weekly psychotherapy appointments.[45] This last point is unfortunate, since poorer functioning and severity of symptoms are more likely to be associated with depression in cancer patients.[111−113] Thus, it is clear that cancer patients who are most in need of treatment for depression have the most difficulty with access to treatment due to problems in pain, physical and social functioning, and disease progression.

Cognitive behavioral psychotherapy in cancer patients. Within the large body of literature demonstrating the efficacy of psychological interventions for cancer patients, most of the studies have used group and individual therapy formats that typically require intensive personal contact with the cancer patient[114] (see Fawzy et al.[115]). Reviews of the literature have identified three efficacious types of psychotherapy in relieving distress: cognitive behavioral therapy, Spiegel's supportive expressive therapy, and Schulberg's interpersonal therapy.[116] Of these, cognitive behavioral therapy may be the most adaptable and acceptable for depressed cancer patients. Supportive expressive group therapy is an intensive psychodynamic therapy, which requires at least a year of participation before psychotherapeutic change occurs.[117] Schulberg's interpersonal therapy is promising[118] but requires doctoral-level therapists to run the intervention, which may inhibit broad acceptance in oncology clinics.

In contrast to these two approaches, cognitive behavioral therapy is highly adaptable to a wide range of patient needs. Its emphasis on the patient's actions and thoughts places more of the control with the patients, compared with supportive expressive and interpersonal therapy, which tend to depend on strong therapeutic alliances either between group members or over the telephone with an experienced therapist. Furthermore, positive effects can begin to be felt relatively quickly in cognitive-behavioral therapy, which helps to establish its credibility with the patient. Finally, there is evidence that cognitive behavioral therapy achieves significant decreases in distress in a relatively brief time, generally 10–12 sessions or less.[119]

The focus of cognitive therapy for depression is to penetrate patients' strongly held distorted thought patterns about themselves and their problems and replace them with a more rational and balanced thought system. With depressed cancer patients, their cognitive distortions may revolve around their losses in functioning, disruption to their family life, or experiences with side effects and pain. For example, since social activities tend to center around eating, head and neck cancer patients often isolate themselves to avoid embarrassment as their diet becomes more restricted to liquid-based or percutaneous endoscopic gastrostomy (PEG) tube feedings. Such patients may find themselves thinking, "I have no life left." According to the model, such thoughts will engender depressed mood and decreased self-esteem. Cognitive therapy teaches, in a step-by-step fashion, how to recognize these types of negative, distorted thoughts, and to counter them with more rational ones. Patients experiencing fatigue, another common major concern, should be encouraged to develop realistic expectations for recovery and pacing during their treatment and postacute phase. To target other concerns, such as hair loss, taste changes, hearing, and cognitive impairment, it is important to address catastrophic thoughts by first distinguishing between temporary symptoms (hair loss and in most cases taste changes) from permanent long-term effects (hearing loss and cognitive changes). With hearing loss and cognitive changes, recognize that it is natural for patients to hope that these issues will improve without intervention and can thus be ignored; however it may be more helpful to replace thoughts related to denial ("I hope it will go away,") with more adaptive thoughts, such as "I need to report any changes in my hearing in case I need to get it tested again."

Behavioral therapy targets the symptoms of depression with various techniques designed to replace maladaptive behaviors with adaptive behaviors. For example, the combination of psychomotor retardation and the loss of pleasure in former activities contribute to depressed people feeling stuck, sometimes to the point that he or she may feel paralyzed. An effective behavioral strategy to counter this inactivity is to help the patient choose and commit to a few achievable activities. Usually, two types of activities are suggested, fun activities and activities that help the patient feel useful again. Patient ratings of satisfaction after the activity help the patient realize that they are able to experience some pleasure, often more pleasure than they expected, and that they are able to contribute to the household, despite their negative assessments of themselves. Although some depressed cancer patients have poor physical functioning, several types of pleasurable and useful activities can be suggested without requiring much exertion. These may include hobbies such as fishing or working with small tools, making a long-distance call to an old friend, taking short walks, writing emails to old friends or family members, reading, or listening to music. Similarly, many useful activities can still be performed with minimal functioning, such as paying bills, running errands such as getting the oil changed or washing dishes.

Speech language and swallowing therapy

Prevention of dysphagia. Prevention of dysphagia is of critical importance for head and neck cancer survivors. Radiation oncology researchers have focused on delivering increasingly targeted radiation to tissues that harbor cancer while avoiding adjacent organs without disease.[120] However, despite improved toxicity profiles, a significant proportion of patients still develop permanent dysphagia.[30,66] Another important approach is to implement intensive, earlier therapies by speech and language pathologists, including preventive swallowing exercises and device-driven exercises (e.g., lingual resistance, expiratory strength trainers).[121,122] Both the National Comprehensive Cancer Network (NCCN)[123] and the American Head and Neck Society recommend that prophylactic swallowing exercises and baseline clinical swallowing exams be delivered at the start of radiation to improve posttreatment function.[62]

Critical barriers to current service delivery: In the US healthcare system, specialized dysphagia prevention services are usually limited to comprehensive cancer centers, where access is limited to narrow insurance plan coverage.[124−126] Since head and neck cancer is relatively rare, community medical centers are not equipped to provide gold-standard radiographic modified barium swallow (MBS) tests for diagnosing dysphagia, nor do they typically employ speech language pathologists (**SLP**s) who specialize in the prevention and treatment of radiation-associated dysphagia. Only 13% of all US speech pathologists work in adult medical settings and even fewer specialize in radiation-associated dysphagia.[127] Furthermore, healthcare systems are slow to adapt a proactive approach to preventing dysphagia. National practice surveys of SLPs working with head and neck cancer patients indicate that between 18.3%[128] and 39%[129] receive proactive referrals from oncologists prior to patients starting radiation.

References

1. ASCO Cancer.Net Editorial Board: Head and neck cancer guide: Statistics. *Statistics Adapted from the American Cancer Society's Publication, Cancer Facts & Figures 2022, and the National Cancer Institute Website.* 2022. All sources accessed January 2022.
2. *American Cancer Society: Cancer Facts & Figures 2023.* 2023.
3. Windon MJ, D'Souza G, Rettig EM, et al. Increasing prevalence of human papillomavirus-positive oropharyngeal cancers among older adults. *Cancer.* 2018; 124:2993−2999.
4. Johnson DE, Burtness B, Leemans CR, et al. Head and neck squamous cell carcinoma. *Nat Rev Dis Prim.* 2020;6:92.
5. Simard EP, Torre LA, Jemal A. International trends in head and neck cancer incidence rates: differences by country, sex and anatomic site. *Oral Oncol.* 2014;50:387−403.
6. Chawla S, Mohanti BK, Rakshak M, et al. Temporal assessment of quality of life of head and neck cancer patients receiving radical radiotherapy. *Qual Life Res.* 1999;8:73−78.
7. Sherman A, Simonton S, Adams D, et al. Coping with head and neck cancer during different phases of treatment. *Head Neck.* 2000;22:787−793.
8. List M, Ritter-Sterr C, Lansky S. A performance status scale for head and neck cancer patients. *Cancer.* 1990;66:564−569.
9. Pourel N, Pieiffert D, Lartigau E, et al. Quality of life in long-term survivors of oropharynx carcinoma. *Int J Radiat Oncol Biol Phys.* 2002;54:742−751.
10. De Boer M, McCormick L, Pruyn J, et al. Physical and psychosocial correlates of head and neck cancer: a review of the literature. *Otolaryngol Head Neck Surg.* 1999;120: 427−436.
11. Zabora J, BrintzenhofeSzoc K, Curbow B, et al. The prevalence of psychological distress by cancer site. *Psycho Oncol.* 2001;10:19−28.
12. Gritz ER, Carmack CL, deMoor C, et al. First year after head and neck cancer: quality of life. *J Clin Oncol.* 1999;17:352−360.
13. Chua K, Reddy S, Lee M, et al. Pain and loss of function in head and neck cancer survivors. *J Pain Symptom Manag.* 1999;18:193−202.
14. Kang D, Kim S, Kim H, et al. Surveillance of symptom burden using the patient-reported outcome version of the common terminology criteria for adverse events in patients with various types of cancers during chemoradiation therapy: real-world study. *JMIR Public Health Surveill.* 2023;9:e44105.
15. Eisbruch A, Schwartz M, Rasch C, et al. Dysphagia and aspiration after chemoradiotherapy for head and neck cancer: which anatomic structures are affected and can they be spared by IMRT? *Int J Radiat Oncol Biol Phys.* 2004;60:1425−1439.
16. Foundation OC. *What Is Trismus?* Oral Cancer Foundation; 2007.
17. Nguyen N, Frank C, Moltz C, et al. Aspiration rate following chemoradiation for head and neck cancer: an underreported occurrence. *Radiother Oncol.* 2006;80:109−274.

18. Lazarus CL, Logemann JA, Pauloski BR, et al. Swallowing and tongue function following treatment for oral and oropharyngeal cancer. *J Speech Lang Hear Res.* 2000;43:1011−1024.

19. Vera-Llonch M, Oster G, Hagiwara M, et al. Oral mucositis in patients undergoing radiation treatment for head and neck carcinoma. *Cancer.* 2006;106:329−336.

20. Li Y, Taylor J, Ten Haken R, et al. The impact of dose on parotid salivary recovery in head and neck cancer patients treated with radiation therapy. *Int J Radiat Oncol Biol Phys.* 2007;67:660−669.

21. Chambers M, Garden A, Rosenthal D, et al. Intensity-modulated radiotherapy: is Xerostomia still prevalent? *Curr Oncol Rep.* 2005;7:131−136.

22. Claus F, Duthoy W, Boterberg T, et al. Intensity modulated radiation therapy for oropharyngeal and oral cavity tumors: clinical use and experience. *Oral Oncol.* 2002;38:597−604.

23. Ang K, Garden A. *Radiotherapy for Head and Neck Cancers. Indications and Techniques.* 3rd ed. Philadelphia: Lippincott Williams & Wilkins; 2006.

24. Sehlen S, Hollenhorst H, Lenk M, et al. Only sociodemographic variables predict quality of life after radiotherapy in patients with head and neck cancer. *Int J Radiat Oncol Biol Phys.* 2002;52:779−783.

25. Hanna EY, Mendoza TR, Rosenthal DI, et al. The symptom burden of treatment-naive patients with head and neck cancer. *Cancer.* 2015;121:766−773.

26. Harrison L, Zelefsky M, Pfister D, et al. Detailed quality of life assessment in patients treated with primary radiotherapy for squamous cell cancer of the base of the tongue. *Head Neck.* 1997;19:169−175.

27. Hassanein K, Musgrove B, Bradbury E. Functional status of patients with oral cancer and its relation to style of coping, social support, and psychological status. *Br J Oral Maxillofac Surg.* 2001;39:340−345.

28. Hutcheson KA, Nurgalieva Z, Zhao H, et al. Two-year prevalence of dysphagia and related outcomes in head and neck cancer survivors: an updated SEER-Medicare analysis. *Head Neck.* 2019;41:479−487.

29. Mortensen H, Jensen K, Aksglaede K, et al. Late dysphagia after IMRT for head and neck cancer and correlation with dose-volume parameters. *Radiother Oncol.* 2013;107:288−294.

30. Caudell J, Schaner P, Meredith R, et al. Factors associated with long-term dysphagia after definitive radiotherapy for locally advanced head-and-neck cancer. *Int J Radiat Oncol Biol Phys.* 2009;73:410−415.

31. Caudell JJ, Schaner PE, Desmond RA, et al. Dosimetric factors associated with long-term dysphagia after definitive radiotherapy for squamous cell carcinoma of the head and neck. *Int J Radiat Oncol Biol Phys.* 2010;76:403−409.

32. Rosenthal DI, Mendoza TR, Fuller CD, et al. Patterns of symptom burden during radiotherapy or concurrent chemoradiotherapy for head and neck cancer: a prospective analysis using the University of Texas MD Anderson Cancer Center Symptom Inventory-Head and Neck Module. *Cancer.* 2014;120:1975−1984.

33. Goepfert RP, Lewin JS, Barrow MP, et al. Grading dysphagia as a toxicity of head and neck cancer: differences in severity classification based on MBS DIGEST and clinical CTCAE grades. *Dysphagia.* 2018;33:185−191.

34. Caglar HB, Tishler RB, Othus M, et al. Dose to larynx predicts for swallowing complications after intensity-modulated radiotherapy. *Int J Radiat Oncol Biol Phys.* 2008;72:1110−1118.

35. Logemann JA, Pauloski BR, Rademaker AW, et al. Swallowing disorders in the first year after radiation and chemoradiation. *Head Neck*. 2008;30:148−158.
36. Eisbruch A, Lyden T, Bradford C, et al. Objective assessment of swallowing dysfunction and aspiration after radiation concurrent with chemotherapy for head and neck cancer. *Int J Radiat Oncol Biol Phys*. 2002;53:23−28.
37. Goepfert RP, Fuller CD, Gunn GB, et al. Symptom burden as a driver of decisional regret in long-term oropharyngeal carcinoma survivors. *Head Neck*. 2017;39:2151−2158.
38. Lazarus C. Management of swallowing disorders in head and neck cancer patients: optimal patterns of care. *Semin Speech Lang*. 2000;21:293−309.
39. Hammerlid E, Taft C. Health-related quality of life in long-term head and neck cancer survivors: a comparison with general population norms. *Br J Cancer*. 2001;84:149−156.
40. De Leeuw JR, De Graeff A, Ros WJ, et al. Negative and positive influences of social support on depression in patients with head and neck cancer: a prospective study. *Psycho Oncol*. 2000;9:20−28.
41. NCI. *NCI/PDQ Physician Statement: Depression*. 2000.
42. Cohen S, Willis tA. Stress, social support, and the buffering hypothesis. *Psychol Bull*. 1985;98:310−357.
43. Hammerlid E, Persson L, Sullivan M, et al. Quality of life effects of psychosocial intervention in patients with head and neck cancer. *Otolaryngol Head Neck Surg*. 1999;120:507−516.
44. deLeeuw J, deGraeff A, Ros W, et al. Prediction of depression 6 months to 3 years after treatment of head and neck cancer. *Head Neck*. 2001;23:892−898.
45. Hutton J, Williams M. An investigation of psychological distress in patients who have been treated for head and neck cancer. *Br J Oral Maxillofac Surg*. 2001;39:333−339.
46. Benazon N, Coyne J. Living with a depressed spouse. *J Fam Psychol*. 2000;14:70−79.
47. Coyne J, Thompson R, Palmer SC. Marital quality, coping with conflict, marital complaints, and affection in couples with a depressed wife. *J Fam Psychol*. 2002;16:26−37.
48. Osazuwa-Peters N, Simpson MC, Zhao L, et al. Suicide risk among cancer survivors: head and neck versus other cancers. *Cancer*. 2018;124:4072−4079.
49. Morton RP, Davies ADM, Baker J, et al. Quality of life in treated head and neck cancer patients: a preliminary report. *Clin Otolaryngol*. 1984;9:181−185.
50. Kugaya A, Akechi T, Okuyama T, et al. Prevalence, predictive factors, and screening for psychologic distress in patients with newly diagnosed head and neck cancer. *Cancer*. 2000;88:2817−2823.
51. Koenig H, George L, Peterson B, et al. Depression in medically ill hospitalized older adults: prevalence, characteristics, and course of symptoms according to six diagnostic schemes. *Am J Psychiatr*. 1997;154:1376−1383.
52. Hammerlid E, Ahlner-Elmqvist M, Bjordal K, et al. A prospective multi-centre study in Sweden and Norway of mental distress and psychiatric morbidity in head and neck cancer patients. *Br J Cancer*. 1999;80:766−774.
53. Bjordal K, Hammerlid E, Ahlner-Elmqvist M, et al. Quality of life in head and neck cancer patients validation of the European organization for research and treatment of cancer quality of life questionnaire-H&N 35. *J Clin Oncol*. 1999;3:1008−1019.
54. Rapoport Y, Kreitler S, Chaitchik S, et al. Psychosocial problems in head and neck cancer patients and their change with time since diagnosis. *Ann Oncol*. 1993;4:69−73.

55. D'Antonio L, Long S, Zimmerman GJ, et al. Relationship between quality of life and depression in patients with head and neck cancer. *Laryngoscope*. 1998;108:806−811.

56. Vijayan M, Joseph S, M Nair H, et al. Can olanzapine preserve life quality in cancer patients undergoing abdominal radiation therapy? *Med Hypotheses*. 2023;171:111014.

57. Kugaya A, Akechi T, Okamura H, et al. Correlates of depressed mood in ambulatory head and neck cancer patients. *Psycho Oncol*. 1999;8:494−499.

58. Manne S, Glassman M. Perceived control, coping efficacy and avoidance coping as mediators between spouses' unsupportive behaviors and cancer patients' psychological distress. *Health Psychol*. 2000;19:155−164.

59. Sellick SCD. Depression and cancer: an appraisal of the literature for prevalence, detection, and practice guideline development for psychological interventions. *Psycho Oncol*. 1999;8:315−333.

60. Balachandra S, Eary RL, Lee R, et al. Substance use and mental health burden in head and neck and other cancer survivors: a National Health Interview Survey analysis. *Cancer*. 2022;128:112−121.

61. Eisbruch A, Kim HM, Feng FY, et al. Chemo-IMRT of oropharyngeal cancer aiming to reduce dysphagia: swallowing organs late complication probabilities and dosimetric correlates. *Int J Radiat Oncol Biol Phys*. 2011;81:e93−e99.

62. Goyal N, Day A, Epstein J, et al. Head and neck cancer survivorship consensus statement from the American Head and Neck Society. *Laryngoscope Investig Otolaryngol*. 2022;7:70−92.

63. Milano M, Vokes E, Kao J, et al. Intensity-modulated radiation therapy in advanced head and neck patients treated with intensive chemoradiotherapy: preliminary experience and future directions. *Int J Oncol*. 2006;28:1141−1151.

64. Paleri V, Roe JW, Strojan P, et al. Strategies to reduce long-term postchemoradiation dysphagia in patients with head and neck cancer: an evidence-based review. *Head Neck*. 2014;36:431−443.

65. Christianen ME, Verdonck-de Leeuw IM, Doornaert P, et al. Patterns of long-term swallowing dysfunction after definitive radiotherapy or chemoradiation. *Radiother Oncol*. 2015;117:139−144.

66. King SN, Dunlap NE, Tennant PA, et al. Pathophysiology of radiation-induced dysphagia in head and neck cancer. *Dysphagia*. 2016;31:339−351.

67. Cooper J, Fu K, Marks J, et al. Late effects of radiation therapy in the head and neck region. *Int J Radiat Oncol Biol Phys*. 1995;31:1141−1164.

68. Nguyen N, Moltz C, Frank C, et al. Dysphagia following chemoradiation for locally advanced head and neck cancer. *Ann Oncol*. 2004;15:383−388.

69. Vainshtein JM, Moon DH, Feng FY, et al. Long-term quality of life after swallowing and salivary-sparing chemo-intensity modulated radiation therapy in survivors of human papillomavirus-related oropharyngeal cancer. *Int J Radiat Oncol Biol Phys*. 2015;91:925−933.

70. Callahan C. Facial disfigurement and sense of self in head and neck cancer. *Soc Work Health Care*. 2004;40:73−87.

71. Nilsen ML, Belsky MA, Scheff N, et al. Late and long-term treatment-related effects and survivorship for head and neck cancer patients. *Curr Treat Options Oncol*. 2020;21:92.

72. Clarke SA, Newell R, Thompson A, et al. Appearance concerns and psychosocial adjustment following head and neck cancer: a cross-sectional study and nine-month follow-up. *Psychol Health Med*. 2014;19:505−518.

73. Teo MFal. *Theoretical Foundations of Body Image, Body Image Care for Cancer Patients.* Oxford University Press; 2018.

74. White CA. Body image dimensions and cancer: a heuristic cognitive behavioural model. *Psycho Oncol.* 2000;9:183−192.

75. Rhoten BA, Murphy B, Ridner SH. Body image in patients with head and neck cancer: a review of the literature. *Oral Oncol.* 2013;49:753−760.

76. Dropkin MJ. Coping with disfigurement and dysfunction after head and neck cancer surgery: a conceptual framework. *Semin Oncol Nurs.* 1989;5:213−219.

77. Fingeret MC, Teo I, Epner DE. Managing body image difficulties of adult cancer patients: lessons from available research. *Cancer.* 2014;120:633−641.

78. Alleva JM, Sheeran P, Webb TL, et al. A meta-analytic review of stand-alone interventions to improve body image. *PLoS One.* 2015;10:e0139177.

79. Semple CJ, Dunwoody L, Kernohan WG, et al. Development and evaluation of a problem-focused psychosocial intervention for patients with head and neck cancer. *Support Care Cancer.* 2009;17:379−388.

80. Chen SC, Huang BS, Lin CY, et al. Psychosocial effects of a skin camouflage program in female survivors with head and neck cancer: a randomized controlled trial. *Psycho Oncol.* 2017;26:1376−1383.

81. Nicoletti G, Sasso A, Malovini A, et al. The role of rehabilitative camouflage after cervicofacial reconstructive surgery: a preliminary study. *Clin Cosmet Invest Dermatol.* 2014;7:43−49.

82. Luckett T, Britton B, Clover K, et al. Evidence for interventions to improve psychological outcomes in people with head and neck cancer: a systematic review of the literature. *Support Care Cancer.* 2011;19:871−881.

83. Chopra D, Shinn E, Teo I, et al. A cognitive behavioral therapy-based intervention to address body image in patients with facial cancers: results from a randomized controlled trial. *Palliat Support Care.* 2023:1−8.

84. Graboyes EM, Maurer S, Park Y, et al. Evaluation of a novel telemedicine-based intervention to manage body image disturbance in head and neck cancer survivors. *Psycho Oncol.* 2020;29:1988−1994.

85. Konradsen H, Kirkevold M, Zoffmann V. Surgical facial cancer treatment: the silencing of disfigurement in nurse-patient interactions. *J Adv Nurs.* 2009;65:2409−2418.

86. Mascarella MA, Morand GB, Hier MP, et al. Dealing with the vicissitudes and abject consequences of head and neck cancer: a vital role for psycho-oncology. *Curr Oncol.* 2022;29:6714−6723.

87. Reynolds LM, Harris L. Stigma in the face of cancer disfigurement: a systematic review and research agenda. *Eur J Cancer Care.* 2021;30:e13327.

88. Bessell A, Brough V, Clarke A, et al. Evaluation of the effectiveness of Face IT, a computer-based psychosocial intervention for disfigurement-related distress. *Psychol Health Med.* 2012;17:565−577.

89. Daut RL, Cleeland CS, Flanery RC. Development of the Wisconsin brief pain questionnaire to assess pain in cancer and other diseases. *Pain.* 1983;17:197−210.

90. Mendoza TR, Wang XS, Cleeland CS, et al. The rapid assessment of fatigue severity in cancer patients. *Cancer.* 1999;85:1186−1196.

91. Basen-Engquist K, Bodurka-Bevers D, Fitzgerald M, et al. Reliability and validity of the functional assessment of cancer therapy - ovarian (FACT-O). *J Clin Oncol.* 2001;19:1809−1817.

92. Bohn MJ, Babor TF, Kranzler HR. The Alcohol Use Disorders Identification Test (AUDIT): validation of a screening instrument for use in medical settings. *J Stud Alcohol*. 1995;56:423−432.

93. Spitzer RL, Kroenke K, Williams JB, et al. Validation and utility of a self-report version of PRIME-MD: the PHQ primary care study. *J Am Med Assoc*. 1999;282:1737−1744.

94. Rost K, Duan N, Rubenstein L, et al. The Quality Improvement for Depression collaboration: general analytic strategies for a coordinated study of quality improvement in depression care. *Gen Hosp Psychiatr*. 2001;23:239−253.

95. Rost K, Nutting P, Smith J, et al. Improving depression outcomes in community primary care practice. *J Gen Intern Med*. 2001;16:143−149.

96. Fechner-Bates S, Coyne J, Schwenk T. The relationship of self-reported distress to depressive disorders and other psychopathology. *J Consult Clin Psychol*. 1994;62:550−559.

97. Gilbody S, House A, Sheldon T. Routinely administered questionnaires for depression and anxiety: a systematic review. *BMJ*. 2001;322:406−409.

98. Kroenke K, Spitzer R. The PHQ-9: a new depression diagnostic and severity measure. *J Gen Intern Med*. 2002;16:606−613.

99. Smith G, Yeo D, Clark J, et al. Measures of health-related quality of life and functional status in survivors of oral cavity cancer who have had defects reconstructed with radial forearm free flaps. *Br J Oral Maxillofac Surg*. 2006;44:187−192.

100. Campbell B, Marbella S, Layde P. Quality of life and recurrence concern in survivors of head and neck cancer. *Laryngoscope*. 2000;110:895−906.

101. Campbell B, Spinelli K, Marbella A, et al. Aspiration, weight loss and quality of life in head and neck cancer survivors. *Arch Otolaryngol Head Neck Surg*. 2004;130:1100−1103.

102. Chen A, Frankowski R, Bishop-Leone J, et al. The development and validation of a dysphagia-specific quality-of-life questionnaire for patients with head and neck cancer. *Arch Otolaryngol Head Neck Surg*. 2001;127:870−876.

103. Burns M, Campbell R, French S, et al. Trajectory of anxiety related to radiation therapy mask immobilization and treatment delivery in head and neck cancer and radiation therapists' ability to detect this anxiety. *Adv Radiat Oncol*. 2022;7:100967.

104. Forbes E, Clover K, Oultram S, et al. Situational anxiety in head and neck cancer: rates, patterns and clinical management interventions in a regional cancer setting. *J Med Radiat Sci*. 2024;71(1):100−109.

105. Fuji H, Fujibuchi T, Tanaka H, et al. Changes in satisfaction and anxiety about radiotherapy for pediatric cancer by two-step audio-visual instruction. *Tech Innov Patient Support Radiat Oncol*. 2023;27.

106. Forbes E, Baker AL, Britton B, et al. A systematic review of nonpharmacological interventions to reduce procedural anxiety among patients undergoing radiation therapy for cancer. *Cancer Med*. 2023;12:20396−20422.

107. Passik S, Dugan W, McDonald M, et al. Oncologists' recognition of depression in their patients with cancer. *J Clin Oncol*. 1998;16:1594−1600.

108. Berard R, Boermeester F, Viljoen G. Depressive disorders in an out-patient oncology setting: prevalence, assessment, and management. *Psycho Oncol*. 1998;7:112−120.

109. Holland J. Cancer's psychological challenges. *Sci Am*. 1996;275:158−161.

110. Berglund G, Bolund C, Gustafsson U, et al. Is the wish to participate in a cancer rehabilitation program an indicator of the need? Comparisons of participants and non-participants in a randomized study. *Psycho Oncol*. 1997;6:35−46.

111. Guidozzi F. Living with ovarian cancer. *Gynecol Oncol*. 1993;50:202−207.

112. Portenoy R, Kornblith A, Wong G, et al. Pain in ovarian cancer patients: prevalence, characteristics, and associated symptoms. *Cancer.* 1994;74:907−915.
113. Kornblith A, Thaler H, Wong G, et al. Quality of life of women with ovarian cancer. *Gynecol Oncol.* 1995;59:231−242.
114. Kissane D, Bloch S, Miach P, et al. Cognitive-existential group therapy for patients with primary breast cancer- techniques and themes. *Psycho Oncol.* 1997;6:25−33.
115. Fawzy F, Fawzy N, Arndt L, et al. Critical review of psychosocial interventions in cancer care. *Arch Gen Psychiatr.* 1995;52:100−113.
116. Compas B, Keefe F, Haaga D, et al. Sampling of empirically supported psychological treatments from health psychology: smoking, chronic pain, cancer, and bulimia nervosa. *J Consult Clin Psychol.* 1998;66:89−112.
117. Spielberg D, Spira J. *Supportive-expressive Group Therapy: A Treatment Manual of Psychosocial Intervention for Women with Recurrent Breast Cancer.* Psychosocial Treatment Laboratory- Stanford University School of Medicine; 1991.
118. Donnelly J, Kornblith A, Fleishman S, et al. A pilot study of interpersonal psychotherapy by telephone with cancer patients and their partners. *Psycho Oncol.* 2000;9:44−56.
119. Dobson KS. A meta-analysis of the efficacy of cognitive therapy for depression. *JCCP.* 1989;57:414−419.
120. Tubiana M, Eschwege F. Conformal radiotherapy and intensity-modulated radiotherapy–clinical data. *Acta Oncol.* 2000;39:555−567.
121. Burkhead LM, Sapienza CM, Rosenbek JC. Strength-training exercise in dysphagia rehabilitation: principles, procedures, and directions for future research. *Dysphagia.* 2007;22:251−265.
122. Lazarus. Tongue strength and exercise in healthy individuals and in head and neck cancer patients. *Semin Speech Lang.* 2006;27:260−267.
123. Pfister DG, Spencer S, Adelstein D, et al. Head and neck cancers, version 2.2020, NCCN clinical practice guidelines in oncology. *J Natl Compr Cancer Netw.* 2020;18:873−898.
124. Arora S, Thornton K, Komaromy M, et al. Demonopolizing medical knowledge. *Acad Med.* 2014;89:30−32.
125. Taplin SH, Anhang Price R, Edwards HM, et al. Introduction: understanding and influencing multilevel factors across the cancer care continuum. *J Natl Cancer Inst.* 2012;2012:2−10.
126. Asch SM, Kerr EA, Keesey J, et al. Who is at greatest risk for receiving poor-quality health care? *N Engl J Med.* 2006;354:1147−1156.
127. U.S. Bureau of Labor Statistics: Occupational employment and Wages. *29-1127 Speech-Language Pathologists.* PBS suite 2135, 2 Massachusetts Ave, Washington, DC 20212-0001. U.S. Bureau of Labor Statistics, Division of Occupational Employment Statistics, 2012; May 2012.
128. Krisciunas GP, Sokoloff W, Stepas K, et al. Survey of usual practice: dysphagia therapy in head and neck cancer patients. *Dysphagia.* 2012;27:538−549.
129. Logan AM, Landera MA. Clinical practices in head and neck cancer: a speech-language pathologist practice pattern survey. *Ann Otol Rhinol Laryngol.* 2021;130:1254−1262.

The role of acupuncture in head and neck cancer

18

Zunli Mo, PhD

Miami Cancer Institute, Miami, FL, United States

Introduction

Cancer is a genetic disease in which some of the human body's cells grow uncontrollably, invade into nearby areas, and spread to other parts of the body. In the US, head and neck cancer (HNC) accounts for about 4% of all cancer. It has been estimated that there are 66,920 new cases and 15,400 deaths from HNC annually.[1]

HNC treatment is very challenging and can vary depending on the type, location, and extent of the cancer, including a combination of surgery, chemotherapy, and radiation therapy. Surgery removes tumors and addresses as much as possible to treat the cancer while maintaining the appearance and physical and sensory function of nearby structures. Chemotherapy is used when tumors cannot be completely removed by surgery or when surgery may cause significant functional impairment. Chemotherapy has also been shown to enhance the effectiveness of radiation therapy. Radiation therapy is very effective in treating HNC especially for inoperable tumors with high-risk factors of local recurrence.[2] Other antineoplastic therapies include immunotherapy, targeted therapy, or hormone therapy.[3] These types of cancer treatments have increased the survival of cancer patients over recent decades. Some individuals receiving cancer treatment experience significant adverse effects during treatment. In addition to the adverse effects caused by cancer treatment, many people diagnosed with cancer suffer from anxiety, depression, and fear of recurrence.[4] Thus, a high proportion of patients use complementary and alternative medicine (CAM), including acupuncture to manage their physical and psychological symptoms.[5,6]

Acupuncture

Acupuncture is an age-old healing practice of traditional Chinese medicine (TCM) which started in China about 3000 years ago. The first documentation of acupuncture that described it as an organized system of diagnosis and treatment is in The Yellow Emperor's Classic of Internal Medicine, which dates to 100 BCE.

Acupuncture has been integrated into many hospital systems across the US. During the past 50 years, acupuncture as an integrative medicine has become a popular therapy to manage adverse effects during cancer treatment.[7] In a 2007 National

Head and Neck Cancer Rehabilitation. https://doi.org/10.1016/B978-0-443-11806-7.00017-5
Copyright © 2025 Elsevier Inc. All rights reserved, including those for text and data mining, AI training, and similar technologies.

Health Interview Survey (NHIS), core interviews were administered to 23,393 adults that revealed that acupuncture users (including former and recent users) increased from 4.2% to 6.3% of the population, representing 8.19 million and 14.01 million users in 2002 and 2007, respectively. People not only used acupuncture as a complementary and alternative approach to conventional treatment for a specific health condition but also used it as a preventive means to promote general health.[8]

Acupuncture is a key component of TCM, which is an integrative medicine approach that provides evidence-based complementary therapies. In acupuncture treatments, fine needles are inserted into specific points on the body, which induce a natural self-healing process to balance the flow of energy (qi) throughout the body. It is based on the theory that many different meridians run throughout the body and represent different organ systems, connected by these points.[9] Acupuncture moves qi and brings balance to the body's organ functions and other systems. Stimulating acupoints by needling, applying pressure or heat can thus treat or cure specific ailments that are caused by dysfunction along the meridians.[10] During an acupuncture treatment session, an infrared light heating lamp (called "Teding Diancibo Pu" (TDP) is used. Loosely translated, TDP is a specific electromagnetic spectrum. A TDP lamp has 33 body essential minerals, which are heated by infrared light to produce therapeutic rays to increase microcirculation. At the completion of the treatment session, most people feel relaxed and energized.[11]

Yin and yang are the underlying principles of acupuncture and TCM. Yin qualities are feminine in nature and are represented by cold, moistness, dark, and the moon. Yang qualities are masculine in nature and manifest as heat, dryness, light, and the sun. The principles of yin and yang are easily observed in everyday natural phenomenon. The harmony and balance of yin and yang forces are displayed in nature.[11] For example, dry mouth manifests when there is an imbalance of yin and yang in the body. Acupuncture rebalances yin and yang, whereby aiding in recovery of bodily function. Studies suggest acupuncture may work through specific neuronal and cortical pathways to cause release of endorphins at the spine and supraspinal levels. Acupuncture stimulates nerves, which transfer the signal to the spinal cord, midbrain, and hypothalamus–pituitary system, triggering release of endorphins and enkephalins.[12-14] Han concluded that low-frequency (2 Hz) electroacupuncture analgesia (EAA) is induced by the activation of mu- and delta-opioid receptors via the release of enkephalin, beta-endorphin, and endomorphin in supraspinal CNS regions, whereas the effects of high-frequency (100 Hz) EAA involve the actions of dynorphin on kappa opioid receptors in the spinal cord.[14]

Although the mechanism of acupuncture is not fully understood, several animal studies have also explored its immunomodulatory effects. They found that acupuncture worked through immunomodulation, with significant changes in cytokines including interleukin (IL)-1, IL-6, IL-8, IL-10, and tumor necrosis factor -alpha.[15,16] Li et al. demonstrated that electroacupuncture's success in alleviating neuropathic pain is at least partially due to inhibition of the activation of spinal microglia cells and downregulation of the expression of brain-derived neurotrophic factor.[17] Another experimental study performed in animals demonstrated that electroacupuncture stimulation could modulate the vagal—adrenal antiinflammatory axis.[18]

Benefits of acupuncture treatment

Applying acupuncture has been examined for managing treatment-related side effects and management of perioperative symptoms associated with cancer surgery. Acupuncture is relatively safe without serious adverse events (AEs) and does not interfere with prescription drugs and treatment plans or cause additional side effects. Recent advances from published clinical trials have shown that acupuncture can alleviate symptoms of adverse effects during and post—cancer treatment.[19] Acupuncture in the preoperative period can relieve anxiety and stress, which can help maintain homeostasis during surgery aiding in success of the operation.[19] Several randomized controlled trials (RCTs) have evaluated acupuncture in the management of adverse effects of cancer treatment and reported beneficial impacts on depression,[20] chemotherapy-induced nausea and vomiting,[21] chemotherapy-related neuropathy,[22] and chemotherapy-related hot flashes.[23] Studies have also demonstrated that acupuncture can reduce fatigue,[24] joint pain and stiffness,[25] and radiation-induced xerostomia.[21] Although these are common side effects of chemotherapy and radiation therapy, acupuncture is not limited to treat only these symptoms. It also improves other ailments and enhances quality of life for survivorship.[26]

Acupuncture treatment session

Before the acupuncture session, the patient completes a medical form and signs a consent form. The acupuncturist reviews the medical record including information regarding the cancer characteristics and treatment and asks the patient pertinent questions about their health status. Patients may be asked to change into a gown (depending upon the clothes worn) and to lie down on a comfortable examining table or to sit in a wheelchair if the patient's condition does not allow him/her to move to lie on the examining table. The acupuncturist then cleans the areas of the skin with alcohol before inserting the needles. Single-use, disposable needles are now the practice standard. The needles that are used are about as thin as hair and most people feel little, if any, discomfort during the procedure.

Approximately 5—20 needles are placed under the skin, and sometimes the acupuncturist will twirl them slightly as they are placed or connected with an electric device for stimulation, based on the patient's symptoms. A combination of various sensations may occur such as pressure, heaviness, numbness, soreness, and/or distension in the needling area. The needles will then be left in place for

15–30 min. Generally, one or two treatments a week is common for a single symptom. The number of treatments will depend on the symptom(s) being treated and its severity. It is common to receive six to eight treatments.

Precautions in acupuncture treatment

Although acupuncture is generally safe for patients of all ages when provided by well-trained practitioners, there are key areas of precaution for cancer patients. Acupuncture is safe while receiving chemotherapy or radiation therapy; however, it is important to note if the patient has a bleeding disorder, abnormal platelet count (<20,000/uL) taking anticoagulants, which may contribute to local bruising as a side effect of acupuncture can occur with needle-induced stimulation. Cancer-related neutropenia (absolute neutrophil count <500/uL) may compromise a patient's immune system and make them more susceptible to infection. Acupuncture treatment is not recommended if a patient has cancer-related neutropenia. Another contraindication to acupuncture is in placement of acupuncture needles in the limbs of patients who had lymph node(s) removed or have lymphedema, which is common practice, however, not noted in scientific studies. In patients with a cardiac pacemaker or intracardiac defibrillator, electroacupuncture should be avoided. Direct insertion of needle into a tumor nodule of ulcerated wound is contraindicated.

Acupuncture has a very low rate of AEs when conducted by licensed and qualified practitioners. A metaanalysis review of acupuncture[27] notes acupuncture can be considered among the safer treatments in healthcare. Although AEs are rare, minor AEs can occur and are usually very mild. Severe AEs requiring medical management are uncommon. Complications of acupuncture are rare, but may include bleeding, infection, bruising, discomfort, and pneumothorax.[28]

Licensed acupuncturists must acquire rigorous training and maintain National Certification Commission for Acupuncture and Oriental Medicine certificate throughout their practice, which reflect the solid medical competence required to manage AEs properly and minimize the risk of malpractice.

Xerostomia

Recent advancement in treatment of HNC has greatly improved the survival rates. However, radiation therapy and chemotherapy often come with significant toxicities and long-term complications. Xerostomia is a common adverse effect of radiation therapy. Patients suffering from xerostomia can complain of difficulty chewing and swallowing due to lack of saliva and have an increased risk of caries, impaired sleep, bad breath, hoarseness, and psychological and social disability.[29]

Acupuncture provides significant reductions in dry mouth for patients after head or neck cancer surgery. It has been demonstrated to reduce xerostomia score and increase saliva volume and density without changing salivary pH in irradiated patients with head and neck squamous cell carcinoma.[30] When combined with medication, it has also been shown to prevent oral mucositis and improve salivary flow rate.[31] Acupuncture has been recommended for the treatment of xerostomia following radiotherapy, inhibiting dry mouth, and promoting salivary secretion and salivary gland dysfunction and improving quality of life for HNC patients.[29,32–35] Acupuncture-like transcutaneous electrical nerve stimulation regimens have also been reported as being safe, well tolerated, and effective for treatment of radiation-induced xerostomia.[36]

Chemotherapy-related peripheral neuropathy

Chemotherapy-induced peripheral neuropathy (CIPN) is a common adverse effect of chemotherapy affecting peripheral nerves of the upper and lower extremities that are often dose dependent and progressive. It can be very distressing to cancer patients and can be a cause of dose-reduction, changes in cancer treatment, or termination of chemotherapy. CIPN begins with numbness of distal extremities and may progress to long-term touch, heat, and cold dysesthesias and severe motor impairment affecting daily functioning. Patients can also complain of pinching, burning, tingling, or electric shock-like sensation in the hands and feet. The morbidity associated with CIPN can lead to pronounced alterations in quality of life and independent performance of activities of daily living.[37–39]

Acupuncture is a well-tolerated, feasible, and effective treatment for CIPN in HNC patients. Preliminary evidence supports the effectiveness of acupuncture in reducing the incidence of high grade CIPN during chemotherapy. A recent controlled trial in patients with CIPN suggested that acupuncture may alleviate CIPN sensory symptoms.[22] Bao et al. reported on a randomized control trial (RCT) comparing acupuncture with sham procedure or usual care of CIPN symptoms with significant improvement in the CIPN symptoms of the acupuncture group.[40] Another RCT pilot study concluded that acupuncture provides a promising intervention for breast cancer survivors with chronic moderate CIPN.[22] There have been several other studies in breast cancer patients that have also demonstrated that acupuncture reduced CIPN severity during neoadjuvant or adjuvant treatment.[22,40–43] Furthermore, 19 RCTs covering 1174 patients also concluded that acupuncture significantly improved CIPN symptoms when compared with medicine and sham acupuncture.[44] Acupuncture was also demonstrated to enhance the recovery of nerve conduction velocity and improving pain.[44]

Pain

Pain is the most common symptom in cancer patients among various stages. Moderate to severe pain has been reported in 40% of patients with early- or intermediate-stage cancer and among 80% of cancer patients at advanced stages.[45,46]

Acupuncture in pain management has been proven useful in several studies.[47,48] An evidence-based clinical practice guideline for management of cancer patients with acupuncture published in 2022,[48] which strongly recommends acupuncture is useful to relieve pain in patients with moderate to severe cancer pain. A combination treatment with acupuncture/acupressure reduces pain intensity, decreases the opioid dose, and alleviates opioid-related side effects in moderate to severe cancer pain patients who are using analgesics.[47]

A metaanalysis of 14 RCTs (with a total of 920 patients) showed acupuncture and acupressure were combined with analgesic therapy to reduce cancer pain intensity in 6 RCTs and decrease opioid dose in 2 RCTs.[48]

Acupuncture is a well-tolerated, feasible, and effective treatment of radiotherapy-related pain among HNC patients, leading to lower usage of mild opioids. The use of acupuncture can have an impact not only on improving the quality of life but also on reducing the side effects and costs of analgesic therapy. Further research is needed for the inclusion of acupuncture in the standard-of-care treatment process in this group of patients.[49] In a systematic review and metaanalysis, data from acupuncture studies indicate that acupuncture can be considered advantageous over conventional treatment for improving shoulder pain and dysfunction in the head and neck patients.[50] A 2021 systematic review and metaanalysis by Dai and colleagues found acupuncture and derived therapies (such as electroacupuncture, laser acupuncture, and transcutaneous electrical nerve stimulation) led to greater reductions in the NRS (numeric rating scale) score than conventional analgesics. For single-arm trials (18 studies, 1084 patients), metaanalysis showed that both the immediate effect and long-term longitudinal effect of acupuncture on analgesia were positive.[51] Another systematic review of acupuncture for palliative cancer pain management suggests that acupuncture may be an effective and safe treatment associated with pain reduction in the palliative care of patients with cancer.[26]

Cancer-related fatigue

Cancer-related fatigue (CRF) is a distressing symptom in cancer patients during/after chemotherapy or radiation therapy that severely affects quality of life. Unfortunately, accurate and effective pharmacological and nonpharmacologic strategies for managing CRF are lacking. Acupuncture treatment has been widely used to treat fatigue. In a systematic review and metaanalysis of 12 studies including a total of 1084 participants, acupuncture treatment had a beneficial effect compared with sham or with usual care on fatigue There were no serious adverse effects, and it was concluded that acupuncture treatment is an effective and safe treatment for CRF.[52] According to the NCCN guidelines, acupuncture can be used to treat several cancer-related symptoms including CRF.[53] A metaanalysis of CRF treatments in several cancer types concluded that acupuncture is effective for CRF management.[54] Recent research reports that acupuncture may also be a useful adjunct for reducing fatigue in cancer palliative care.[55]

Anxiety

Anxiety disorders are one of the most common mental health concerns in cancer patients. Pharmacology and psychotherapy are the conventional treatment for anxiety disorders. However, these present limited efficacies, especially in the case of chronic anxiety, with high relapse rates and adverse side effects. Acupuncture has been studied as a potential treatment of anxiety. Several studies have suggested that acupuncture may be effective in reducing symptoms of anxiety.

A systematic review of the clinical research published in 2018 found that different methodologies (different acupoints, design, duration, type of acupuncture) lead to similar results of decreased levels of anxiety.[56] Other systematic reviews also identified the beneficial effects of acupuncture in the treatment of various symptoms in breast cancer patients including anxiety.[57,58]

Summary

The current evidence for using acupuncture to treat symptoms commonly seen in HNC patients is encouraging. Acupuncture is a well-established, generally safe technique in integrative medicine that is well tolerated with low physical risks to HNC patients.

References

1. Cancer.Net. *Head and Neck Cancer: Statistics*. February 2023.
2. Chen YP, Ismaila N, Chua MLK, et al. Chemotherapy in combination with radiotherapy for definitive-intent treatment of stage II-IVA nasopharyngeal carcinoma: CSCO and ASCO guideline. *J Clin Oncol*. March 1, 2021;39(7):840−859. https://doi.org/10.1200/JCO.20.03237.
3. Masarwy R, Kampel L, Horowitz G, Gutfeld O, Muhanna N, et al. Neoadjuvant PD-1/PD-L1 inhibitors for resectable head and neck cancer: a systematic review and meta-analysis. *JAMA Otolaryngol Head Neck Surg*. October 1, 2021;147(10):871−878. https://doi.org/10.1001/jamaoto.2021.2191.
4. Richardson AE, Broadbent E, Morton RP, et al. A systematic review of psychological interventions for patients with head and neck cancer. *Support Care Cancer*. June 2019; 27(6):2007−2021. https://doi.org/10.1007/s00520-019-04768-3.
5. Calcagni N, Gana K, Quintard B, et al. A systematic review of complementary and alternative medicine in oncology: psychological and physical effects of manipulative and body-based practices. *PLoS One*. October 17, 2019;14(10):e0223564. https://doi.org/10.1371/journal.pone.0223564.
6. Oh B, Butow P, Mullan B, Mullan B, et al. Patient-doctor communication: the use of complementary and alternative medicine by adult patients with cancer. *J Soc Integr Oncol*. 2010;8:56−64.
7. Mao JJ, Witt. Acupuncture as an evidence-based treatment for cancer pain management: the joint society for integrative oncology-American society for clinical oncology

guideline. *J Integr Complement Med*. April 2023;29(4):209–211. https://doi.org/10.1089/jicm.2023.0018. Epub 2023 Feb 27.

8. Zhang Y, Lao LX, Chen HY, Ceballos R. Acupuncture use among American adults: what acupuncture practitioners can learn from National Health Interview Survey 2007? *Evid Based Complement Alternat Med*. February 22, 2012. https://doi.org/10.1155/2012/710750.

9. Zhou W, Benharash P. Effects and mechanisms of acupuncture based on the principle of meridians. *J Acupunct Meridian Stud*. 2014;7(4):190–193. https://doi.org/10.1016/j.jams.2014.02.007.

10. Longhurst JC. Defining meridians: a modern basis of understanding. *J Acupunct Meridian Stud*. 2010;3(2):67–74. https://doi.org/10.1016/S2005-2901(10)60014-3.

11. Chen FI, Antochi AD, Barbilian AG, et al. Acupuncture and the retrospect of its modern research. *Rom J Morphol Embryol*. 2019;60(2):411–418.

12. NIH consensus conference. Acupuncture. *JAMA*. 1998;280(17):1518–1524.

13. Mayer DJ. Biological mechanisms of acupuncture. *Prog Brain Res*. 2000;122:457–477. https://doi.org/10.1016/s0079-6123(08)62157-3.

14. Han JS. Acupuncture: neuropeptide release produced by electrical stimulation of different frequencies. *Trends Neurosci*. January 2003;26(1):17–22. https://doi.org/10.1016/s0166-2236(02)00006-1.

15. Joos S, Schott C, Zhou H, Martin E, et al. Immunomodulatory effects of acupuncture in the treatment of allergic asthma: a randomized controlled study. *J Alternative Compl Med*. December 2000;6(6):519–525. https://doi.org/10.1089/acm.2000.6.519.

16. Petti FB, Liguori A, Ippoliti F. Study on cytokines IL-2, IL-6, IL-10 in patients of chronic allergic rhinitis treated with acupuncture. *J Tradit Chin Med*. June 2002;22(2):104–111.

17. Li S, Gu P, Tu WZ, et al. Effects of electroacupuncture on activation of microglia cells in spinal cord in rats with neuropathic pain. *Zhongguo Zhen Jiu*. 2017;37(4):411–416. 22. https://doi.org/10.13703/j.0255-2930.2017.04.016.

18. Liu SB, Wang ZF, Su YS, et al. A neuroanatomical basis for electroacupuncture to drive the vagal-adrenal axis. *Nature*. October 2021;598(7882):641–645. https://doi.org/10.1038/s41586-021-04001-4. Epub 2021 Oct 13.

19. Zhang XW, Hou WB, Pu FL, et al. Acupuncture for cancer-related conditions: an overview of systematic reviews. *Phytomedicine*. November 2022;106:154430. https://doi.org/10.1016/j.phymed.2022.154430.

20. Tu M, Jiang Y, et al. Acupuncture for treating chronic stable angina pectoris associated anxiety and depression: a systematic review and meta-analysis. *J Complement Ther Clin Pract*. November 2021;45:101484. https://doi.org/10.1016/j.ctcp.2021.101484.

21. Shen J, Wenger N, Glaspy J, et al. Electroacupuncture for control of myeloablative chemotherapy-induced emesis: a randomized controlled trial. *JAMA*. 2000;284:2755–2761. https://doi.org/10.1001/jama.284.21.2755.

22. Lu W, Giobbie-Hurder A, Freedman RA, et al. Acupuncture for chemotherapy-induced peripheral neuropathy in breast cancer survivors: a randomized controlled pilot trial. *Oncologist*. April 2020;25(4):310–318. https://doi.org/10.1634/theoncologist.2019-0489.

23. Lu W, Giobbie-Hurder A, Tanasijevic A, et al. Acupuncture for hot flashes in hormone receptor-positive breast cancer, a coordinated multinational study: rationale and design of the study protocol. *Contemp Clin Trials*. October 2022;121:106885. https://doi.org/10.1016/j.cct.2022.106885.

24. Yin ZH, Wang LJ, Cheng Y, et al. Acupuncture for chronic fatigue syndrome: an overview of systematic reviews. *Chin J Integr Med*. December 2021;27(12):940−946. https://doi.org/10.1007/s11655-020-3195-3.

25. Hershman DL, Unger JM, Greenlee H, et al. Comparison of acupuncture vs sham acupuncture or waiting list control in the treatment of aromatase inhibitor-related joint pain: a randomized clinical trial. *JAMA Netw Open*. November 1, 2022;5(11): e2241720. https://doi.org/10.1001/jamanetworkopen.2022.41720.

26. Yang J, Wahner-RoedlerD, Zhou X, et al. Acupuncture for palliative cancer pain management: systematic review. *BMJ Support Palliat Care*. September 2021;11(3): 264−270. https://doi.org/10.1136/bmjspcare-2020-002638.

27. Bäumler P, Zhang W, Stubinger T, Irnich D. Acupuncture-related adverse events: systematic review and meta-analyses of prospective clinical studies. *BMJ Open*. September 6, 2021;11(9). https://doi.org/10.1136/bmjopen-2020-045961.

28. Lesi G, Razzini G, Musti MA, et al. Acupuncture as an integrative approach for the treatment of hot flashes in women with breast cancer: a prospective multicenter randomized controlled trial (AcCliMaT). *J Clin Oncol*. 2016;34:1795−1802. https://doi.org/10.1200/JCO.2015.63.2893.

29. Ni X, Tian T, Chen D, et al. Acupuncture for radiationinduced xerostomia in cancer patients: a systematic review and meta-analysis. *Integr Cancer Ther*. January−Decemder 2020;19:1534735420980825. https://doi.org/10.1177/1534735420980825.

30. Menezes A, Sanchos G, gomes ESN, et al. The combination of traditional and auricular acupuncture to prevent xerostomia and anxiety in irradiated patients with HNSCC: a preventive, parallel, single-blind, 2-arm controlled study. *Oral Surg Oral Med Oral Pathol Oral Radiol*. June 2021;131(6):675−683. https://doi.org/10.1016/j.oooo.2021.02.016.

31. Wu T, Fu C, Deng YR, Huang WP, Wang JY, Jiao Y. Acupuncture therapy for radiotherapy-induced adverse effect: a systematic review and network meta-analysis. *Front Public Health*. December 15, 2022;10:1026971. https://doi.org/10.3389/fpubh.2022.1026971.

32. Johnstone PA, Niemtzow RC, Riffenburgh RH. Acupuncture for xerostomia: clinical update. *Cancer*. 2002;94:1151−1156.

33. Garcia MK, Meng Z, Rosenthal DI, et al. Effect of true and sham acupuncture on radiation-induced xerostomia among patients with head and neck cancer: a randomized clinical trial. *JAMA Netw Open*. 2019;2:16910. https://doi.org/10.1001/jamanetworkopen.2019.16910.

34. Zhang SQ, Chen HB, Liu J, Dai WJ, Lu QQ, Li JC. Research status and prospects of acupuncture for prevention and treatment of chemo- and radiotherapy-induced salivary gland dysfunction in head and neck cancer. *Anat Rec*. 2021;304(11):2381−2396. https://doi.org/10.1002/ar.24784.

35. Cohen L, Danhauer S, Rosenthal DI, et al. A phase III, randomized, sham-controlled trial of acupuncture for treatment of radiation-induced xerostomia (RIX) in patients with head and neck cancer: Wake Forest NCI Community Oncology Research Program Research Base (WF NCORP RB) trial WF-97115. *J Clin Oncol*. 2022;40:12004.

36. Iovoli AJ, Ostrowski A, Rivers CI, et al. Two- versus four-times weekly acupuncture-like transcutaneous electrical nerve stimulation for treatment of radiation-induced xerostomia: a pilot study. *J Altern Complement Med*. 2020;26:323−328. https://doi.org/10.1089/acm.2019.0131.

37. Hausheer FH, Schilsky RL, Bain S, Berghorn EJ, Lieberman F. Diagnosis, management, and evaluation of chemotherapy-induced peripheral neuropathy. *Semin Oncol*. February 2006;33(1):15–49. https://doi.org/10.1053/j.seminoncol.2005.12.010.

38. Park SB, Goldstein D, Krishnan AV, et al. Chemotherapy-induced peripheral neurotoxicity: a critical analysis. *CA A Cancer J Clin*. 2013;63(6):419–437. https://doi.org/10.3322/caac.21204.

39. Goldstein N, Obaid A. Management of peripheral neuropathy induced by chemotherapy in adults with cancer: a review. *Int J Palliat Nurs*. 2017;23(1):13–17. https://doi.org/10.12968/ijpn.2017.23.1.13.

40. Bao T, Patil S, Chen C, Chen C, et al. Effect of acupuncture vs sham procedure on chemotherapy-induced peripheral neuropathy symptoms: a randomized clinical trial. *JAMA Netw Open*. March 2020;3(3):e200681. https://doi.org/10.1001/jamanetworkopen.2020.0681.

41. Iravani S, Kazemi Motlagh AH, Razavi SZE, el at. Effectiveness of acupuncture treatment on chemotherapy-induced peripheral neuropathy: a pilot, randomized, assessor-blinded, controlled trial. *Pain Res Manag*. June 29, 2020. https://doi.org/10.1155/2020/2504674.

42. Molassiotis A, Suen LKP, Cheng HL, et al. A randomized assessor-blinded wait-list-controlled trial to assess the effectiveness of acupuncture in the management of chemotherapy-induced peripheral neuropathy. *Integr Cancer Ther*. 2019;18. https://doi.org/10.1177/1534735419836501.

43. Han X, Wang L, Shi HF, et al. Acupuncture combined with methylcobalamin for the treatment of chemotherapy-induced peripheral neuropathy in patients with multiple myeloma. *BMC Cancer*. 2017;17:40. https://doi.org/10.1186/s12885-016-3037-z.

44. Jin Y, Wang Y, Zhang JY, Xiao X, Zhang Q, et al. Efficacy and safety of acupuncture against chemotherapy-induced peripheral neuropathy: a systematic review and meta-analysis. *Evid Based Complement Alternat Med*. November 9, 2020. https://doi.org/10.1155/2020/8875433.

45. Bruera E, Kim HN. Cancer pain. *JAMA*. November 12, 2003;290(18):2476–2479. https://doi.org/10.1001/jama.290.18.2476.

46. Laird B, Colvin L, Fallon M. Management of cancer pain: basic principles and neuropathic cancer pain. *Eur J Cancer*. May 2008;44(8):1078–1082. https://doi.org/10.1016/j.ejca.2008.03.022.

47. Ge L, Wang Q, He Y, et al. Acupuncture for cancer pain: an evidence-based clinical practice guideline. *Chin Med*. January 5, 2022;17(1):8. https://doi.org/10.1186/s13020-021-00558-4.

48. He YH, Guo XF, May BH, et al. Clinical evidence for association of acupuncture and acupressure with improved cancer pain: a systematic review and meta-analysis. *JAMA Oncol*. February 1, 2020;6(2):271–278. https://doi.org/10.1001/jamaoncol.2019.5233.

49. Dymackova R, Selingerova I, Kazda T, et al. Effect of acupuncture in pain management of head and neck cancer radiotherapy: prospective randomized unicentric study. *J Clin Med*. March 7, 2021;10(5):1111. https://doi.org/10.3390/jcm10051111.

50. Almeida KAM, Rocha AP, Carvas N, Pinto ACPN. Rehabilitation interventions for shoulder dysfunction in patients with head and neck cancer: systematic review and meta-analysis. *Phys Ther*. October 30, 2020;100(11):1997–2008. https://doi.org/10.1093/ptj/pzaa147.

51. Dai L, Liu Y, Ji G, Xu Y. Acupuncture and derived therapies for pain in palliative cancer management: systematic review and meta-analysis based on single-arm and controlled

trials. *J Palliat Med.* July 2021;24(7):1078−1099. https://doi.org/10.1089/jpm.2020. 0405.

52. Choi TY, Ang L, Jun JH, et al. Acupuncture for managing cancer-related fatigue in breast cancer patients: a systematic review and meta-analysis. *Cancers.* September 11, 2022; 14(18):4419. https://doi.org/10.3390/cancers14184419.

53. Halámková J, Dymáčková R, Krakorova DA. Acupuncture from the perspective of evidence-based medicine—options of clinical use based on National Comprehensive Cancer Network (NCCN) guidelines. *Klin Onkol.* 2022;35:94−99. https://doi.org/ 10.48095/ccko202294.

54. Zhang Y, Lin L, Li H, Hu Y, Tian L. Effects of acupuncture on cancer-related fatigue: a meta-analysis. *Support Care Cancer.* 2018;26:415−425. https://doi.org/10.1007/s00520-017-3955-6.

55. Arring NM, Barton DL, Brooks T, Zick SM. Integrative therapies for cancer-related fatigue. *Cancer J.* 2019;25:349−356. https://doi.org/10.1097/PPO.0000000000000396.

56. Amorim D, Amado J, Brito I, et al. Acupuncture and electroacupuncture for anxiety disorders: a systematic review of the clinical research. *J Complement Ther Clin Pract.* May 2018;31:31−37. https://doi.org/10.1016/j.ctcp.2018.01.008.

57. Tola YO, Chow KM, et al. Effects of non-pharmacological interventions on preoperative anxiety and postoperative pain in patients undergoing breast cancer surgery: a systematic review. *J Clin Nurs.* December 2021;30(23−24):3369−3384. https://doi.org/10.1111/ jocn.15827.

58. Zhang Y, Sun Y, Li D, et al. Acupuncture for breast cancer: a systematic review and meta-analysis of patient-reported outcomes. *Front Oncol.* June 10, 2021. https://doi.org/ 10.3389/fonc.2021.646315.

Index

'Note: Page numbers followed by "f" indicate figures, "t" indicate tables and "b" indicate boxes.'

Printed and bound by CPI Group (UK) Ltd, Croydon, CR0 4YY

03/10/2024

01040349-0005